A Supplement to New Frontiers in Geriatrics Research

A Supplement to New Frontiers in Geriatrics Research

An Agenda for Surgical and Related Medical Specialties

Joseph LoCicero III, MD, FACS, Editor

Ronnie A. Rosenthal, MD, FACS, Associate Editor

Mark R. Katlic, MD, FACS, Associate Editor

Peter Pompei, MD, Associate Editor

A Project of
The American Geriatrics Society
and
The John A. Hartford Foundation

PUBLISHED BY THE AMERICAN GERIATRICS SOCIETY
New York, NY, USA

This publication was prepared by the American Geriatrics Society as a service to health care providers involved in the care of older persons. Funding provided by The John A. Hartford Foundation made the development of this publication possible.

A Supplement to New Frontiers in Geriatrics Research is independently prepared and published. All decisions regarding its content are solely the responsibility of the authors and editors. Their decisions are not subject to any form of approval by other interests or organizations.

No responsibility is assumed by the authors or the American Geriatrics Society for any injury or damage to persons or property, as a matter of product liability, negligence, warrant, or otherwise, arising out of the use or application of any methods, products, instructions, or ideas contained herein. No guarantee, endorsement, or warranty of any kind, express or implied (including specifically no warrant of merchantability or fitness for a particular purpose) is given by the Society in connection with any information contained herein. Independent verification of any diagnosis, treatment, or drug use or dosage should be obtained. No test or procedure should be performed unless, in the judgment of an independent, qualified physician, it is justified in the light of the risk involved.

Citation: LoCicero J 3rd, Rosenthal RA, Katlic MR, Pompei P, eds.
A Supplement to New Frontiers in Geriatrics Research:
An Agenda for Surgical and Related Medical Specialties. 2007.

ISBN 1–886775–11–7
Printed in the U.S.A.

To David H. Solomon, MD, MACP, whose dedication to older patients and to extending the knowledge of geriatrics into surgical and related medical specialties is unbounded and inspiring

CONTENTS

CONTENTS

ACKNOWLEDGMENTS

THE JOHN A. HARTFORD FOUNDATION

We are indebted to The John A. Hartford Foundation for their unswerving commitment to "improving the quality and financing of health care and assisting the health care system to accommodate the nation's aging population." The innovative programs developed with their support will provide better health care for current and future generations of older adults.

Founded in 1929, The John A. Hartford Foundation is a committed champion of training, research, and service system innovations that promote the health and independence of America's older adults. Through its grantmaking, the Foundation seeks to strengthen the nation's capacity to provide effective, affordable care to this rapidly increasing older population by educating "aging-prepared" health professionals (physicians, nurses, social workers) and developing innovations that improve and better integrate health and supportive services. The Foundation was established by John A. Hartford. Mr. Hartford and his brother, George L. Hartford, both former chief executives of the Great Atlantic & Pacific Tea Company, left the bulk of their estates to the Foundation upon their deaths in the 1950s. Additional information about the Foundation and its programs is available at www.jhartfound.org.

PROJECT PARTICIPANTS

Many talented and knowledgeable people continue to collaborate to make the updating of the research agenda possible. Each has made a substantial contribution to the development of the research agenda, and we thank the following people for dedicating their time and effort to complete the tasks that made this volume possible:

Anesthesiology

Christopher J. Jankowski, MD, *Content Expert*
Assistant Professor of Anesthesiology
Mayo Clinic College of Medicine
Consultant in Anesthesiology
Mayo Clinic
Rochester, MN

David J. Cook, MD, *Senior Writer*
Professor of Anesthesiology
Mayo Clinic and Foundation
Rochester, MN

Emergency Medicine

Christopher R. Carpenter, MD, MSc, FACEP, *Content Expert*
Assistant Professor
Division of Emergency Medicine
Washington University School of Medicine
St. Louis, MO

Lowell W. Gerson, PhD, *Senior Writer*
Professor Emeritus of Epidemiology
Northeastern Ohio Universities College of Medicine
Senior Scientist
Emergency Medicine Research Center
Summa Health System
Akron, OH

General Surgery

Sandhya Lagoo-Deenadayalan, MD, PhD, *Content Expert*
Department of Surgery
Duke University Medical Center
Durham, NC

Walter J. Pories, MD, FACS, *Senior Writer*
Professor of Surgery and Biochemistry
Department of Surgery
Brody School of Medicine
East Carolina University
Greenville, NC

Gynecology

Erin Duecy, MD, *Content Expert*
Assistant Professor, Department of Obstetrics and Gynecology
University of Rochester Medical Center
Rochester, NY

Morton A. Stenchever, MD, *Senior Writer*
Professor and Chairman Emeritus
Department of Obstetrics and Gynecology
University of Washington School of Medicine
Seattle, WA

Ophthalmology

David S. Friedman, MD, MPH, PhD, *Content Expert*
Associate Professor
Department of Ophthalmology
The Wilmer Eye Institute
The Johns Hopkins University
Baltimore, MD

Andrew G. Lee, MD, *Senior Writer*
Professor of Ophthalmology, Neurology, and Neurosurgery
University of Iowa Hospitals and Clinics
Iowa City, IA

Orthopedic Surgery

Susan Day, MD, *Content Expert*
Clinical Instructor
Michigan State University
Grand Rapids Orthopaedic Residency Program
Grand Rapids, MI

Robert Karpman, MD, *Senior Writer*
Vice-President of Medical Affairs
Caritas Holy Family Hospital
Methuen, MA

Otolaryngology

Michael M. Johns, MD, *Content Expert*
Assistant Professor of Otolaryngology
Director of Emory Voice Center
Emory University School of Medicine
Atlanta, GA

Sarah Wise, MD, *Chapter Contributor*
Assistant Professor of Otolaryngology
Emory University School of Medicine
Atlanta, GA

Steven M. Parnes, MD, *Senior Writer*
Chairman of Otolaryngology–Head and Neck Surgery
Albany Medical College
Albany, NY

Physical Medicine and Rehabilitation

Laura W. Lee, MD, MBA, *Content Expert*
Assistant Professor
Department of Physical Medicine and Rehabilitation
University of Virginia Health Systems
Charlottesville, VA

Hilary C. Siebens, MD, *Senior Writer*
Professor of Clinical Physical Medicine and Rehabilitation
University of Virginia
Charlottesville, VA

Thoracic Surgery

Joseph C. Cleveland, Jr., MD, *Content Expert*
Associate Professor of Surgery
Surgical Director, Cardiac Transplantation and MCS
Department of Surgery
Division of Cardiothoracic Surgery
University of Colorado at Denver and Health Sciences Center
Denver, CO

Thomas A. D'Amico, MD, *Content Expert*
Professor of Surgery
Program Director
Division of Thoracic Surgery
Department of Surgery
Duke University Medical Center
Durham, NC

Nicola Francalancia, MD, FACS, *Content Expert*
Cardiac Surgery Associates
St. Francis Heart Center
Indianapolis, IN

Joseph LoCicero III, MD, FACS, *Senior Writer and Editor*
Director of Surgical Oncology
Chief of General Thoracic Surgery
Maimonides Medical Center
Brooklyn, NY

Urology

Badinrath Konety, MD, MBA, *Content Expert*
Associate Professor
Departments of Urology, Epidemiology, and Biostatistics
University of California at San Francisco
San Francisco, CA

George W. Drach, MD, *Senior Writer*
Professor of Urology
Division of Urology
University of Pennsylvania
Philadelphia, PA

Geriatrics for Specialists Initiative (GSI)

John R. Burton, MD
Project Co-Director 1998–2003, Project Director 2003–2007
Mason F. Lord Professor of Medicine
Division of Geriatric Medicine and Gerontology
The Johns Hopkins University School of Medicine
Baltimore, MD

David H. Solomon, MD, MACP, *Consultant Project Director 1997–2003*
Professor Emeritus of Medicine/Geriatrics
David Geffen School of Medicine at UCLA
Los Angeles, CA

Dennis W. Jahnigen, MD, *(deceased)*
Project Director 1994–1998
Goodstein Professor of Geriatric Medicine
Director of the Center on Aging
University of Colorado Health Sciences Center
Denver, CO

Publications Consultants

Sue Radcliff, *Research Consultant*
Denver, CO

Barbara B. Reitt, PhD, ELS(D), *Medical Editor*
Reitt Editing Services
Northampton, MA

L. Pilar Wyman, *Indexer*
Wyman Indexing
Annapolis, MD

American Geriatrics Society

Janis Eisner, *Administrative Director, Geriatrics for Specialists*
American Geriatrics Society
The Empire State Building
New York, NY

Elizabeth Haranas, *Health Coordinator*
American Geriatrics Society
The Empire State Building
New York, NY

Nancy Lundebjerg, MPA, *Deputy Executive Vice President*
American Geriatrics Society
The Empire State Building
New York, NY

Rachael Edberg Silverman, *Senior Health Coordinator*
American Geriatrics Society
The Empire State Building
New York, NY

AGS COUNCIL OF THE SECTION ON SURGICAL AND RELATED MEDICAL SPECIALTIES

We thank the members of the Council (formerly the Interdisciplinary Leadership Group) for their wise guidance of the overall Geriatrics for Specialists project. Members in 2007:

American Academy of Ophthalmology (AAO)
Andrew G. Lee, MD
Gwen Sterns, MD

American Academy of Orthopaedic Surgeons (AAOS)
Thomas P. Sculco, MD
Charles Weiss, MD

American Academy of Otolaryngology—Head and Neck Surgery (AAO-H&NS)
Ara Chalian, MD
Steven M. Parnes, MD

American Academy of Physical Medicine and Rehabilitation (AAPM&R)
Hilary C. Siebens, MD
Dale C. Strasser, MD

American College of Emergency Physicians (ACEP)
Teresita Hogan, MD

American College of Obstetricians and Gynecologists (ACOG)
Ira Golditch, MD
Sterling Williams, MD

American College of Surgeons
Ajit Sachdeva, MD
James C. Thompson, MD

American Society of Anesthesiologists (ASA)
Sheila Barnett, MBBC
Jeffrey Silverstein, MD

American Urological Association (AUA)
George W. Drach, MD
Allen Seftel, MD

Association of Program Directors in Surgery (APDS)
J. Patrick O'Leary, MD
Walter J. Pories, MD

Society of Thoracic Surgeons (STS)
Joseph C. Cleveland, Jr., MD
Joseph LoCicero III, MD, FACS

Society for Academic Emergency Medicine (SAEM)
Lowell W. Gerson, PhD

1

INTRODUCTION

*Joseph LoCicero III, MD, FACS; Ronnie A. Rosenthal, MD, FACS; Mark R. Katlic, MD, FACS; Peter Pompei, MD**

Welcome to the supplement to update the only research agenda that addresses the quality of care for elderly patients who may require a surgical procedure and who are cared for by specialists in surgical disciplines and related medical fields. The original research agenda, entitled *New Frontiers in Geriatrics Research: An Agenda for Surgical and Related Medical Specialties,* [1] was written by specialists in selected surgical and medical disciplines who reviewed the scientific knowledge of each discipline that is focused on the perioperative experience of older adults and made recommendations about what new research would best advance our knowledge of common surgical conditions in elderly patients, influence surgical outcomes, and improve perioperative management. The proposed research questions ranged from simple observational studies to complex randomized trials. The agenda revealed that we have only a minimal understanding of the basic physiology of certain surgical diseases in the older adult. The three main objectives of the research agenda and its supplement are to fill obvious gaps in knowledge in each specialty area, clarify inconsistencies in the existing literature, and point to possible resolutions of ongoing controversies.

THE SCOPE OF THIS RESEARCH AGENDA

As in the original agenda, the ten specialties addressed herein include five surgical specialties: general surgery, orthopedics, otolaryngology, thoracic surgery (separated into cardiac issues and general thoracic issues), and urology. Two other specialties are included that are predominantly surgical but have a significant element of medical practice: gynecology and ophthalmology. Three related medical specialties are also included: anesthesiology, emergency medicine, and physical medicine and rehabilitation (physiatry). Altogether, these ten specialties encompass the perioperative course of most surgical patients.

THE AGS–HARTFORD FOUNDATION PROJECT

New Frontiers describes in detail the development of this project and its many accomplishments since its inception in 1994 (see pp. 2–5). In brief, The John A. Hartford Foundation of New York (Hartford Foundation) awarded an initial planning grant to the American Geriatrics Society (AGS) in 1992. The successful project that grew out of that seed money, Increasing Geriatrics Expertise in Surgical and Related Medical Specialties (Geriatrics for Specialists), entered its fourth funding phase on July 1, 2005, with a grant that runs through June 30, 2009.

---

* LoCicero: Director of Surgical Oncology and Chief of Thoracic Surgery, Maimonides Medical Center, Brooklyn, NY; Rosenthal: Associate Professor of Surgery, Yale University School of Medicine, Chief of Surgical Service, VA Connecticut Healthcare System, New Haven, CT; Katlic: Director of Thoracic Surgery, Geisinger Health System, Wilkes Barre, PA; Pompei: Associate Professor, Department of Medicine, Stanford University, Stanford, CA.

In planning this project, the AGS and The Hartford Foundation were guided by the belief that the most effective way to help all surgical and related medical specialists do a better job of caring for older patients was not to contribute to the further fragmentation of the target specialties by creating subspecialties in geriatrics. Rather, Geriatrics for Specialists made a commitment to the following broad objectives, which continue to guide the project today:

- To improve the amount and quality of education in geriatrics received by medical and surgical residents.
- To identify and support specialty faculty interested in promoting geriatrics training and research within their own professional disciplines.
- To assist professional certifying bodies and professional societies in improving the ability of their constituencies to care for elderly patients.
- To enhance the knowledge and expertise of practicing surgeons and related medical specialists in the geriatrics aspects of the care of their older patients through maintenance of certification and continuing medical education.

This project was launched at the right moment. Several factors combined to require a concentrated focus on the geriatrics components of the surgical and related medical specialties. These included the rapid expansion of the older population and particularly the oldest-old segment, the increasing ability of surgeons to operate successfully on older patients, the unique vulnerability of older people under stress, the surgeon's traditional role as the primary responsible physician for surgical patients, and, finally, insufficient education regarding geriatrics in medical schools and residencies.

The success of phases I and II of the project was due largely to its deliberately multilevel, "customized" approach, which sought to stimulate geriatrics-related activity among both established leaders and younger "grassroots" faculty in anesthesiology, emergency medicine, general surgery, gynecology, ophthalmology, orthopedics, otolaryngology, physical medicine and rehabilitation, thoracic surgery, and urology by employing the following strategies:

- Identifying and developing leadership,
- Developing and disseminating curriculum and training materials,
- Supporting educational symposia and special interest groups,
- Supporting resident research seed grants and senior investigator awards,
- Encouraging change of Residency Review Committee special requirements and board certifying examinations.

In Phase III, Geriatrics for Specialists established the Section for Surgical and Related Medical Specialties and introduced the Dennis W. Jahnigen Career Development Awards Program and the Geriatrics Education for Specialty Residents Program. In Phase IV, Geriatrics for Specialists is maintaining and strengthening the successful programs of Phases I, II, and III, which worked toward long-term collaboration between geriatrics and the specialties, including the following:

The AGS Section for Surgical and Related Medical Specialties. Past programs include The Surgical Patient: Strategies for Improving Outcomes; Challenges in the Care of the Geriatric Surgical Patient; The Pre-Surgical Evaluation and Management of the Older Patient; Surgical Issues in Older Adults: Research Updates from the Specialties and Clinical Case-Based Discussions; Insights into the Difficult World of Surgery for Older Adults; and From Bench to Bedside, Adventures in Perioperative Geriatrics. The 2008 program will be presented on May 3, 2008, in Washington, DC.

Council of the Section. This group, a working unit of national specialty leaders committed to improving care of the elderly patient, was originally formed as the Interdisciplinary Leadership Group (ILG) in 1998. In 2000, the ILG issued the Statement of Principles: Toward Improved Care of Older Patients in Surgical and Medical Specialties, which has been published in the *Journal of the American Geriatrics Society*[2] and in journals of several of the specialties. The ILG has evolved into the Council of a new Section for Surgical and Related Medical Specialties in the AGS. The Council provides governance for the Section. Leadership of the Council is now moving into the hands of the specialists.

Jahnigen Career Development Scholars Program. These competitive 2-year awards of $75,000 per year (plus a required minimum institutional support of $25,000 per year) are designed to support education and research training for specialty faculty who seek to launch academic careers in the geriatrics aspect of their specialty. These emerging leaders are vital to developing knowledge of geriatrics and improving geriatrics education in the specialties. Developing such scholars is a continuing investment that is critical to the viability of all that has been accomplished to date. For informational purposes the latest awards, supported by The John A. Hartford Foundation and The Atlantic Philanthropies, are posted online at http://www.americangeriatrics.org/hartford/jahnigen.shtml.

Geriatrics Education for Specialty Residents Program. This initiative provides important opportunities for residency program directors to enrich their curricula through collaborations with geriatricians from their own institutions. This program has been expanded to provide support for 25 programs in years 2007, 2008, and 2009. Although the deadline for the next set of awards has passed, the request for proposals remains online, for information only, at http://www.americangeriatrics.org/specialists/gsr_program.shtml.

***Geriatrics Syllabus for Specialists*.**[3] A short, useful guide geared toward surgeons caring for older patients, this publication was designed to provide vital information easily and quickly. Although it is currently not available, an update is under consideration.

Maintenance of Certification (MOC). This initiative was added to the mission since the publication of *New Frontiers.* It was recognized that the majority of physicians involved in perioperative care of older patients fall into the category of practitioners trained before this educational effort began. Incorporating geriatrics into MOC programs is a fitting and logical next objective for the initiative, given the number of physicians already in practice.

New Frontiers in Geriatrics Research: An Agenda for Surgical and Related Medical Specialties.[1] The first research agenda assists faculty in the specialties who have decided to pursue academic careers focused on the geriatric aspects of their specialty by clarifying the state of knowledge at present and pointing out wide-open opportunities for valuable research. This supplement is a logical extension of the first research agenda.

USING THIS BOOK

CHAPTER STRUCTURE

In *New Frontiers*, each chapter presents the key elements of the literature review for that specialty, and the reports discussed are listed in the references section at the end of the chapter. Chapters are organized in sections, each devoted to a major clinical topic. At the end of each topic, the pertinent research agenda items are gathered and highlighted; each item has a unique number to facilitate cross-referencing and citation. Each chapter ends with a discussion that focuses on the issues of greatest concern in the care of older patients by practitioners in the discipline. Three Key Questions are identified, that is, those having the highest priority in the opinion of the experts participating in the project, and examples of hypothesis-generating and hypothesis-testing research needed to address each Key Question are provided.

In this supplement, the specialty authors began with the research questions, including the Key Questions, posed in *New Frontiers* and critically reviewed the relevant literature that was published subsequently. They looked for general and specific studies addressing questions, studies that fully or partially answered the questions, and studies that raised additional questions or that highlighted the need for additional data. With this information, the authors of supplement chapters make recommendations about keeping, eliminating, or modifying the original research questions. In addition, because many developments have occurred since the literature searches for *New Frontiers* were completed, the authors were also asked to address the need to add new questions to the agenda.

In *New Frontiers*, a junior author worked as content expert with a senior author within each specific specialty field to produce cogent research questions. In this supplement, many of the junior authors have acted as the senior author, and new content experts, who were Jahnigen research scholars, were enlisted, bringing a force to the project not previously possible.

THE LITERATURE REVIEWS

The basic approach for all the literature reviews is described here. Unique features of individual literature reviews are presented in a methods section in each specialty chapter. Because the objective was to define the current knowledge base, the focus was on recent literature. The general plan was to conduct an English-language search, limited to the human, using MEDLINE (through PubMed). All searches included the terms *65 or older* or *aged* or *geriatric*, followed by a list of content topics of importance in each specialty. In *New Frontiers*, the time period covered was from January 1982 to October 2002, though the earliest year searched varied, from 1980 to 1994. For this supplement, the search was from October 2002 to December 2005; for some topics, important research findings that are more recent are also included. The full list of titles of papers resulting from the initial search was sent to the content expert, who selected titles meeting relevance criteria and then obtained abstracts of them. Following this, the content experts chose the papers to examine in full. In general, case reports and letters were excluded at this stage.

AGENDA ITEMS

Each agenda item is tagged with an abbreviation that indicates the specialty field (eg, "Ophth" for ophthalmology, "GenSurg" for general surgery) and a number, starting with the Arabic 1 in each chapter. The number is not meant to indicate importance or priority; it is provided simply to allow for easy cross-reference and citation. Agenda items from *New Frontiers* are discussed first in each chapter under headings referring to "Progress" in the topic in question. New agenda items added with this supplement are gathered at the ends of chapters under the heading "New Horizons" in the topic; the numbering of new agenda items in any chapter starts with the next Arabic number after the last item from that chapter in *New Frontiers.* In a few chapters, new Key Questions or modifications in original ones are proposed. The new Key Questions are assigned unique numbers.

Immediately following its identifying tag, each agenda item is also labeled with a letter from A to D, designating the type of research design and the clinical priority or importance of the proposed study. The word *level* is decidedly not intended to imply degrees of quality. The definitions for A-level through D-level studies, as explained in *New Frontiers,* are as follows:

- **Level A** identifies important studies with hypothesis-testing intent, using such designs as randomized controlled trials, certain nonrandomized controlled trials, or those cohort studies that focus on a single hypothesis.
- **Level B** identifies important studies with hypothesis-generating intent. Designs would include exploratory, multi-targeted cohort and case-control studies; retrospective or prospective analysis of large databases; cross-sectional observational studies; time series; outcome studies; retrospective case series; or post hoc analyses of randomized controlled trials.
- **Level C** identifies hypothesis-testing studies judged by the content experts to be of lesser importance and priority than those labeled A.
- **Level D** identifies hypothesis-generating studies judged to be of lesser importance than studies labeled B.

Proposed A (or C) studies generally must be preceded by B (or D) studies since research literature on geriatrics aspects of the specialties is today generally deficient in information that would allow for construction of the most efficient and cost-effective controlled trials. The research agenda items are almost entirely focused on clinical research. Where basic science investigations are critically needed to precede any clinical investigation, we have indicated that, but we have not suggested details regarding the design and execution of such studies.

Cross-Cutting Issues

New Frontiers ended with a chapter entitled "Cross-Cutting Issues," which covered topics that are relevant to many if not all the other chapters. (See *New Frontiers,* pp. 369–419.) This supplement does not cover these questions (agenda items CCI 1 through CCI 73). A second supplement is planned that will review recent research in these issues (physiologic changes in aging, stress response in aging, wound healing, pharmacology, outcomes assessment, preoperative assessment, perioperative clinical pathways, health-related quality of life, and models of care delivery).

Index

All elements in *New Frontiers* and this supplement are thoroughly indexed by topic: discussions of the literature in all the specialty fields and for each cross-cutting issue, specific studies by name; tables and figures; the agenda items and Key Questions, descriptions of research design, project history and methods, and more. Wherever the reference in the index is to an agenda item, the page number is bolded, which allows readers to look up a specific topic of particular interest (eg, postoperative delirium) and find all the agenda items in the book that relate to that topic. Index references to tables are signaled by the letter t after the page number; figures are likewise referenced with the letter f after the page number. The indexes for *New Frontiers* and its supplement have been merged. All index references to text, tables, figures, and agenda items in this supplement are followed by the tag S1. When a topic might be referred to by any one of several synonyms, we index it under all the various terms.

REFERENCES

1. Solomon DH, LoCicero J, 3rd, Rosenthal RA (eds). New Frontiers in Geriatrics Research: An Agenda for Surgical and Related Medical Specialties. New York: American Geriatrics Society, 2004 (online at http://www.frycomm/ags/rasp).
2. The Interdisciplinary Leadership Group of the American Geriatrics Society Project to Increase Geriatrics Expertise in Surgical and Medical Specialties. A statement of principles: toward improved care of older patients in surgical and medical specialties. J Am Geriatr Soc. 2000; 48:699-701.
3. Katz PR, Grossberg GT, Potter JF, Solomon DH. Geriatrics Syllabus for Specialists. New York: American Geriatrics Society, 2002.

2

GERIATRIC ANESTHESIA

*Christopher J. Jankowski, MD; David J. Cook, MD**

With the aging of the US population, issues related to surgical care of older patients have considerable public health significance. The elderly age group requires health care resources at a per capita rate that is higher than for any other age group. Perioperative care of older patients generates a variety of challenges. Age-related disease and declining physiologic functional reserve limit the ability of elderly surgical patients to withstand the stresses of anesthesia, surgery, and recovery. Elderly surgical patients have more perioperative complications than younger patients.[1] Complicating the issue is the difficulty of establishing the functional reserve of the older patients because of deconditioning, age-related disease, and cognitive impairment. Even determining who is an appropriate surgical candidate can be difficult. Further, the paucity of well-designed, definitive research concerning elderly surgical patients has provided clinicians with little guidance.

The chapter on geriatric anesthesia in *New Frontiers in Geriatrics Research* noted that geriatrics issues affect all areas of anesthesiology: preoperative evaluations, intraoperative management, postoperative care, and chronic pain management.[2] The chapter began with a review of age-related physiologic changes in the nervous, cardiovascular, respiratory, and urinary systems (see *New Frontiers,* pp. 10–14). In addition, it provided a synopsis of alterations in pharmacokinetics and pharmacodynamics seen in the elderly patient (see p. 14). This information provided a framework for the discussion of existing research and the development of recommendations for needed research. The result was 41 agenda items pertinent to anesthesiology, management of pain, and the perioperative care of the elderly patient. In addition, three issues were defined as Key Questions:

> ***Anes KQ1*: What preoperative assessments are useful in developing patient management plans for surgeries common in the elderly population?**
>
> ***Anes KQ2*: Can proper choice of postoperative analgesic techniques reduce postoperative morbidity or improve functional status at discharge?**
>
> ***Anes KQ3*: How can postoperative pulmonary complications in the elderly patient be reduced?**

The Key Questions specifically address the pre- and postoperative care of the older patient. The literature reviewed for *New Frontiers* suggested that there is no substantive difference in outcome between general anesthesia and regional anesthesia. It has been argued that this is the most significant choice anesthesiologists can make regarding intraoperative care. Thus, investigations regarding other intraoperative management issues were thought likely to be of low yield. Given limited research funding, the decision was made to focus the research agenda on areas more likely to be fruitful.

* Jankowski: Assistant Professor of Anesthesiology, Mayo Clinic, Consultant in Anesthesiology, Mayo Clinic, Rochester, MN; Cook: Professor of Anesthesiology, Mayo Clinic and Foundation, Rochester, MN.

This review updates the literature review of *New Frontiers* and identifies progress since the initial review of 2004. It also addresses emerging areas of research that warrant further investigation with regard to the perioperative care of the elderly person. *New Frontiers* laid out a broad agenda for research into issues of perioperative care of elderly surgical patients. That several of the questions have yet to be answered is not discouraging. To be answered satisfactorily, many of the issues require large multicenter clinical trials. Several years are required to conceive and design such trials, obtain funding, collect and analyze data, and publish the results. Thus, the number of publications addressing items in the research agenda put forward in *New Frontiers* is encouraging. It indicates that researchers already are aware of areas requiring more investigation.

This update identifies two emerging areas that require further study: perioperative glucose control and the role of intra- and postoperative anesthetic and analgesic management, specifically, regional versus general anesthesia. Two new agenda items have therefore been added to the research agenda in geriatric anesthesiology. (See the section New Horizons in Geriatric Anesthesia at the end of the chapter.)

As more data regarding these and issues previously identified by the project become available, information can be incorporated into clinical pathways aimed at improving medical and functional outcomes in elderly surgical patients. Anesthesiologists are involved throughout the continuum of care for every older surgical patient and will have a key role in investigating and implementing interventions to ensure that older patients have optimal surgical outcomes.

METHODS

A literature search was performed on the National Library of Medicine's PubMed database in July 2005. *Anesthesiology* and *intraoperative care* were searched as major MeSH headings and combined with various MeSH terms denoting advanced age: *age*, *geriatric assessment*, *aged*, *aged 80 and over*, *frail elderly*, *longevity*, and *geriatrics*. The following limits were placed on all searches: aged: 65+ years, the English language, humans, and the years 2000–2005. The anesthesiology portion of the search yielded 62 articles, and the intraoperative care segment resulted in 200 articles.

A separate search of the PubMed database was performed in June 2005. In this search, the topic *anesthesiology* was combined with the following terms for advanced age: *65 or older*, *aged*, and *geriatric*. Limits placed on the search included: the English language, core clinical journals, and the years 2000–2005. This search located 107 articles.

Additionally, reference lists from review articles included in the search results were examined for relevant articles.

Finally, separate searches were performed for each individual agenda item, using appropriate search terms and limiting the search as described.

All articles obtained in the various search strategies were reviewed to determine their relevance to the research agenda set forth in the 41 agenda items and three Key Questions in the anesthesiology chapter of *New Frontiers*. Papers that are relevant to the research agenda are briefly summarized herein, and recommendations are made as to whether any original agenda items need to be altered or omitted in light of recent findings.

PROGRESS IN PREOPERATIVE ASSESSMENT OF THE ELDERLY PATIENT

RISK ASSESSMENT

See *New Frontiers,* pp. 16–17.

FUNCTIONAL ASSESSMENT

See *New Frontiers,* pp. 17–18.

PREOPERATIVE TESTING

See *New Frontiers,* pp. 18–21.

PREOPERATIVE OPTIMIZATION

See *New Frontiers,* p. 21.

THE PREOPERATIVE RESEARCH AGENDA

Anes 1 (Level B): **Prospective epidemiologic studies are needed to describe the relative frequency of various outcomes characteristic of older surgical patients for the most common types of surgery.**

New Research Addressing This Question: No research published since the initial literature review was found.

Modification of This Question in Light of New Research: This question remains vital. Descriptions of the outcomes of older surgical patients will be the cornerstone for the design, testing, and implementation of strategies for appropriate preoperative evaluation of and intervention for aged patients (see Anes 3).

Anes 2 (Level B): **Once better understanding of characteristic outcomes of specific types of surgery for older patients is attained, patient- and surgery-specific risk factors for geriatric complications should be identified by multivariate analysis that would stratify surgical risk as low, intermediate, or high, depending on type of surgery.**

New Research Addressing This Question: No research published since the initial literature review was found.

Modification of This Question in Light of New Research: Anes 2 should remain on the research agenda. Information obtained from these types of studies will be invaluable in the design, testing, and implementation of preoperative testing and interventional strategies for improving outcome in geriatric surgical patients.

Anes 3 (Level B): **The positive predictive value of preoperative assessment instruments should be determined in prospective nonrandomized or prospective cohort trials.**

New Research Addressing This Question: The ongoing growth of the elderly age group has serious implications for preoperative evaluation clinics. Elderly patients are the most frequent users of surgical services and often require more extensive preoperative evaluation than younger patients having equivalent procedures. Thus, the challenge is to evaluate increasing numbers of patients needing relatively thorough examinations in a manner that is both cost-efficient and able to correctly identify conditions that may influence perioperative management. The use of questionnaires is one method by which this may be achieved. Ideally, these instruments could differentiate between patients whose medical status dictates a detailed preoperative medical evaluation and those who require a less extensive evaluation. Patients identified as needing an extensive preoperative work-up could be referred directly to a physician. Others could be sent first to a midlevel provider and referred to a physician only if pertinent issues were identified.

Hilditch et al developed a screening questionnaire to determine which patients need to be evaluated by an anesthesiologist before the day of surgery. The 17-question instrument contained closed-end questions regarding general health, exercise tolerance, family history, and previous anesthetic history. Patient responses to the items in the questionnaire were compared with the history obtained by an anesthesiologist. All questions except those regarding kidney disease and previous personal and family anesthetic history had at least good validity as determined by κ-coefficients or percentage agreement with the anesthesiologist's assessment, or both. [3]

Another approach to preoperative evaluation is to have allied health personnel screen patients to determine those who need to be examined by an anesthesiologist before going to surgery. A study by van Klei et al assessed the accuracy of specially trained nurses in preoperative health assessment. In this study, experienced postanesthesia care unit nurses received training in medical history taking and physical examination and attended lectures on a variety of medical subjects related to perioperative care, including those concerning the elderly patient. Patients (N = 4540) were first assessed by a trained nurse and then by an anesthesiologist. The nurses were asked to determine whether a patient was ready for surgery or required further evaluation. The nurse's assessment was compared with that of the anesthesiologist. Nurses were able to identify patients who were not ready for surgery with a sensitivity of 83% (95% confidence interval [CI]: 79% to 87%), a specificity of 87% (86% to 88%), a positive predictive value of 34% (31% to 38%), and a negative predictive value of 98% (98% to 99%). Therefore, although nurses often incorrectly identified patients as being not ready for surgery and referred them for further evaluation when none was needed, they rarely incorrectly classified patients requiring more extensive work-up as being ready for surgery. Although there was some inefficiency to this approach (anesthesiologists still needed to see patients who needed minimal assessment), it nonetheless provided for more efficient resource utilization than the traditional model by eliminating the need for a physician-conducted preoperative evaluation in certain patients. Most importantly, patients who required physician-conducted preoperative examinations rarely were misidentified. [4]

Given the importance of malnutrition in predicting adverse surgical outcomes, [5] it is vital to preoperatively identify malnourished patients, since this information may influence surgical decision making. [6] The Mini Nutritional Assessment (MNA) tool can be used to evaluate nutritional status during a preoperative evaluation. [7–9] However, because it requires anthropomorphic measurements and the completion of a questionnaire, it is time-consuming and may not be appropriate in the setting of a focused preoperative examination. The Mini Nutritional Assessment–Short Form (MNA–SF) consists of six items extracted from the original MNA: five questions and body mass index. [10] The MNA–SF can be administered quickly and has a sensitivity and specificity of 100% and 69.5%, respectively, for determining the absence of overt malnutrition in elderly surgical patients. Although the positive predictive value is only 19.4%, the negative predictive value was 100% (if the MNA–SF is negative, the patient does not have overt malnutrition).[11]

Modification of This Question in Light of New Research: The MNA–SF successfully identifies patients with overt malnutrition. Given that this condition may alter surgical planning,[6] it would be reasonable to evaluate the MNA–SF in a prospective trial to determine whether its application improves perioperative outcomes in older surgical patients (see Anes 4).

The Hilditch questionnaire and nurse evaluation studies are encouraging. However, neither approach focused on the elderly age group. Given the complexity of older surgical patients, these instruments need to be validated in elderly cohorts. Further, taken together, the results of the two studies suggest that a third approach may be viable: the use of a questionnaire to triage patients requiring extensive evaluation directly to a physician. Others would be seen by a midlevel provider and referred to a physician only if relevant issues were identified. Therefore, Anes 3 should neither be modified nor eliminated.

Anes 4 (Level A): **Following evaluation of preoperative assessment instruments (Anes 3), prospective randomized trials should be performed to determine whether the application of these metrics could improve outcomes for elderly surgical patients by altering perioperative intervention, surgical timing, the type or extent of surgery, or postoperative management.**

New Research Addressing This Question: No research published since the initial literature review was found.

Modification of This Question in Light of New Research: Development of instruments described in Anes 3 will be beneficial only if they result in interventions to improve outcomes. Therefore, Anes 4 should remain unchanged.

Anes 5 (Level B): **Prospective cohort studies are needed to determine whether assessment of the older surgical patient's preoperative functional status affects surgical decision making or perioperative care.**

New Research Addressing This Question: A prospective cohort study of 544 patients examined the relative contributions of preoperative health status and intraoperative factors on the incidence of complications in older surgical patients. Multivariate analysis demonstrated that decreased functional status (defined as ≥ 3, where 1 = no limitation of activities, 2 = intermittent limitation, 3 = mild limitation, 4 = moderate limitation, and 5 = severe limitation) is an independent risk factor for adverse postoperative neurologic events.[12] In a prospective cohort study of elderly patients having hip and knee arthroplasty, even subtle declines in preoperative functional status was found to predict postoperative delirium.[13] However, our search strategy uncovered no studies addressing whether baseline functional status affects surgical decision making or perioperative care. No specific recommendations regarding functional status of the heart, pulmonary system, kidneys, mobility, or cognitive status are yet available.

Modification of This Question in Light of New Research: No modification of Anes 5 is recommended. Altering surgical care in light of predictors of adverse outcome is a reasonable approach to the care of older surgical patients. The advent of newer, less invasive alternatives to traditional open procedures offers options where none were previously available.[14] Assessing whether preoperative functional status leads to alterations in perioperative care lays a foundation for the studies proposed in Anes 6. In addition, studies proposed in Anes 5 will provide a measure of the value that those involved in the surgical decision-making process and providing perioperative care place on functional assessment. If the predictive value of functional status on perioperative outcomes is shown not to be appreciated, there will be opportunities to improve care through educational efforts emphasizing its importance.

> *Anes 6 (Level A)*: **Depending on findings of prospective cohort studies (Anes 5), randomized trials should be performed to determine whether preoperative functional status assessment of elderly patients changes decisions about type or timing of surgery, or pre- or postoperative care strategies and outcomes.**

New Research Addressing This Question: No research published since the initial literature review was found.

Modification of This Question in Light of New Research: In an era of limited health care resources, studies such as those suggested by Anes 6 are vitally important. As more options for less invasive surgical procedures evolve (see Anes 5), selecting the correct procedure for a given patient will become more complicated. A key public health issue will be to select procedures in order to maximize improvement in functional status while minimizing the risk of complications and resource utilization. For example, is there a level of preoperative functional status at which the risk of complications for a given orthopedic procedure is sufficiently high such that it would better to perform a less invasive or temporizing procedure? Conversely, is there a subgroup of patients for whom more heroic operations are indicated? The goal of these studies would be to quantify this information for various elderly surgical populations and develop metrics that would enable surgical decision making to relate more directly to current and predicted functional status.

> *Anes 7 (Level B)*: **Cross-sectional or prospective cohort studies are needed to determine by multivariate analysis whether there is an association between pre-existing cognitive impairment, depression, or alcohol abuse and adverse outcomes in geriatric patients.**

New Research Addressing This Question: It is well known that significant pre-existing cognitive impairment, depression, or alcohol abuse predict delirium in elderly medical patients.[15,16] Alcohol abuse and significant cognitive impairment also predict postoperative delirium in elderly noncardiac surgical patients.[17] However, these issues have not been extensively studied in elderly surgical patients. This is important because, unlike medical patients, older surgical patients are generally not acutely ill at the time of surgery. Also, the physiologic stresses imposed by anesthesia and surgery differ from those of medical illness. Thus, studies in this area are essential.

A prospective cohort study examining predictors of postoperative delirium in 427 elderly total hip and total knee arthroplasty patients demonstrated that even subtle preoperative cognitive impairment predicts postoperative delirium. Forty six (10.8%) developed postoperative delirium. Preoperative verbal intelligence as measured by the American National Adult Reading Test [18] and gross cognitive status as measured by the Mini-Mental State Examination (MMSE) [19] were similar between those who did and did not develop postoperative delirium. However, as a group, patients who subsequently developed postoperative delirium were found to have decreased verbal fluency (as measured by the Controlled Oral Word Association Test [20]), verbal learning (as measured by the Auditory Verbal Learning Test [21]), and concentration (as measured by the Stroop Color-Word Test [22]). [13] Gruber-Baldini et al performed a multicenter longitudinal cohort study in 674 elderly hip fracture patients that examined the outcomes associated with cognitive impairment. This group found that that prefracture or in-hospital cognitive impairment as indicated by an MMSE score lower than 24 or the presence of delirium predicted poor functional outcome at 2 and 12 months postoperatively. In addition, incident cognitive dysfunction predicted later functional and social impairment. [23]

Modification of This Question in Light of New Research: Although these studies provide some guidance with regard to cognitive impairment, further work needs to be done to make sure that the results are applicable across a wide range of surgical procedures. In addition, further research is required to determine which tests are most useful for the preoperative evaluation of cognitive function (see Anes 33). Finally, given the prevalence of depression and alcohol abuse in the elderly age group, it is vital to examine the role they play in postoperative outcomes. [24–30]

> *Anes 8 (Level A)*: **For any association that is established by cross-sectional cohort studies between cognitive impairment, depression, or alcohol abuse and adverse outcomes in elderly surgical patients (Anes 7), prospective randomized trials should be performed to determine the effect of pre- or postoperative interventions on these adverse outcomes.**

New Research Addressing This Question: No research published since the initial literature review was found.

Modification of This Question in Light of New Research: No modification of Anes 8 is recommended.

PROGRESS IN INTRAOPERATIVE MANAGEMENT

Regional Versus General Anesthesia

See *New Frontiers,* pp. 23–25.

Physiologic Management

See *New Frontiers,* pp. 25–26.

The Intraoperative Research Agenda

> *Anes 9 (Level B)*: **Cross-sectional or retrospective case-control studies are needed to identify the incidence of adverse cardiac or**

thrombotic-embolic complications in elderly patients undergoing surgery with and without preoperative β-blockade, antithrombotic or antiplatelet therapy, or with a hematocrit above a target value. These studies should be in surgeries identified as having an intermediate or high risk for related complications.

New Research Addressing This Question: A large multicenter prospective observational study addressed the effects of perioperative aspirin for patients undergoing coronary artery bypass grafting. Aspirin (650 mg) administered within 48 hours after revascularization was found to be independently associated with a lower incidence of death, nonfatal myocardial infarction, stroke, renal failure, and bowel infarction. Multivariate analysis did not reveal any other factors to be associated with the reductions of these adverse outcomes. In addition, discontinuation of aspirin use before surgery was found to be an independent risk factor for mortality (odds ratio [OR] = 1.79, 95% CI: 1.18 to 2.69). The risk of hemorrhage, gastritis, infection, and impaired wound healing was not increased with aspirin use.[31]

No studies addressing the issue of perioperative aspirin therapy in a noncardiac surgical population were identified.

A number of previously published prospective studies demonstrate an association between perioperative β-blockade and improved cardiac outcomes, particularly in high-risk patients undergoing high-risk procedures.[32–35] However, in a recent large retrospective study involving nearly 800,000 patients, perioperative β-adrenergic blockade was found to be associated with an increase in in-hospital mortality in patients who had a low a priori risk of cardiac morbidity and mortality (OR = 1.43, 95% CI: 1.29 to 1.58) (see Figure 2.1).[36] Ongoing studies will refine understanding of the role of perioperative β-blockade in elderly surgical patients.[37–39]

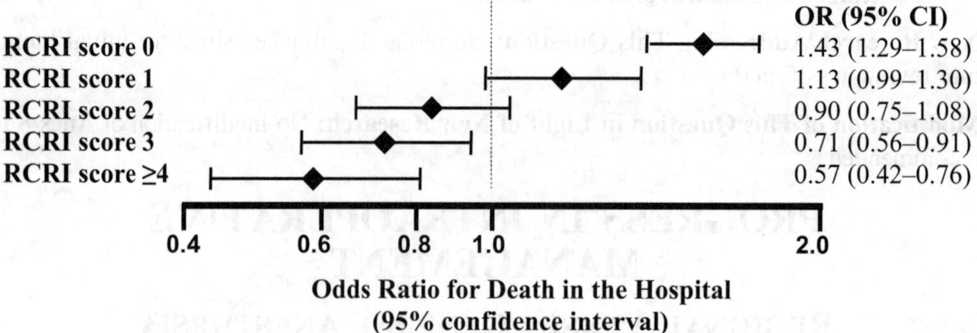

Figure 2.1—Odds ratios for in-hospital deaths for patients who received perioperative β-blocker therapy versus those who did not, stratified by cardiac risk as determined by the Relative Cardiac Risk Index or RCRI (Lee TH, Marcantonio ER, Mangione CM, et al. Derivation and prospective validation of a simple index for prediction of cardiac risk of major noncardiac surgery. Circulation 1999;100:1043–1049). Components of the RCRI include diabetes mellitus, ischemic heart disease, cerebrovascular disease, renal insufficiency, and high-risk surgery. (Source: Adapted with permission from Lindenauer PK, Pekow P, Wang K, et al. Perioperative beta-blocker therapy and mortality after major noncardiac surgery. N Engl J Med 2005;353:349–361. Copyright © 2005 Massachusetts Medical Society. All rights reserved.)

Postoperative thromboembolic complications are common and an area of active study (see Anes 10). A retrospective case-control study demonstrated that enoxaparin is superior to warfarin monotherapy for early venous thromboprophylaxis following hip and knee arthroplasty in postmenopausal women (OR 8.6, $P < .0001$ for any thrombosis, OR 11.3, $P < .0001$ for proximal thrombosis).[40] However, in another retrospective case-control study, thomboprophylaxis with tinzaparin was found to be associated with an increased incidence of serious postoperative bleeding.[41] Thus, although low-molecular-weight heparins may be more effective than warfarin therapy in preventing venous thromboembolism, they carry the risk of hemorrhagic complications. Multimodal thromboprohylaxis may offer a way to minimize thrombotic complications and bleeding associated with prophylactic measures. In a large retrospective case series, extensive multimodal thromboprophylaxis (preoperative discontinuation of procoagulant medications, autologous blood donation, hypotensive epidural anesthesia, intravenous heparin during surgery and before femoral preparation, aspiration of intramedullary contents, pneumatic compression, thigh-high stockings, early mobilization, and chemoprophylaxis with aspirin or warfarin for 4 to 6 weeks postoperatively) decreased the incidence of thrombosis and pulmonary embolism in hip arthroplasty patients in comparison with historical controls.[42]

No studies were identified regarding hematocrit value.

Modification of This Question in Light of New Research: There is little question that in high-risk patients undergoing high-risk surgery, perioperative β-blockade reduces adverse cardiac outcomes. Extant studies will help determine its role in patients with lower risk.[37–39]

Perioperative antiplatelet therapy in the form of aspirin has a salutary effect on patients undergoing coronary artery bypass grafting. However, the role of aspirin and other antiplatelet therapy in elderly noncardiac surgical patients still needs to be defined.

Although the efficacy and safety of various antithrombotic strategies have been studied in large prospective randomized trials (see Anes 10), none focused exclusively on elderly patients. This is significant, given the frequency of polypharmacy in older patients and the drug interactions associated with warfarin.[43] Clearly, there is a need for investigations in this area. In addition to retrospective case-control studies, one option for obtaining hypotheses-generating data might be to perform post hoc analyses on data from the elderly patients who participated in the randomized trials. These studies should examine the incidence of adverse reactions as closely as prevention of thrombosis. Subsequent prospective randomized trials could be designed on the basis of these results. Further, there is a need for well-designed retrospective studies examining the utility of multimodal approaches to thromboprophylaxis. This approach is especially attractive for geriatric patients, given that it minimizes pharmacologic intervention.

Alternative medicines are used by a large proportion of the population, and many are associated with excessive bleeding.[44,45] However, to date, no larger studies have associated them with increased perioperative blood loss, transfusion, or bleeding complications. In an era of limited research funding, investigations into the perioperative implications of the use of these substances should have low priority.

A more appropriate use of research resources might be to examine ways to improve administration of known therapies for preventing thrombotic complications. Despite evidence of their efficacy, they are not used universally. For example, although the Netherlands has national guidelines for thromboprophylaxis, compliance is not optimal.[46] Computerized alerts and other systems changes may improve delivery of thromboprophylaxis,[47,48] and there is a need to evaluate the feasibility of broad application of these measures.

Finally, research is still required to determine appropriate target hemoglobin levels in older surgical patients. The American Society of Anesthesiologists Practice Guidelines for Perioperative Blood Transfusion and Adjuvant Therapies states that patients usually should receive transfusions for hemoglobin levels of $\leq$ 6 g/dL and rarely for levels $>$ 10.[49] However, this guideline does not specifically consider elderly patients. Further, higher hemoglobin levels may be beneficial in the elderly patient.[50] Therefore, there is a critical need for studies in this area.

Anes 10 (Level A): **For any association in elderly patients of cardiac thrombotic-embolic complications with a specific preoperative therapy or hematocrit level, prospective cohort or randomized studies are needed to determine if pre- or intraoperative therapies would reduce the complications.**

New Research Addressing This Question: A number of recent large prospective randomized trials have examined the efficacy of a variety of thromboprophylactic strategies, including newer agents such as factor Xa and thrombin inhibitors.[51–60] However, as noted (see Anes 9), none focused solely on older patients.

Modification of This Question in Light of New Research: Prospective studies regarding cardiac complications and β-blockers have been completed (see Anes 9).
As noted how-
ever, questions remain. Ongoing studies may clarify the issue.[37–39]

Although there has been active investigation of various thromboprophylactic therapies, these studies have not addressed older patients per se. Therefore, more research is required to assure that these interventions have acceptable risk-benefit ratios in this highly vulnerable population.

Studies regarding hematocrit levels and antiplatelet therapy are still needed.

As a whole, studies suggested by Anes 10 address a broad range of critical issues in elderly surgical patients. Although they will be difficult to design and execute, these studies will provide information that could significantly alter surgical care for older patients.

Anes 11 (Level D): **Prospective nonrandomized investigation of the effect of perioperative temperature management on surgical morbidity in the geriatric population is needed. These investigations should be conducted under conditions where either the surgery is physiologically very challenging or the older patient carries a high burden of comorbidity. Cardiac, respiratory, bleeding, and renal outcomes would be the primary focus of these investigations.**

New Research Addressing This Question: The search did not locate any articles that directly addressed Anes 11. However, two studies addressed other outcomes related to perioperative temperature management. In one study, 338 mostly elderly patients were randomized to either aggressive forced-air intraoperative warming therapy or standard care during a variety of noncardiac procedures. Patients who were randomized to aggressive intraoperative warming had relative risk reduction of 46% for the development of pressure ulcers.[61]

In an interesting study, Yucel et al performed a post hoc analysis of a cohort of patients with colorectal cancer who were randomized to normothermic versus hypothermic (34.5°C) temperature management during primary resection. The groups were demographically similar, including information on tumor grade and stage.[62] With up to 9 years of follow-up, there was no difference in cancer-free or overall survival. However, in the original study, hypothermia was associated with increased incidence of infection, decreased wound collagen deposition, and increases in days to first solid food, suture removal, and hospital discharge.[63] Given the strong evidence of other adverse outcomes associated with it,[63–68] the results of this study should not be viewed as an endorsement of perioperative hypothermia. That said, the authors are to be commended for evaluating long-term outcomes associated with perioperative hypothermia. Across the spectrum of geriatric surgical care, more studies addressing the long-term implications of perioperative management are needed.

Modification of This Question in Light of New Research: As noted, no studies have been published directly addressing Anes 11 since *New Frontiers* was published. In addition, recent evidence suggests that advanced age is a risk for developing intraoperative hypothermia.[69] Thus, Anes 11 should remain on the research agenda. However, relevant outcomes should be expanded to include surgical site infections.[63]

> *Anes 12 (Level D)*: **Retrospective or cross-sectional research studies should be conducted to identify any relationship between the use or timing of perioperative antibiotic therapy and postoperative pneumonia or wound infection. Differences, if any, between younger and older patients undergoing the same type of surgery should also be examined.**

New Research Addressing This Question: A retrospective study examined the effect of intraoperative redosing of prophylactic cefazolin on surgical site infection in cardiac surgery lasting more than 240 minutes after the first dose was given. Most of the 1548 patients were elderly. The overall risk of surgical site infection was similar between those who had intraoperative redosing (9.4%) and those who did not (9.3%) (OR 1.01, 95% CI: 0.70 to 1.47). However, redosing reduced the incidence of surgical site infection in patients whose procedures lasted longer than 400 minutes (7.7% versus 16.0%, OR 0.44, 95% CI: 0.23 to 0.86).[70]

Modification of This Question in Light of New Research: This study is an encouraging start. However, its results may not be generalizable to the noncardiac surgical population. Further, no studies have addressed prophylactic antibiotic use and the risk of pneumonia. Likewise, there have been no studies to determine what, if any, differences exist between younger and older patients. Anes 12 should remain on the research agenda unchanged.

> *Anes 13 (Level C)*: **Depending on the findings in Anes 12, prospective randomized studies should be used to determine whether preoperative or postoperative antibiotic therapies reduce complications related to infections in elderly surgical patients.**

New Research Addressing This Question: No research published since the initial literature review was found.

Modification of This Question in Light of New Research: Surgical site infections are a major source of postoperative morbidity and mortality and may be responsible for ~$1.6 billion in excess hospital charges annually in the United States.[71] Determining effective strategies to prevent complications from perioperative infections will have important public health and patient care implications. Anes 13 should not be altered.

> *Anes 14 (Level D)*: **Multicenter case-control or prospective cohort studies should be performed to determine whether receiving or not receiving blood in the perioperative period affects the incidence of perioperative infection and immunosuppression in elderly patients. Multivariate analysis would be required to separate the effect of homologous blood transfusion from the comorbid conditions making transfusion more likely.**

New Research Addressing This Question: The search revealed two articles related to Anes 14. The first was a small retrospective analysis of 56 patients undergoing repair of ruptured abdominal aortic aneurysms. Respiratory complications (prolonged ventilation, infection, or respiratory distress) occurred in 40.0% of patients receiving salvaged autologous blood and in 12.5% patients who did not ($P = .047$). However, the analysis did not consider whether this may have been a function of comorbid conditions. Also, 95% of patients who received salvaged autologous blood had suprarenal aortic cross-clamping, compared with only 63% in the group that did not receive salvaged blood. These, among other reasons, limit the applicability of this study to a general elderly surgical population.[72]

The results from the second study may be more broadly applicable. Tang et al performed a single-center prospective cohort study of 2809 patients undergoing elective resection of the colon and rectum to determine the risk factors for surgical site infection. Most patients were older than 56 years. By the use of multivariate analysis, homologous blood transfusion was found to be an independent risk factor for overall surgical infection (OR = 2.0, 95% CI: 1.1 to 3.3 for 1 to 3 units transfused, OR = 6.2, 95% CI: 4.2 to 10.2 for $\geq$ 4 units transfused). Interestingly, of the 14 risk factors found to be significant via multivariate analysis, only blood transfusion was a significant risk factor for all surgical site infections examined (incisional and organ-space with and without anastomotic leakage).[73]

Modification of This Question in Light of New Research: The study by Tang et al is well done. Nevertheless, more research is needed, specifically, studies more closely examining the effects of age and including other populations for whom surgical site infections may be devastating, such as orthopedic and cardiac surgical patients. In addition, the studies must be designed and analyzed with a view toward specific implications for improving practice.

> *Anes 15 (Level C)*: **If perioperative infection and immunosuppression in older surgical patients are shown to be associated with receiving blood in the preoperative period (Anes 14), alternative strategies such as delaying surgery or erythropoietin therapy should then be compared with blood transfusion in prospective cohort studies, because a randomized trial could not be justified.**

New Research Addressing This Question: No research published since the initial literature review was found.

Modification of This Question in Light of New Research: An aging population places strain on health care resources. Therefore, it is essential to examine simple, inexpensive strategies such as delaying surgery to improve outcome. Anes 15 should remain on the research agenda unchanged.

> *Anes 16 (Level D)*: **Cohort or case-control studies are needed to determine the relationship in older surgical patients between perioperative termination of anticoagulation and thromboembolic or bleeding risk.**

New Research Addressing This Question: No research published since the initial literature review was found.

Modification of This Question in Light of New Research: Given the frequency with which older surgical patients require long-term anticoagulation for mechanical heart valves, chronic congestive heart failure, and history of thrombosis, as well as the variability of perioperative anticoagulant bridging therapy, studies of this nature are imperative. Anes 16 should remain on the research agenda unchanged.

> *Anes 17 (Level C)*: **The effect of timing of termination and resumption as well as the temporizing use of antiplatelet agents in older surgical patients should be compared in case-control or prospective cohort studies.**

New Research Addressing This Question: No research published since the initial literature review was found.

Modification of This Question in Light of New Research: Anes 17 should remain on the research agenda unchanged.

> *Anes 18 (Level B)*: **In prospective cohort studies the incidence of perioperative hypotension, aspiration, and renal insufficiency should be compared in elderly patients undergoing standard nothing-by-mouth orders before surgery and in elderly patients who would be allowed clear liquids closer to the time of surgery. This study would need to be conducted in:**

- **patients undergoing specific types of procedures where liberalization of fluid intake is not contraindicated for surgical reasons,**
- **patients undergoing procedures that place them at greater risk for developing hypovolemia (eg, bowel prep), and**
- **instances where preoperative hypovolemia may contribute to complications (eg, angiographic procedures).**

New Research Addressing This Question: No research published since the initial literature review was found.

Modification of This Question in Light of New Research: Cardiac catheterizations are common in the United States, and most are performed on elderly patients. Aging is associated with both chronic dehydration and reduced creatinine clearance, and these two factors are fundamental determinants of contrast nephropathy.[74] Prevention of contrast nephropathy is an area of active investigation, but those studies have not reached specific conclusions or recommendations regarding care of the elderly patient in angiographic procedures.[74]

In January 1999 the American Society of Anesthesiologist Task Force on Preoperative Fasting issued new guidelines for preoperative fasting and the use of pharmacologic agents to reduce the risk of pulmonary aspiration.[75] The revised guidelines call for preoperative fasts of 6, 4, and 2 hours for solids, nonclear liquids, and clear liquids, respectively. In theory, the preoperative fast may now have a lesser effect on volume status and may reduce the incidence of perioperative hypotension and renal insufficiency. That said, chronic dehydration is common in the elderly patient; its incidence increases with age, and it is often misdiagnosed.[76–78] Given the frequency of baseline chronic dehydration, it is unlikely that the new preoperative fasting guidelines will have a significant effect on the incidence of hypotension and renal insufficiency. However, there remains need for studies examining this issue. Further, the new guidelines may increase the incidence of aspiration in elderly surgical patients, a group that already is at high risk.[79,80] It is critical that the effect of the new preoperative fasting guideline on the incidence of aspiration be examined.

PROGRESS IN POSTOPERATIVE MANAGEMENT

POSTOPERATIVE RESPIRATORY INSUFFICIENCY

See *New Frontiers,* pp. 28–29.

ACUTE PAIN MANAGEMENT

See *New Frontiers,* p. 29.

PAIN AND ADVERSE OUTCOMES

See *New Frontiers,* pp. 30–32.

DELIRIUM AND COGNITIVE DECLINE

See *New Frontiers,* pp. 32–34.

THE POSTOPERATIVE RESEARCH AGENDA

Anes 19 (Level B): **Prospective studies that better identify patient and procedural risk factors for respiratory failure, aspiration, and pneumonia in elderly surgical patients are needed.**

New Research Addressing This Question: No research published since the initial literature review was found.

Modification of This Question in Light of New Research: Pulmonary complications are common after surgery.[81,82] Although patient and procedural risk factors have been studied, little is known about them in the elderly age group. Recent awareness of the role of obstructive sleep apnea in postoperative pulmonary complications, along with its prevalence and the unreliability of traditional markers for the syndrome in the elderly patient,[83,84] make studies suggested by Anes 19 even more important. Therefore, it should remain on the research agenda unchanged.

Anes 20 (Level A): **Randomized trials are needed to determine if respiratory monitoring or O_2 therapy can reduce the incidence of respiratory failure in elderly surgical patients.**

New Research Addressing This Question: Though there are ongoing studies addressing this issue,[85] none have been published to date.

Modification of This Question in Light of New Research: The interventions suggested by Anes 20 require little effort or expense. If proved to be effective, they will provide an elegant solution to a significant problem. Therefore, Anes 20 should not be altered or eliminated.

Anes 21 (Level A): **Randomized studies of prophylactic antibiotics, changes in pharyngeal instrumentation, or the way feeding is advanced are needed to determine whether practice changes reduce aspiration and postoperative pneumonia in elderly surgical patients. (See also the Key Questions at the beginning of the chapter.)**

New Research Addressing This Question: No research published since the initial literature review was found.

Modification of This Question in Light of New Research: Anes 21 should remain on the research agenda unchanged. The trend toward earlier discharge and feeding in abdominal surgery patients makes studies regarding the effects of early advancement of feeding even more pertinent.

Anes 22 (Level B): **Cross-sectional studies capable of identifying any relationship in elderly surgical patients between intensive nutritional support in high-risk surgery and functional status on discharge (eg, chronic respiratory failure, ambulation, independent living) are needed.**

New Research Addressing This Question: No research published since the initial literature review was found.

Modification of This Question in Light of New Research: Functional status may be the most significant outcome measure for elderly surgical patients. Therefore, studies examining the association between perioperative interventions and functional status are especially important. Anes 22 should remain on the research agenda unchanged.

Anes 23 (Level A): **Data from studies of associations between nutritional support and postoperative functional status after high-risk surgery in elderly patients (Anes 22) should be used to design prospective cohort or randomized controlled trials comparing feeding strategies in elderly patients at risk for malnutrition and muscle wasting following major surgery.**

New Research Addressing This Question: No research published since the initial literature review was found.

Modification of This Question in Light of New Research: Anes 23 should remain on the research agenda unchanged.

Anes 24 (Level C): **Randomized trials of interventions that might attenuate postoperative catabolism or facilitate the transition to anabolism in the elderly patient are needed.**

New Research Addressing This Question: No research published since the initial literature review was found.

Modification of This Question in Light of New Research: Anes 24 should remain on the research agenda unchanged.

Anes 25 (Level C): **Large cross-sectional studies describing analgesic practice and its complications in the elderly surgical patient are needed.**

New Research Addressing This Question: Frasco et al examined the effect of the Pain Initiative of the Joint Commission for Accreditation of Healthcare Organizations (JCAHO) on perioperative analgesic care. [86] The JCAHO Pain Initiative standards recognize that pain is often undertreated in surgical patients and are an attempt to enhance perioperative analgesic care by improving assessment and promoting aggressive treatment of pain. [87] In the Frasco study, 541 patients treated by the use of the JCAHO Pain Initiative guidelines were compared with matched historical controls who had surgery in the period immediately before the JCAHO Pain Initiative was implemented. Mean age (± S.D.) in the treatment group was 63.1 (± 14.3) years and 63.9 (± 13.8) years in the historical controls. However, patients ranged from 15 to 93 years of age. Those whose care was delivered according to the guidelines received more opiates, but also required more treatment for postoperative nausea and vomiting. There was no difference between groups in the incidence of respiratory depression requiring intervention. [86]

Modification of This Question in Light of New Research: Anes 25 should remain on the research agenda unchanged. The study described did not focus on elderly surgical patients. Given the alterations in baseline opiate sensitivity [88,89] and decreases in metabolism and elimination capacity in the elderly patient (see *New Frontiers,* pp. 13–14), the studies suggested in Anes 25 remain vitally important and will form the cornerstone for studies based on Anes 26.

Anes 26 (Level B): **Depending in part on findings of large, descriptive studies of analgesia in elderly patients (Anes 25), prospective cohort studies are needed to determine the effect of analgesic modes (patient-controlled versus as-needed versus scheduled dosing), route of administration, the role of nonopioid adjunctive drugs, and nonpharmacologic interventions. These investigations must define a balance between adequate analgesia and reduction of the incidence of adverse drug events in the elderly patient.**

New Research Addressing This Question: No research published since the initial literature review was found.

Modification of This Question in Light of New Research: The information provided by studies related to this question will provide important preliminary data for trials outlined in Anes 27. Anes 26 should remain on the research agenda unchanged.

Anes 27 (Level A): **Prospective randomized controlled trials comparing outcomes with analgesic programs specific to types of surgery are needed to determine whether analgesic regimes designed for the elderly patient reduce in-hospital morbidity or improve functional status on discharge. (See also the Key Questions at the beginning of the chapter.)**

New Research Addressing This Question: In a prospective observational study to determine the risk factors for postoperative delirium in elderly patients undergoing total hip and knee arthroplasty, patients whose postoperative analgesic regimen consisted of continuous perineural infusions of local anesthetics supplemented with small amounts of opiates were found to have a 59% lower incidence of postoperative delirium than those who received patient-controlled analgesia intravenous opiates alone.[90] The study did not address the issue of functional status on discharge.

Modification of This Question in Light of New Research: Though the study described was not a randomized trial, its results suggest that investigations in this area may be fruitful. Future trials should be randomized and consider hospital resource utilization and long-term functional status as well as in-hospital morbidity and functional status on discharge. Further, the utility of multimodal analgesic approaches and novel analgesic adjuncts, such as dexmedetomidine,[91,92] should be examined in trials involving operations that are not amenable to regional anesthetic and analgesic techniques.

Anes 28 (Level D): **Improved tools for the assessment of pain in the cognitively impaired elderly patient should be developed.**

New Research Addressing This Question: Pain is often inadequately treated in the cognitively impaired elderly patient.[93] It is a subjective experience, and significant cognitive impairment limits patients' abilities to complete self-report measures.[94,95] Therefore, the development of appropriate measures of pain in elderly patients with cognitive impairment is imperative. The challenge is to develop tools that do not rely on self-report of symptoms.

Several new instruments for the assessment of pain in cognitively impaired older patients have been introduced recently. The first is the DOLOPLUS 2. It consists of 10 items across three domains: somatic reactions (somatic complaints, protective body postures at rest, protection of sore areas, expression, sleep pattern), psychomotor reactions (washing and/or dressing, mobility), and psychosocial reactions (communication, social life, and behavioral problems). Although this scale is recommended for use only in noncommunicative patients, several items rely on the patient's ability to communicate.[96] The only validation study for the instrument compared it with the Visual Analog Scale (VAS), a self-report tool.[97] Thus, its utility is unclear.

The Pain Assessment in Advanced Dementia (PAINAD) scale is an observational metric based on five items: breathing, vocalization, facial expression, body language, and consolability.[98] The PAINAD scale was validated in a cohort of severely demented nursing home patients. Reliability (consistency across time and different raters) and validity (ability to measure pain and not other conditions [eg, depression] and to accurately reflect changes in pain experience) are adequate.[99]

Fisher et al developed the Proxy Pain Questionnaire (PPQ) to investigate the association in nursing home patients between caregiver reports and Minimum Data Set (MDS) reports of pain.[100] The MDS is a quarterly assessment of nursing home patients that evaluates a variety of parameters, including pain.[101,102] The attractiveness of the PPQ lies in its simplicity. It consists of three questions: (1) Within the last week has this resident experienced pain? (2) How often does this resident experience pain? (3) In general, when this patient is in pain, how would you describe the extent of the pain? Despite the straightforward nature of the instrument, it is very reliable. Unfortunately, it was found to be only weakly valid in comparison with the MDS.[99] However, pain may be under-reported by use of the MDS.[103] Thus, further validation is necessary to determine the utility of the PPQ.

The Pain Assessment for the Dementing Elderly (PADE) is another instrument designed for use by non-research-trained staff. It consists of 24 brief questions and takes about 5 minutes to complete.[104] It is highly reliable, but weakly valid.[99]

Modification of This Question in Light of New Research: A key aspect of perioperative care is excellent pain control. Pain is associated with a variety of adverse outcomes.[105–111] Satisfactory postoperative analgesia depends on the ability to assess level of pain. With an aging population, increasing numbers of cognitively impaired patients will require surgery. For these patients, traditional self-reported measures of pain, such as the VAS and the Numeric Pain Scale scores, clearly are inadequate.[112] In addition, existing tools are underutilized.[113] Development of instruments to assess pain in this population is essential. Although the studies described are encouraging, none was tested in a surgical population. Future development of such metrics needs to include postoperative patients in the validation cohort. In addition, when possible, instruments should be designed to be used by caregivers rather than specially trained researchers or clinicians in order to increase vastly the utility of future assessments.

***Anes 29 (Level C)*: Improved tools for assessing pain in cognitively impaired elderly patients (Anes 28) should be used to determine the adequacy of pain management strategies in this group of patients.**

New Research Addressing This Question: As noted in Anes 28, no sufficient tools have been developed.

Modification of This Question in Light of New Research: The use of new tools for evaluating pain in this population to test pain management strategies will be crucial to improving perioperative care in this vulnerable population. Anes 29 should remain on the research agenda unchanged.

***Anes 30 (Level D)*: A retrospective review is needed to determine the incidence of polypharmacy with combinations of drugs that might contribute to complications (hypotension, bradycardia, falls, confusion, bleeding diathesis, constipation, and urinary retention) in geriatric surgical patients.**

New Research Addressing This Question: No research published since the initial literature review was found.

Modification of This Question in Light of New Research: The baseline frequency of polypharmacy in the elderly person,[114,115] combined with the large number of medications administered in the perioperative period, makes answering this question important. Anes 30 should not be altered or eliminated.

Anes 31 (Level A): **The effect on outcomes for elderly surgical patients of simplifying drug regimens in hospital or of communicating that information to primary care physicians should be examined in a randomized controlled trial.**

New Research Addressing This Question: No research published since the initial literature review was found.

Modification of This Question in Light of New Research: Acute hospitalization provides an excellent opportunity to review and appropriately adjust the often complicated medication regimens of elderly surgical patients and thus to minimize the risks associated with polypharmacy. However, a program to do so would require a great deal of effort on the part of health care providers. Therefore, there must be studies evaluating the efficacy of this approach before it is implemented.

Anes 32 (Level B): **Cross-sectional studies, with multivariate analysis, are needed to determine whether the risk factors for delirium in elderly surgical patients are the same as those for elderly medical patients.**

New Research Addressing This Question: A single-center prospective cohort study addressing this issue in elective orthopedic surgical patients has recently been completed. Results are forthcoming.[116]

Modification of This Question in Light of New Research: The ongoing study may clarify this issue. However, further investigations will be necessary to confirm its results and test its applicability across a broad range of elderly surgical patients.

Anes 33 (Level B): **Studies are needed on the utility of the Confusion Assessment Method (CAM) for serial testing of elderly patients before and after surgery to facilitate the diagnosis of postoperative delirium. The CAM should be compared with other tests of cognitive function and with the clinical diagnosis for delirium. At the same time, since dementia is the leading predisposing factor for delirium, the utility of short mental status tests to make the preoperative diagnosis of early dementia should be tested, using a full psychiatric examination as the gold standard.**

New Research Addressing This Question: The literature search did not reveal any studies assessing the utility of the CAM in a purely surgical population. This is significant for two reasons: First, the CAM was developed by the use of patients in a general medicine ward and an outpatient population.[117] Applying the instrument in a surgical population may be difficult. For example, using it in the early postoperative period may identify patients as delirious when they are still under the influence of anesthetic agents. It is unclear whether delirium in that circumstance is prognostic of outcome in the same way as delirium that occurs after the effects of anesthetics have abated. However, there is evidence that, in hip fracture surgery patients, a positive CAM 60 minutes after discontinuation of volatile anesthetic agents predicts later postoperative delirium.[118] And second, the CAM already has been used as the endpoint for a number of studies examining postoperative delirium.[13,17,23,50,90,105,118–137] Without validation and agreement on the appropriate time at which to begin screening for delirium, it is difficult to interpret the findings of studies applying the CAM in surgical patients.

The CAM has been compared with other screening tests for delirium. Gaudreau et al compared the Nursing Delirium Screening Scale (Nu-DESC) with the CAM, the Memorial Delirium Assessment Scale (MDAS), [138] and the criteria from the *Diagnostic and Statistical Manual of Mental Disorders,* 4th edition (DSM-IV). The Nu-DESC is a brief, five-item observational instrument based on the DSM-IV criteria for delirium. In a comparison with the CAM, the Nu-DESC was found to be 85.7% sensitive and 86.8% specific. However, CAM results, not DSM-IV criteria, were considered the gold standard for the diagnosis of delirium in this study. [139] Adamis et al compared the Delirium Rating Scale, [140] a 10-item clinician-rated symptom rating scale for delirium, with the CAM and found good to very good agreement between the two instruments in acutely ill hospitalized patients, but, again, no gold standard for diagnosis was used for comparison. [141] Other studies have the same methodologic flaw. [142–144]

Regarding preoperative cognitive screening, the MMSE [19] is a widely accepted screen for dementia; however, it is too cumbersome and time-consuming for use in busy clinical practices. Because of this, short tests of cognition have been developed. [145–148] The Mini-Cog is a more recently developed screening tool for dementia and is considered to be among the most useful. [149,150] It consists of three-item recall and a clock-drawing test and is to be performed in 2 to 4 minutes, rather than the 5 to 12 minutes necessary for the MMSE. It is similar in sensitivity and specificity to the MMSE and formal neuropsychologic testing for detecting dementia. [151] No studies were identified that used the Mini-Cog in a surgical population.

Modification of This Question in Light of New Research: There remains a need for studies examining the use of the CAM in elderly surgical patients. Research is needed not only to validate its usefulness in this population but also to determine the optimal time at which to apply it in relation to emergence from anesthesia. Studies comparing other delirium assessment instruments with the CAM must utilize gold standard clinical criteria, such as those in the updated text revision of DSM-IV (the DSM-IV-TR). These projects are essential to improving understanding of issues regarding postoperative delirium because without valid, standardized instruments to determine the presence of delirium, it will be difficult to interpret the results of studies.

Although research into the Mini-Cog is encouraging, there remains a need for further investigation into the utility of this and other instruments for surgical populations.

***Anes 34 (Level A)*: Prospective controlled (nonrandomized; ie, by ward or unit) trials in patients at moderate to high risk for delirium should be performed to determine the effect of preoperative or postoperative interventions on the incidence of delirium.**

New Research Addressing This Question: A longitudinal prospective sequential study examined the effect of a nurse-led interdisciplinary intervention for delirium. [136] The intervention consisted of nursing education, systematic screening for delirium using the NEECHAM Confusion Scale, [152] consultation with a trained geriatric care provider, and use of a scheduled pain medication protocol. A cohort of 60 elderly patients admitted for hip fracture treatment received standard care; 60 subsequent patients (median age 80 years, interquartile range 12 years) received the intervention. The incidence of delirium was similar in the control and intervention cohorts (23.3% versus 20.0%, respectively, P = .82). However, the duration of delirium was shorter in the intervention cohort (P = .03). Severity of delirium was reduced in the intervention group as well. In addition, cognitive function measured by the memory subdimension of the MMSE [19] was better in the delirious patients than in the interventional group. Unfortunately, the intervention did not result in improved rehabilitation or functional status.

In a prospective trial Marcantonio et al randomized 126 hip fracture patients to either usual care or to receive a proactive geriatrics consultation. [50] In the intervention group, a geriatrician made daily rounds and made recommendations based on a structured protocol (see Table 2.1). The number of recommendations was limited to five on the initial visit and three in subsequent visits in order to improve compliance. Mental status and incidence and severity of delirium were assessed daily by blinded observers using validated scales. [19,117,138,153,154] The incidence of delirium was reduced in the intervention group (32% versus 50%, $P = .04$, relative risk 0.64, 95% CI: 0.37 to 0.98). Delirium severity was reduced as well. This study is encouraging because the recommendations used for the intervention group could, by and large, be implemented through education of surgical care

***TABLE 2.1*—Content of the Structured Geriatrics Consultation to Prevent Postoperative Delirium**

1. Adequate CNS oxygen delivery:
   a. Supplemental oxygen to keep saturation > 90%, preferably > 95%
   b. Treatment to raise systolic blood pressure > 2/3 baseline or > 90 mmHg
   c. Transfusion to keep hematocrit > 30%
2. Fluid/electrolyte balance:
   a. Treatment to restore serum sodium, potassium, glucose to normal limits (glucose < 300 mg/dL for diabetics)
   b. Treat fluid overload or dehydration as appropriate
3. Treatment of severe pain:
   a. Around-the-clock acetaminophen (1 gram four times daily)
   b. Early-stage breakthrough pain: low-dose morphine, avoid meperidine
   c. Late-stage break-through pain: oxycodone as needed
4. Elimination of unnecessary medicine:
   a. Discontinue/minimize benzodiazepines, anticholinergics, antihistamines
   b. Eliminate drug interactions, adverse effects; modify drugs accordingly
   c. Eliminate medication redundancies
5. Regulation of bowel/bladder function:
   a. Bowel movement by postoperative day 2 and every 48 hours
   b. Discontinue urinary catheter by postoperative day 2, screen for retention or incontinence
   c. Skin care program for patients with established incontinence
6. Adequate nutritional intake:
   a. Dentures used properly, proper positioning for meals, assist as needed
   b. Nutritional supplements as needed
   c. If unable to take food orally, feed via temporary nasogastric tube
7. Early mobilization and rehabilitation:
   a. Out of bed on postoperative day 1 and several hours daily

***Table 2.1*—Content of the Structured Geriatrics Consultation to Prevent Postoperative Delirium—Cont'd**

b. Mobilize/ambulate by nursing staff as tolerated
c. Daily physical therapy; occupational therapy if needed

8. Prevention, early detection, and treatment of major postoperative complications:
   a. Myocardial infarction/ischemia—electrocardiogram, cardiac enzymes if needed
   b. Supraventricular arrhythmias/atrial fibrillation—appropriate rate control, electrolyte adjustments, anticoagulation
   c. Pneumonia/chronic obstructive pulmonary disease—screening, treatment, including chest therapy
   d. Pulmonary embolus—appropriate anticoagulation
   e. Screening for and treatment of urinary tract infection
9. Appropriate environmental stimuli:
   a. Appropriate use of glasses and hearing aids
   b. Provision of clock and calendar
   c. If available, use of radio, tape recorder, and soft lighting
10. Treatment of agitated delirium:
    a. Appropriate diagnostic workup/management
    b. For agitation, calm reassurance, family presence, and/or sitter
    c. For agitation, if absolutely necessary, low-dose haloperidol 0.25–0.5 mg every 4 hours as needed; if contraindicated, use lorazepam at same dose

SOURCE: Marcantonio ER, Flacker JM, Wright RJ, et al. Reducing delirium after hip fracture: a randomized trial. J Am Geriatr Soc 2001;49:516–522. Adapted and reprinted with permission.

providers and adapted into care protocols for geriatric surgical patients without significant increase of health care resource utilization.

In addition to studies examining altered paradigms of perioperative care for geriatric surgical patients, pharmacologic prevention of delirium has been examined. In a study examining the use of low-dose haloperidol for the prevention of delirium, 430 hip surgery patients ≥ 70 years old were randomized to receive 1.5 mg per day of haloperidol or placebo starting preoperatively and continuing for up to 3 days after surgery.[155] Though there was no difference in the incidence of delirium, severity and duration were reduced in those receiving haloperidol. Importantly, hospital length of stay also was reduced (mean difference = 5.5 days, 95% CI: 1.4 to 2.3 days, $P < .001$). Again, this study demonstrates that a relatively simple and inexpensive intervention can markedly influence perioperative outcome.

Modification of This Question in Light of New Research: The studies described show that pre- and postoperative interventions can improve delirium-related outcomes in elderly hip fracture patients. However, they were performed only in hip surgery patients, a group at relatively high risk for postoperative delirium. Further work is required to determine whether these interventions are effective in other high- and moderate-risk surgical populations. In addition, studies are needed that address the relative contribution of each component of multimodal delirium prevention programs, such as those in the studies by Marcantonio and Milisen.[135,136] Subsequent studies can examine the efficacy of optimized multimodal protocols that are based on projects identifying the most effective individual interventions for preventing delirium. Finally, it is crucial to assess whether the recommendations provided by the geriatric consultation service in the Marcantonio study can be successfully incorporated into the routine care of geriatric surgical patients without the necessity of separate geriatric consultation. This goal is especially important, given the increasing numbers of older patients undergoing surgery and the relatively limited number of geriatricians and hospitalists available to provide such services.

PROGRESS IN CHRONIC PAIN

See *New Frontiers,* pp. 36–37.

Anes 35 (Level B): **The first priority in chronic pain trials is large cross-sectional studies that are powered to identify any relationship between pain intervention and functional outcomes.**

New Research Addressing This Question: No research published since the initial literature review was found.

Modification of This Question in Light of New Research: Anes 35 should remain on the research agenda unchanged. Although efforts have been made to demonstrate improvements in functional status in elderly chronic pain patients that are related to opiate therapy (see Anes 36), there remains a need for hypothesis-generating studies that examine other therapies, including implantable spinal cord stimulators, pain blocks, physical and psychological rehabilitation therapy, and complementary therapies such as acupuncture.

Anes 36 (Level A): **With the establishment of any relationship between intervention for chronic pain and functional outcomes in elderly patients (Anes 35), it must be determined prospectively if specific chronic pain therapies can improve functional outcomes in treatment groups relative to a historical or concurrent nonrandomized control.**

New Research Addressing This Question: Although no hypothesis-generating studies as suggested in Anes 35 have been published, there have been a number of reports examining the effects of pain intervention on functional outcome. Specifically, these studies evaluated the impact of opiate therapy. Eight studies [156–163] published since 2001 that enrolled a total of 2640 patients were included in a recent systematic review that included three other studies, for a total of 2877 patients. The quality of the included studies ranged from low to moderate or high, but overall, opiates were associated with significant improvements in functional status, including quality of life.[164]

No studies examining functional status outcomes as they relate to other pain management strategies in elderly patients were identified.

Modification of This Question in Light of New Research: Further studies are needed and should be based on outcomes from studies to address Anes 35. Here, too, a variety of therapeutic modalities should be examined.

Anes 37 (Level C): **Given the high incidence rate of herpes zoster in the geriatric population, further prospective studies are needed to determine if antiviral, analgesic, or anti-inflammatory therapies during acute zoster can reduce, relative to standard care, the development of chronic postherpetic neuralgia.**

New Research Addressing This Question: Postherpetic neuralgia (PHN) is common in the elderly age group.[165,166] The pain associated with it is associated with significant functional disability.[167] Thus, studies aimed at the prevention of PHN have considerable public health significance.

The literature search did not identify any trials published since *New Frontiers* comparing the use of antiviral therapy versus standard care for the prevention of PHN. A systematic review concluded that oral acyclovir provided a modest reduction in pain 1 to 3 months after zoster onset.[168]

No studies exploring the use of steroids and analgesics were identified.

For theoretical reasons, combination therapy may be more effective in preventing PHN. Pasqualucci et al randomized 600 patients with acute herpes zoster to receive either intravenous acyclovir for 9 days combined with prednisolone for 21 days or epidural bupivacaine (boluses given every 6 to 12 hours) combined with epidural prednisolone every 3 to 4 days. Treatment duration in the epidural group ranged from 7 to 21 days. The incidence of PHN pain at 1 year was 22.2% and 1.6% in the acyclovir and epidural groups, respectively ($P < .001$).[169]

Because this approach requires hospitalization and extensive use of health care resources, van Wijck et al compared oral antivirals and analgesics with a single epidural injection of methylprednisolone and bupivacaine. Although the incidence of pain at 1 month was modestly reduced in the epidural group (48% versus 58%, relative risk 0.38, 95% CI: 0.71 to 0.97, $P = .02$), there were no differences at 3 and 6 months.[170]

A more recent approach to the prevention of PHN is the use of vaccines. With age, there is a progressive decline in cell-mediated immunity to varicella zoster virus; the incidence and severity of herpes zoster and PHN are associated with this decline.[171–179] That recurrence of herpes zoster is rare in immunocompetent individuals, presumably as a result of an immunizing effect, suggests that strategies to increase cell-mediated immunity would be useful in the prevention of PHN.[171–173,180,181]

In a multicenter randomized, double-blind, and placebo-controlled trial of over 38,000 patients aged 60 years and older, Oxman et al tested an investigational live attenuated varicella zoster vaccine for the prevention of PHN. The results were promising. In patients who received the vaccine, the herpes zoster and PHN were reduced by 51.3% and 66.5%, respectively (for both $P < .001$). There was a low incidence of side effects.[182]

Modification of This Question in Light of New Research: Given the lack of definitive answers regarding other strategies for its prevention, there remains a need for further prospective studies examining the role of antiviral, analgesic, and anti-inflammatory therapies during acute zoster in the prevention of PHN. Special consideration should be given to combination therapies and examining resource utilization. Moreover, Anes 37 should be designated as an A-level agenda item because PHN is both common and associated with significant functional disability among older persons.

As promising as vaccines may be for the prevention of PHN, in their current form they are not 100% effective in preventing PHN. Clearly, more research regarding this therapy is needed.

Anes 38 (Level D): **Cross-sectional studies documenting the association of chronic pain therapy with the incidence of complications like confusion, postural hypotension, falls, urinary retention, and constipation in the elderly population are needed.**

New Research Addressing This Question: No research published since the initial literature review was found.

Modification of This Question in Light of New Research: Elderly persons have diminished physiologic functional reserve that affects all organ systems. (See *New Frontiers,* pp. 17–18.) This makes them more prone to adverse side effects from chronic pain treatment modalities. Information provided by Anes 38 will allow for more rational approach to treatment decision making. This is analogous to the possibility of using functional status to assist in surgical planning (see Anes 6). For example, patients with a high propensity for confusion may not be appropriate candidates for chronic opiate therapy.

> *Anes 39 (Level D)*: **Cross-sectional studies that describe pain management in cognitively impaired patients, relative to a nonimpaired population, are needed.**

New Research Addressing This Question: No research published since the initial literature review was found.

Modification of This Question in Light of New Research: Anes 39 should remain unaltered. Given the diminished functional reserve capacity in cognitively impaired patients and potential for pain therapies (eg, opiates) to alter cognitive function, this question remains vital.

> *Anes 40 (Level D)*: **Pain assessment tools for chronic pain in the cognitively impaired elderly patient must be compared prospectively with standard assessment methods.**

New Research Addressing This Question: No research published since the initial literature review was found.

Modification of This Question in Light of New Research: Assessment of chronic pain includes evaluating the effects of pain, including functional status and altered mood. However, in chronic pain clinical practice and research, the same tools used to assess acute pain are used for chronic pain. Therefore, information derived in Anes 28 could be applied to Anes 40.

> *Anes 41 (Level C)*: **Prospective trials comparing different analgesic strategies with regard to clinical and functional outcomes are needed.**

New Research Addressing This Question: A study by Wong et al is an example of the usefulness of the research proposed in Anes 41. In this prospective, randomized, double-blind trial, 100 patients with pancreatic cancer were assigned to receive either neurolytic celiac plexus block with systemic analgesic therapy as needed or optimized systemic analgesic therapy along with a sham block. Patients were followed for 1 year or until death. Pain control ($P \leq .01$) and quality of life ($P < .001$) improved 1 week after randomization in both groups, but there was a larger decrease in pain in those who received the block ($P = .005$). Pain control was better in the block group over time, as well ($P = .01$). However, opiate consumption, opiate side effects, and quality of life were similar between groups. There was no difference in survival between groups.[183]

Modification of This Question in Light of New Research: More studies, such as the one described but focusing on elderly patients, are needed across the spectrum of chronic pain conditions and therapies. This is especially crucial because many current invasive and implantable pain therapies are costly. If they cannot be shown to confer significant clinical and functional benefit, there will be little justification for their use in treating elderly patients.

NEW HORIZONS IN GERIATRIC ANESTHESIA

Since publication of *New Frontiers*, two areas of study have emerged—one new, one old—that bear further research in geriatric patients.

PERIOPERATIVE GLUCOSE CONTROL

Diabetes mellitus is associated with adverse perioperative outcomes. [184–190] Even in patients without diabetes, hyperglycemia is associated with increased mortality, incidence of postoperative infection, and resource utilization in surgical patients. [191,192] Because of this, a number of recent studies have examined the role of glucose control in critically ill and surgical patients. [191,193–202] In 2001, van den Berghe et al published a landmark study examining the effect of intensive insulin therapy on mortality, morbidity, and resource utilization in critically ill patients. In this prospective study, patients admitted to a surgical intensive care unit were randomized to receive either intensive insulin therapy (maintenance of blood glucose between 80 and 110 mg/dL) or conventional treatment (insulin only for blood glucose > 215 mg/dL and subsequent maintenance of blood glucose between 180 and 200 mg/dL). Overall, intensive care unit mortality was 4.6% and 8.0% ($P > .04$) in the intensive insulin and conventional treatment groups, respectively. The adjusted reduction in mortality was 32% (95% CI: 2% to 55%). [202] Intensive insulin therapy is associated with better immune system function, [203] reduced inflammation, [204] improved lipid profiles, [205] preservation of endothelial function, [206] and protected mitochondrial structure and function. [207] However, it appears that the clinical benefit of this therapy is due to blood glucose levels independently of insulin dose. [208,209]

Therefore, studies addressing the role of intra- and postoperative glucose management in elderly surgical patients are imperative. However, hypoglycemia is associated with mortality in elderly patients, [210] and the incidence of hypoglycemia is high with intensive insulin therapy. [202] Given that glucose would not likely be as well controlled outside of a study situation, [211] studies examining morbidity and mortality associated with various glucose levels should also address morbidity caused by strategies to lower perioperative glucose.

> *Anes 42 (Level A)*: **Large prospective randomized studies addressing the role of intraoperative and postoperative glucose management in elderly surgical patients are needed, to include assessment of associations of specific glucose levels or specific glucose control strategies with morbidity and mortality.**

REGIONAL VERSUS GENERAL ANESTHESIA

New Frontiers concluded that research on the impact of intraoperative anesthetic management on perioperative outcomes in the elderly was unlikely to be fruitful. (See *New Frontiers,* pp. 23–25.) Well-designed investigation into the effects on the perioperative outcomes of regional versus general anesthesia—arguably the most substantively dissimilar choices regarding intraoperative anesthetic management—failed to demonstrate clinically significant differences in outcomes between the two techniques.[212] Given the equivalency in outcome between these two vastly different techniques, it was felt that further research into this area was unlikely to yield clinically useful information and should not be pursued, especially given limited funds for research. However, recent studies suggest that anesthetic management may indeed affect cognitive outcome.

For example, in vivo studies demonstrate that exposing neurons to volatile anesthetic gases increases oligomerization and toxicity of Alzheimer-like proteins.[213] Further, in an animal model, exposure to clinically relevant concentrations of volatile anesthetics leads to impaired memory and learning.[214–216]

Design issues may be why previous studies of regional versus general anesthesia failed to show differences in cognitive outcomes. In theory, the advantage of regional anesthetic techniques is that they minimize exposure to medications that act on the central nervous system and block the neuroendocrine stress response to surgery.[217] A major weakness of previous studies examining the effect of regional versus general anesthesia on cognitive outcomes was that postoperative analgesic management was not controlled.[135,218,219] Thus, patients were exposed to pharmacologic agents that may have affected cognitive outcomes (eg, opiates). It is possible that improvements in cognitive outcome related to anesthetic or analgesic technique require that those techniques be continued into the postoperative period. Recently, postoperative analgesic techniques have been developed which employ indwelling perineural catheters to deliver continuous infusions of local anesthetics. These techniques are associated with significant reductions in parenteral opiate requirements and excellent analgesia.[220] Preliminary evidence suggests that, by themselves, these techniques are associated with reduced incidence of postoperative delirium. In addition, these techniques may lead to improved cognitive outcomes when patients also receive regional instead of general anesthesia.[90]

In light of the development of peripheral nerve catheter techniques and these data, prospective randomized trials should be performed that examine the effect of intravenous patient-controlled opiate analgesia versus central neuraxial or peripheral nerve catheter analgesia, or both, on cognitive outcomes in the setting of both regional versus general anesthesia. These studies will be difficult and expensive to perform, but they are exceedingly important, as the results may have a profound impact on the perioperative care of elderly surgical patients.

Anes 43 (Level A): **Prospective randomized trials are needed to determine the effect of intravenous patient-controlled opiate analgesia versus central or peripheral nerve catheter analgesia, or both, on cognitive outcomes in the setting of both regional versus general anesthesia.**

REFERENCES

1. Tiret L, Desmonts JM, Hatton F, Vourc'h G. Complications associated with anaesthesia—a prospective survey in France. Can Anaesth Soc J 1986;33:336-344.
2. Cook DJ. Geriatric anesthesia. In Solomon DH, LoCicero J, 3rd, Rosenthal RA (eds): New Frontiers in Geriatrics Research: An Agenda for Surgical and Related Medical Specialties. New York: American Geriatrics Society, 2004, pp. 9-52 (online at http://www.frycomm.com/ags/rasp).
3. Hilditch WG, Asbury AJ, Jack E, McGrane S. Validation of a pre-anaesthetic screening questionnaire. Anaesthesia 2003;58:874-877.

4. van Klei WA, Hennis PJ, Moen J, et al. The accuracy of trained nurses in pre-operative health assessment: results of the OPEN study. Anaesthesia 2004;59:971-978.
5. Gibbs J, Cull W, Henderson W, et al. Preoperative serum albumin level as a predictor of operative mortality and morbidity: results from the National VA Surgical Risk Study. Arch Surg 1999;134:36-42.
6. Perioperative total parenteral nutrition in surgical patients. The Veterans Affairs Total Parenteral Nutrition Cooperative Study Group. N Engl J Med 1991;325:525-532.
7. Guigoz Y, Vellas BJ. [Malnutrition in the elderly: the Mini Nutritional Assessment (MNA)]. Ther Umsch 1997;54:345-350.
8. Guigoz Y, Vellas B, Garry PJ. Assessing the nutritional status of the elderly: the Mini Nutritional Assessment as part of the geriatric evaluation. Nutr Rev 1996;54:S59-S65.
9. Cohendy R, Gros T, Arnaud-Battandier F, et al. Preoperative nutritional evaluation of elderly patients: the Mini Nutritional Assessment as a practical tool. Clin Nutr 1999;18:345-348.
10. Rubenstein LZ, Harker JO, Salva A, et al. Screening for undernutrition in geriatric practice: developing the short-form mini-nutritional assessment (MNA-SF). J Gerontol A Biol Sci Med Sci 2001;56:M366-M372.
11. Cohendy R, Rubenstein LZ, Eledjam JJ. The Mini Nutritional Assessment-Short Form for preoperative nutritional evaluation of elderly patients. Aging (Milano) 2001;13:293-297.
12. Leung JM, Dzankic S. Relative importance of preoperative health status versus intraoperative factors in predicting postoperative adverse outcomes in geriatric surgical patients. J Am Geriatr Soc 2001;49:1080-1085.
13. Jankowski CJ, Cook DJ, Schroeder DR, Warner DO. Mild reductions in preoperative cognitive and functional status are associated with postoperative delirium [abstract]. Anesth Analg 2005;100:S178.
14. Law WL, Chu KW, Tung PH. Laparoscopic colorectal resection: a safe option for elderly patients. J Am Coll Surg 2002;195:768-773.
15. Pompei P, Foreman M, Rudberg MA, et al. Delirium in hospitalized older persons: outcomes and predictors. J Am Geriatr Soc 1994;42:809-815.
16. Inouye SK, Viscoli CM, Horwitz RI, et al. A predictive model for delirium in hospitalized elderly medical patients based on admission characteristics. Ann Intern Med 1993;119:474-481.
17. Marcantonio ER, Goldman L, Mangione CM, et al. A clinical prediction rule for delirium after elective noncardiac surgery. JAMA 1994;271:134-139.
18. Taylor KI, Salmon DP, Rice VA, et al. Longitudinal examination of American National Adult Reading Test (AMNART) performance in dementia of the Alzheimer type (DAT): validation and correction based on degree of cognitive decline. J Clin Exp Neuropsychol 1996;18:883-891.
19. Folstein MF, Robins LN, Helzer JE. The Mini-Mental State Examination. Arch Gen Psychiatry 1983;40:812.
20. Loonstra AS, Tarlow AR, Sellers AH. COWAT metanorms across age, education, and gender. Appl Neuropsychol 2001;8:161-166.
21. Steinberg BA, Bieliauskas LA, Smith GE, et al. Mayo's Older Americans Normative Studies: Age- and IQ-Adjusted Norms for the Auditory Verbal Learning Test and the Visual Spatial Learning Test. Clin Neuropsychol 2005;19:464-523.
22. Jensen AR, Rohwer WD, Jr. The Stroop color-word test: a review. Acta Psychol (Amst) 1966;25:36-93.
23. Gruber-Baldini AL, Zimmerman S, Morrison RS, et al. Cognitive impairment in hip fracture patients: timing of detection and longitudinal follow-up. J Am Geriatr Soc 2003;51:1227-1236.
24. Liberto JG, Oslin DW, Ruskin PE. Alcoholism in older persons: a review of the literature. Hosp Community Psychiatry 1992;43:975-984.

25. Rocca WA, Grossardt BR, Peterson BJ, et al. The Mayo Clinic cohort study of personality and aging: design and sampling, reliability and validity of instruments, and baseline description. Neuroepidemiology 2006;26:119-129.
26. Licht-Strunk E, van der Kooij KG, van Schaik DJ, et al. Prevalence of depression in older patients consulting their general practitioner in The Netherlands. Int J Geriatr Psychiatry 2005;20:1013-1019.
27. Ostbye T, Kristjansson B, Hill G, et al. Prevalence and predictors of depression in elderly Canadians: The Canadian Study of Health and Aging. Chronic Dis Can 2005;26:93-99.
28. Harris T, Cook DG, Victor C, et al. Onset and persistence of depression in older people—results from a 2-year community follow-up study. Age Ageing 2006;35:25-32.
29. Hybels CF, Blazer DG. Epidemiology of late-life mental disorders. Clin Geriatr Med 2003;19:663-696, v.
30. Blazer DG. Depression in late life: review and commentary. J Gerontol A Biol Sci Med Sci 2003;58:M249-M265.
31. Mangano DT. Aspirin and mortality from coronary bypass surgery. N Engl J Med 2002;347:1309-1317.
32. Wallace A, Layug B, Tateo I, et al. Prophylactic atenolol reduces postoperative myocardial ischemia. McSPI Research Group. Anesthesiology 1998;88:7-17.
33. Mangano DT, Layug EL, Wallace A, Tateo I. Effect of atenolol on mortality and cardiovascular morbidity after noncardiac surgery. Multicenter Study of Perioperative Ischemia Research Group. N Engl J Med 1996;335:1713-1720.
34. Poldermans D, Boersma E, Bax JJ, et al. Bisoprolol reduces cardiac death and myocardial infarction in high-risk patients as long as 2 years after successful major vascular surgery. Eur Heart J 2001;22:1353-1358.
35. Poldermans D, Boersma E, Bax JJ, et al. The effect of bisoprolol on perioperative mortality and myocardial infarction in high-risk patients undergoing vascular surgery. Dutch Echocardiographic Cardiac Risk Evaluation Applying Stress Echocardiography Study Group. N Engl J Med 1999;341:1789-1794.
36. Lindenauer PK, Pekow P, Wang K, et al. Perioperative beta-blocker therapy and mortality after major noncardiac surgery. N Engl J Med 2005;353:349-361.
37. Devereaux PJ, Yusuf S, Yang H, et al. Are the recommendations to use perioperative beta-blocker therapy in patients undergoing noncardiac surgery based on reliable evidence? CMAJ 2004;171:245-247.
38. Schouten O, Poldermans D, Visser L, et al. Fluvastatin and bisoprolol for the reduction of perioperative cardiac mortality and morbidity in high-risk patients undergoing non-cardiac surgery: rationale and design of the DECREASE-IV study. Am Heart J 2004;148:1047-1052.
39. Silverstein JH. Personal communication (study in progress): Elder surgery—functional recovery after beta blockade. NIH Grant #5R01AG018772-05. Abstract available at http://crisp.cit.nih.gov.
40. Brotman DJ, Jaffer AK, Hurbanek JG, Morra N. Warfarin prophylaxis and venous thromboembolism in the first 5 days following hip and knee arthroplasty. Thromb Haemost 2004;92:1012-1017.
41. Cook G, Depares J, Singh M, McElduff P. Readmission after hysterectomy and prophylactic low molecular weight heparin: retrospective case-control study. BMJ 2006;332:819-820.
42. Gonzalez Della Valle A, Serota A, Go G, et al. Venous thromboembolism is rare with a multimodal prophylaxis protocol after total hip arthroplasty. Clin Orthop Relat Res 2006;444:146-153.
43. Holbrook AM, Pereira JA, Labiris R, et al. Systematic overview of warfarin and its drug and food interactions. Arch Intern Med 2005;165:1095-1106.

44. Tsen LC, Segal S, Pothier M, Bader AM. Alternative medicine use in presurgical patients. Anesthesiology 2000;93:148-151.
45. Hodges PJ, Kam PC. The peri-operative implications of herbal medicines. Anaesthesia 2002;57:889-899.
46. Ettema HB, Hoppener MR, Henny CP, et al. Compliance of Dutch orthopedic departments with national guidelines on thromboprophylaxis: a survey of Dutch orthopedic thromboprophylaxis. Acta Orthop 2005;76:99-103.
47. Kucher N, Koo S, Quiroz R, et al. Electronic alerts to prevent venous thromboembolism among hospitalized patients. N Engl J Med 2005;352:969-977.
48. Mosen D, Elliott CG, Egger MJ, et al. The effect of a computerized reminder system on the prevention of postoperative venous thromboembolism. Chest 2004;125:1635-1641.
49. Practice guidelines for perioperative blood transfusion and adjuvant therapies: an updated report by the American Society of Anesthesiologists Task Force on Perioperative Blood Transfusion and Adjuvant Therapies. Anesthesiology 2006;105:198-208. Online at: http://www.asahq.org/publicationsAndServices/BCTGuidesFinal.pdf.
50. Marcantonio ER, Flacker JM, Wright RJ, Resnick NM. Reducing delirium after hip fracture: a randomized trial. J Am Geriatr Soc 2001;49:516-522.
51. Bauer KA, Eriksson BI, Lassen MR, Turpie AG. Fondaparinux compared with enoxaparin for the prevention of venous thromboembolism after elective major knee surgery. N Engl J Med 2001;345:1305-1310.
52. Eriksson BI, Agnelli G, Cohen AT, et al. The direct thrombin inhibitor melagatran followed by oral ximelagatran compared with enoxaparin for the prevention of venous thromboembolism after total hip or knee replacement: the EXPRESS study. J Thromb Haemost 2003;1:2490-2496.
53. Francis CW, Berkowitz SD, Comp PC, et al. Comparison of ximelagatran with warfarin for the prevention of venous thromboembolism after total knee replacement. N Engl J Med 2003;349:1703-1712.
54. Colwell CW, Jr., Berkowitz SD, Davidson BL, et al. Comparison of ximelagatran, an oral direct thrombin inhibitor, with enoxaparin for the prevention of venous thromboembolism following total hip replacement: a randomized, double-blind study. J Thromb Haemost 2003;1:2119-2130.
55. Eriksson BI, Bergqvist D, Kalebo P, et al. Ximelagatran and melagatran compared with dalteparin for prevention of venous thromboembolism after total hip or knee replacement: the METHRO II randomised trial. Lancet 2002;360:1441-1447.
56. Eriksson BI, Dahl OE, Buller HR, et al. A new oral direct thrombin inhibitor, dabigatran etexilate, compared with enoxaparin for prevention of thromboembolic events following total hip or knee replacement: the BISTRO II randomized trial. J Thromb Haemost 2005;3:103-111.
57. Agnelli G, Bergqvist D, Cohen AT, et al. Randomized clinical trial of postoperative fondaparinux versus perioperative dalteparin for prevention of venous thromboembolism in high-risk abdominal surgery. Br J Surg 2005;92:1212-1220.
58. Eriksson BI, Borris L, Dahl OE, et al. Oral, direct factor Xa inhibition with BAY 59-7939 for the prevention of venous thromboembolism after total hip replacement. J Thromb Haemost 2006;4:121-128.
59. Turpie AG, Fisher WD, Bauer KA, et al. BAY 59-7939: an oral, direct factor Xa inhibitor for the prevention of venous thromboembolism in patients after total knee replacement. A phase II dose-ranging study. J Thromb Haemost 2005;3:2479-2486.
60. Samama CM, Vray M, Barre J, et al. Extended venous thromboembolism prophylaxis after total hip replacement: a comparison of low-molecular-weight heparin with oral anticoagulant. Arch Intern Med 2002;162:2191-2196.

61. Scott EM, Leaper DJ, Clark M, Kelly PJ. Effects of warming therapy on pressure ulcers—a randomized trial. AORN J 2001;73:921-927, 929-933, 936-938.
62. Yucel Y, Barlan M, Lenhardt R, et al. Perioperative hypothermia does not enhance the risk of cancer dissemination. Am J Surg 2005;189:651-655.
63. Kurz A, Sessler DI, Lenhardt R. Perioperative normothermia to reduce the incidence of surgical-wound infection and shorten hospitalization. Study of Wound Infection and Temperature Group. N Engl J Med 1996;334:1209-1215.
64. Just B, Delva E, Camus Y, Lienhart A. Oxygen uptake during recovery following naloxone: relationship with intraoperative heat loss. Anesthesiology 1992;76:60-64.
65. Frank SM, Fleisher LA, Breslow MJ, et al. Perioperative maintenance of normothermia reduces the incidence of morbid cardiac events: a randomized clinical trial. JAMA 1997;277:1127-1134.
66. Schmied H, Kurz A, Sessler DI, et al. Mild hypothermia increases blood loss and transfusion requirements during total hip arthroplasty. Lancet 1996;347:289-292.
67. Carli F, Emery PW, Freemantle CA. Effect of perioperative normothermia on postoperative protein metabolism in elderly patients undergoing hip arthroplasty. Br J Anaesth 1989;63:276-282.
68. Sessler DI, Sessler AM. Experimental determination of heat flow parameters during induction of general anesthesia. Anesthesiology 1998;89:657-665.
69. Macario A, Dexter F. What are the most important risk factors for a patient's developing intraoperative hypothermia? Anesth Analg 2002;94:215-220, table of contents.
70. Zanetti G, Giardina R, Platt R. Intraoperative redosing of cefazolin and risk for surgical site infection in cardiac surgery. Emerg Infect Dis 2001;7:828-831.
71. Martone WJ, Nichols RL. Recognition, prevention, surveillance, and management of surgical site infections: introduction to the problem and symposium overview. Clin Infect Dis 2001;33 Suppl 2:S67-S68.
72. Posacioglu H, Apaydin AZ, Islamoglu F, et al. Adverse effects of cell saver in patients undergoing ruptured abdominal aortic aneurysm repair. Ann Vasc Surg 2002;16:450-455.
73. Tang R, Chen HH, Wang YL, et al. Risk factors for surgical site infection after elective resection of the colon and rectum: a single-center prospective study of 2,809 consecutive patients. Ann Surg 2001;234:181-189.
74. Barrett BJ, Parfrey PS. Clinical practice. Preventing nephropathy induced by contrast medium. N Engl J Med 2006;354:379-386.
75. Practice guidelines for preoperative fasting and the use of pharmacologic agents to reduce the risk of pulmonary aspiration: application to healthy patients undergoing elective procedures: a report by the American Society of Anesthesiologist Task Force on Preoperative Fasting. Anesthesiology 1999;90:896-905. Online at: http://www.asahq.org/publicationsAndServices/NPO.pdf.
76. Thomas DR, Tariq SH, Makhdomm S, et al. Physician misdiagnosis of dehydration in older adults. J Am Med Dir Assoc 2003;4:251-254.
77. Volkert D, Kreuel K, Stehle P. Fluid intake of community-living, independent elderly in Germany—a nationwide, representative study. J Nutr Health Aging 2005;9:305-309.
78. Bennett JA, Thomas V, Riegel B. Unrecognized chronic dehydration in older adults: examining prevalence rate and risk factors. J Gerontol Nurs 2004;30:22-28; quiz 52-53.
79. de Larminat V, Montravers P, Dureuil B, Desmonts JM. Alteration in swallowing reflex after extubation in intensive care unit patients. Crit Care Med 1995;23:486-490.
80. Marik PE. Aspiration pneumonitis and aspiration pneumonia. N Engl J Med 2001;344:665-671.
81. Warner DO. Preventing postoperative pulmonary complications: the role of the anesthesiologist. Anesthesiology 2000;92:1467-1472.

82. Lawrence VA, Hilsenbeck SG, Mulrow CD, et al. Incidence and hospital stay for cardiac and pulmonary complications after abdominal surgery. J Gen Intern Med 1995;10:671-678.
83. Bixler EO, Vgontzas AN, Ten Have T, et al. Effects of age on sleep apnea in men: I. Prevalence and severity. Am J Respir Crit Care Med 1998;157:144-148.
84. Young T, Peppard PE, Gottlieb DJ. Epidemiology of obstructive sleep apnea: a population health perspective. Am J Respir Crit Care Med 2002;165:1217-1239.
85. Gali B, Plevak DJ, Morganthaler T, Gay P. Identification and perioperative management of patients presumed at risk for obstructive sleep apnea. [abstract #0599]. Sleep 2005;28:A202.
86. Frasco PE, Sprung J, Trentman TL. The impact of the joint commission for accreditation of healthcare organizations pain initiative on perioperative opiate consumption and recovery room length of stay. Anesth Analg 2005;100:162-168.
87. Curtiss CP. JCAHO: meeting the standards for pain management. Orthop Nurs 2001;20:27-30, 41.
88. Minto CF, Schnider TW, Shafer SL. Pharmacokinetics and pharmacodynamics of remifentanil. II. Model application. Anesthesiology 1997;86:24-33.
89. Scott JC, Stanski DR. Decreased fentanyl and alfentanil dose requirements with age: a simultaneous pharmacokinetic and pharmacodynamic evaluation. J Pharmacol Exp Ther 1987;240:159-166.
90. Jankowski CJ, Cook DJ, Trenerry MR, et al. Continuous peripheral nerve block analgesia and central neuraxial anesthesia are associated with reduced incidence of postoperative delirium in the elderly [abstract]. Anesthesiology 2005;103:A1467.
91. Arain SR, Ruehlow RM, Uhrich TD, Ebert TJ. The efficacy of dexmedetomidine versus morphine for postoperative analgesia after major inpatient surgery. Anesth Analg 2004;98:153-158, table of contents.
92. Cortinez LI, Hsu YW, Sum-Ping ST, et al. Dexmedetomidine pharmacodynamics: Part II: Crossover comparison of the analgesic effect of dexmedetomidine and remifentanil in healthy volunteers. Anesthesiology 2004;101:1077-1083.
93. Marzinski LR. The tragedy of dementia: clinically assessing pain in the confused nonverbal elderly. J Gerontol Nurs 1991;17:25-28.
94. Merskey H, Bogduk M. Classification of Chronic Pain: Descriptions of Chronic Pain Syndromes and Definitions of Pain Syndromes. Seattle, WA: IASP Press, 1994.
95. Krulewitch H, London MR, Skakel VJ, et al. Assessment of pain in cognitively impaired older adults: a comparison of pain assessment tools and their use by nonprofessional caregivers. J Am Geriatr Soc 2000;48:1607-1611.
96. DOLOPLUS 2: behavioral pain assessment scale for elderly subjects presenting with verbal communication disorders. 2001. Accessed: March 2, 2006. Online at http://www.doloplus.com/versiongb/index.htm.
97. Lefebvre-Chapiro S. The Doloplus 2 scale—evaluating pain in the elderly. Eur J Palliat Care 2001;8:191-194.
98. Warden V, Hurley AC, Volicer L. Development and psychometric evaluation of the Pain Assessment in Advanced Dementia (PAINAD) scale. J Am Med Dir Assoc 2003;4:9-15.
99. Stolee P, Hillier LM, Esbaugh J, et al. Instruments for the assessment of pain in older persons with cognitive impairment. J Am Geriatr Soc 2005;53:319-326.
100. Fisher SE, Burgio LD, Thorn BE, et al. Pain assessment and management in cognitively impaired nursing home residents: Association of Certified Nursing Assistant pain report, Minimum Data Set pain report, and analgesic medication use. J Am Geriatr Soc 2002;50:152-156.
101. Lawton MP, Casten R, Parmelee PA, et al. Psychometric characteristics of the minimum data set II: validity. J Am Geriatr Soc 1998;46:736-744.
102. Casten R, Lawton MP, Parmelee PA, Kleban MH. Psychometric characteristics of the minimum data set I: confirmatory factor analysis. J Am Geriatr Soc 1998;46:726-735.

103. Cohen-Mansfield J. The adequacy of the minimum data set assessment of pain in cognitively impaired nursing home residents. J Pain Symptom Manage 2004;27:343-351.
104. Villanueva MR, Smith TL, Erickson JS, et al. Pain Assessment for the Dementing Elderly (PADE): reliability and validity of a new measure. J Am Med Dir Assoc 2003;4:1-8.
105. Lynch EP, Lazor MA, Gellis JE, et al. The impact of postoperative pain on the development of postoperative delirium. Anesth Analg 1998;86:781-785.
106. Thoren T, Sundberg A, Wattwil M, et al. Effects of epidural bupivacaine and epidural morphine on bowel function and pain after hysterectomy. Acta Anaesthesiol Scand 1989;33:181-185.
107. Scheinin B, Asantila R, Orko R. The effect of bupivacaine and morphine on pain and bowel function after colonic surgery. Acta Anaesthesiol Scand 1987;31:161-164.
108. Liu S, Angel JM, Owens BD, et al. Effects of epidural bupivacaine after thoracotomy. Reg Anesth 1995;20:303-310.
109. Liu SS, Carpenter RL, Mackey DC, et al. Effects of perioperative analgesic technique on rate of recovery after colon surgery. Anesthesiology 1995;83:757-765.
110. Gelman S, Feigenberg Z, Dintzman M, Levy E. Electroenterography after cholecystectomy: the role of high epidural analgesia. Arch Surg 1977;112:580-583.
111. Bonica JJ. The Management of Pain. Philadelphia, PA: Lea & Febiger, 1953.
112. DeLoach LJ, Higgins MS, Caplan AB, Stiff JL. The visual analog scale in the immediate postoperative period: intrasubject variability and correlation with a numeric scale. Anesth Analg 1998;86:102-106.
113. Cadogan MP. Assessing pain in cognitively impaired nursing home residents: the state of the science and the state we're in. J Am Med Dir Assoc 2003;4:50-51.
114. Simons LA, Tett S, Simons J, et al. Multiple medication use in the elderly: use of prescription and non-prescription drugs in an Australian community setting. Med J Aust 1992;157:242-246.
115. Stewart RB, Moore MT, May FE, et al. A longitudinal evaluation of drug use in an ambulatory elderly population. J Clin Epidemiol 1991;44:1353-1359.
116. Jankowski CJ. Personal communication. 2005.
117. Inouye SK, van Dyck CH, Alessi CA, et al. Clarifying confusion: the confusion assessment method. A new method for detection of delirium. Ann Intern Med 1990;113:941-948.
118. Sharma PT, Sieber FE, Zakriya KJ, et al. Recovery room delirium predicts postoperative delirium after hip-fracture repair. Anesth Analg 2005;101:1215-1220, table of contents.
119. Marcantonio E, Ta T, Duthie E, Resnick NM. Delirium severity and psychomotor types: their relationship with outcomes after hip fracture repair. J Am Geriatr Soc 2002;50:850-857.
120. Zakriya KJ, Christmas C, Wenz JF, Sr., et al. Preoperative factors associated with postoperative change in confusion assessment method score in hip fracture patients. Anesth Analg 2002;94:1628-1632, table of contents.
121. Galanakis P, Bickel H, Gradinger R, et al. Acute confusional state in the elderly following hip surgery: incidence, risk factors and complications. Int J Geriatr Psychiatry 2001;16:349-355.
122. Kudoh A, Takahira Y, Katagai H, Takazawa T. Small-dose ketamine improves the postoperative state of depressed patients. Anesth Analg 2002;95:114-118, table of contents.
123. Clayer M, Bruckner J. Occult hypoxia after femoral neck fracture and elective hip surgery. Clin Orthop Relat Res 2000:265-271.
124. Brauer C, Morrison RS, Silberzweig SB, Siu AL. The cause of delirium in patients with hip fracture. Arch Intern Med 2000;160:1856-1860.
125. Zakriya K, Sieber FE, Christmas C, et al. Brief postoperative delirium in hip fracture patients affects functional outcome at three months. Anesth Analg 2004;98:1798-1802, table of contents.
126. Shigeta H, Yasui A, Nimura Y, et al. Postoperative delirium and melatonin levels in elderly patients. Am J Surg 2001;182:449-454.

127. Kagansky N, Rimon E, Naor S, et al. Low incidence of delirium in very old patients after surgery for hip fractures. Am J Geriatr Psychiatry 2004;12:306-314.
128. Kudoh A, Takase H, Takahira Y, Takazawa T. Postoperative confusion increases in elderly long-term benzodiazepine users. Anesth Analg 2004;99:1674-1678, table of contents.
129. Formiga F, Lopez-Soto A, Sacanella E, et al. Mortality and morbidity in nonagenarian patients following hip fracture surgery. Gerontology 2003;49:41-45.
130. Bickel H, Gradinger R, Kochs E, et al. [Incidence and risk factors of delirium after hip surgery]. Psychiatr Prax 2004;31:360-365.
131. Agnoletti V, Ansaloni L, Catena F, et al. Postoperative delirium after elective and emergency surgery: analysis and checking of risk factors: a study protocol. BMC Surg 2005;5:12.
132. Kudoh A, Katagai H, Takase H, Takazawa T. Effect of preoperative discontinuation of antipsychotics in schizophrenic patients on outcome during and after anaesthesia. Eur J Anaesthesiol 2004;21:414-416.
133. Adunsky A, Levy R, Heim M, et al. Meperidine analgesia and delirium in aged hip fracture patients. Arch Gerontol Geriatr 2002;35:253-259.
134. Liptzin B, Laki A, Garb JL, et al. Donepezil in the prevention and treatment of post-surgical delirium. Am J Geriatr Psychiatry 2005;13:1100-1106.
135. Marcantonio ER, Goldman L, Orav EJ, et al. The association of intraoperative factors with the development of postoperative delirium. Am J Med 1998;105:380-384.
136. Milisen K, Foreman MD, Abraham IL, et al. A nurse-led interdisciplinary intervention program for delirium in elderly hip-fracture patients. J Am Geriatr Soc 2001;49:523-532.
137. Jankowski CJ, Keegan MT, Bolton CF, Harrison BA. Neuropathy following axillary brachial plexus block: is it the tourniquet? Anesthesiology 2003;99:1230-1232.
138. Breitbart W, Rosenfeld B, Roth A, et al. The Memorial Delirium Assessment Scale. J Pain Symptom Manage 1997;13:128-137.
139. Gaudreau JD, Gagnon P, Harel F, et al. Fast, systematic, and continuous delirium assessment in hospitalized patients: the nursing delirium screening scale. J Pain Symptom Manage 2005;29:368-375.
140. Trzepacz PT, Baker RW, Greenhouse J. A symptom rating scale for delirium. Psychiatry Res 1988;23:89-97.
141. Adamis D, Treloar A, MacDonald AJ, Martin FC. Concurrent validity of two instruments (the Confusion Assessment Method and the Delirium Rating Scale) in the detection of delirium among older medical inpatients. Age Ageing 2005;34:72-75.
142. McNicoll L, Pisani MA, Ely EW, et al. Detection of delirium in the intensive care unit: comparison of confusion assessment method for the intensive care unit with confusion assessment method ratings. J Am Geriatr Soc 2005;53:495-500.
143. Schuurmans MJ, Shortridge-Baggett LM, Duursma SA. The Delirium Observation Screening Scale: a screening instrument for delirium. Res Theory Nurs Pract 2003;17:31-50.
144. McCusker J, Cole MG, Dendukuri N, Belzile E. The delirium index, a measure of the severity of delirium: new findings on reliability, validity, and responsiveness. J Am Geriatr Soc 2004;52:1744-1749.
145. Buschke H, Kuslansky G, Katz M, et al. Screening for dementia with the memory impairment screen. Neurology 1999;52:231-238.
146. Teng EL, Hasegawa K, Homma A, et al. The Cognitive Abilities Screening Instrument (CASI): a practical test for cross-cultural epidemiological studies of dementia. Int Psychogeriatr 1994;6:45-58; discussion 62.
147. Leopold NA, Borson AJ. An alphabetical 'WORLD'. A new version of an old test. Neurology 1997;49:1521-1524.
148. Watson YI, Arfken CL, Birge SJ. Clock completion: an objective screening test for dementia. J Am Geriatr Soc 1993;41:1235-1240.

149. Lorentz WJ, Scanlan JM, Borson S. Brief screening tests for dementia. Can J Psychiatry 2002;47:723-733.
150. Borson S, Scanlan J, Brush M, et al. The Mini-Cog: a cognitive 'vital signs' measure for dementia screening in multi-lingual elderly. Int J Geriatr Psychiatry 2000;15:1021-1027.
151. Borson S, Scanlan JM, Chen P, Ganguli M. The Mini-Cog as a screen for dementia: validation in a population-based sample. J Am Geriatr Soc 2003;51:1451-1454.
152. Neelon VJ, Champagne MT, Carlson JR, Funk SG. The NEECHAM Confusion Scale: construction, validation, and clinical testing. Nurs Res 1996;45:324-330.
153. Albert MS, Levkoff SE, Reilly C, et al. The delirium symptom interview: an interview for the detection of delirium symptoms in hospitalized patients. J Geriatr Psychiatry Neurol 1992;5:14-21.
154. Blessed G, Tomlinson BE, Roth M. The association between quantitative measures of dementia and of senile change in the cerebral grey matter of elderly subjects. Br J Psychiatry 1968;114:797-811.
155. Kalisvaart KJ, de Jonghe JF, Bogaards MJ, et al. Haloperidol prophylaxis for elderly hip-surgery patients at risk for delirium: a randomized placebo-controlled study. J Am Geriatr Soc 2005;53:1658-1666.
156. Allan L, Hays H, Jensen NH, et al. Randomised crossover trial of transdermal fentanyl and sustained release oral morphine for treating chronic non-cancer pain. BMJ 2001;322:1154-1158.
157. Allan L, Richarz U, Simpson K, Slappendel R. Transdermal fentanyl versus sustained release oral morphine in strong-opioid naive patients with chronic low back pain. Spine 2005;30:2484-2490.
158. Babul N, Noveck R, Chipman H, et al. Efficacy and safety of extended-release, once-daily tramadol in chronic pain: a randomized 12-week clinical trial in osteoarthritis of the knee. J Pain Symptom Manage 2004;28:59-71.
159. Boureau F, Legallicier P, Kabir-Ahmadi M. Tramadol in post-herpetic neuralgia: a randomized, double-blind, placebo-controlled trial. Pain 2003;104:323-331.
160. Franco ML, Seoane A, Franco ML. Usefulness of transdermal fentanyl in the management of nonmalignant chronic pain: a prospective, observational, multicenter study. Pain Clinic 2002;14:99-112.
161. Milligan K, Lanteri-Minet M, Borchert K, et al. Evaluation of long-term efficacy and safety of transdermal fentanyl in the treatment of chronic noncancer pain. J Pain 2001;2:197-204.
162. Mystakidou K, Parpa E, Tsilika E, et al. Long-term management of noncancer pain with transdermal therapeutic system-fentanyl. J Pain 2003;4:298-306.
163. Tassain V, Attal N, Fletcher D, et al. Long term effects of oral sustained release morphine on neuropsychological performance in patients with chronic non-cancer pain. Pain 2003;104:389-400.
164. Devulder J, Richarz U, Nataraja SH. Impact of long-term use of opioids on quality of life in patients with chronic, non-malignant pain. Curr Med Res Opin 2005;21:1555-1568.
165. Portenoy RK, Duma C, Foley KM. Acute herpetic and postherpetic neuralgia: clinical review and current management. Ann Neurol 1986;20:651-664.
166. Stankus SJ, Dlugopolski M, Packer D. Management of herpes zoster (shingles) and postherpetic neuralgia. Am Fam Physician 2000;61:2437-2444, 2447-2438.
167. Oster G, Harding G, Dukes E, et al. Pain, medication use, and health-related quality of life in older persons with postherpetic neuralgia: results from a population-based survey. J Pain 2005;6:356-363.
168. Alper BS, Lewis PR. Does treatment of acute herpes zoster prevent or shorten postherpetic neuralgia? J Fam Pract 2000;49:255-264.

169. Pasqualucci A, Pasqualucci V, Galla F, et al. Prevention of post-herpetic neuralgia: acyclovir and prednisolone versus epidural local anesthetic and methylprednisolone. Acta Anaesthesiol Scand 2000;44:910-918.
170. van Wijck AJ, Opstelten W, Moons KG, et al. The PINE study of epidural steroids and local anaesthetics to prevent postherpetic neuralgia: a randomised controlled trial. Lancet 2006;367:219-224.
171. Weller TH. Varicella and herpes zoster: changing concepts of the natural history, control, and importance of a not-so-benign virus. N Engl J Med 1983;309:1434-1440.
172. Ragozzino MW, Melton LJ, 3rd, Kurland LT, et al. Population-based study of herpes zoster and its sequelae. Medicine (Baltimore) 1982;61:310-316.
173. Donahue JG, Choo PW, Manson JE, Platt R. The incidence of herpes zoster. Arch Intern Med 1995;155:1605-1609.
174. Choo PW, Galil K, Donahue JG, et al. Risk factors for postherpetic neuralgia. Arch Intern Med 1997;157:1217-1224.
175. Galil K, Choo PW, Donahue JG, Platt R. The sequelae of herpes zoster. Arch Intern Med 1997;157:1209-1213.
176. Miller AE. Selective decline in cellular immune response to varicella-zoster in the elderly. Neurology 1980;30:582-587.
177. Berger R, Florent G, Just M. Decrease of the lymphoproliferative response to varicella-zoster virus antigen in the aged. Infect Immun 1981;32:24-27.
178. Burke BL, Steele RW, Beard OW, et al. Immune responses to varicella-zoster in the aged. Arch Intern Med 1982;142:291-293.
179. Levin MJ, Murray M, Rotbart HA, et al. Immune response of elderly individuals to a live attenuated varicella vaccine. J Infect Dis 1992;166:253-259.
180. Hope-Simpson RE. The nature of herpes zoster: a long-term study and a new hypothesis. Proc R Soc Med 1965;58:9-20.
181. Oxman MN. Immunization to reduce the frequency and severity of herpes zoster and its complications. Neurology 1995;45:S41-S46.
182. Oxman MN, Levin MJ, Johnson GR, et al. A vaccine to prevent herpes zoster and postherpetic neuralgia in older adults. N Engl J Med 2005;352:2271-2284.
183. Wong GY, Schroeder DR, Carns PE, et al. Effect of neurolytic celiac plexus block on pain relief, quality of life, and survival in patients with unresectable pancreatic cancer: a randomized controlled trial. JAMA 2004;291:1092-1099.
184. Zerr KJ, Furnary AP, Grunkemeier GL, et al. Glucose control lowers the risk of wound infection in diabetics after open heart operations. Ann Thorac Surg 1997;63:356-361.
185. Latham R, Lancaster AD, Covington JF, et al. The association of diabetes and glucose control with surgical-site infections among cardiothoracic surgery patients. Infect Control Hosp Epidemiol 2001;22:607-612.
186. Pomposelli JJ, Baxter JK, 3rd, Babineau TJ, et al. Early postoperative glucose control predicts nosocomial infection rate in diabetic patients. JPEN J Parenter Enteral Nutr 1998;22:77-81.
187. Eagle KA, Berger PB, Calkins H, et al. ACC/AHA guideline update for perioperative cardiovascular evaluation for noncardiac surgery—executive summary a report of the American College of Cardiology/American Heart Association Task Force on Practice Guidelines (Committee to Update the 1996 Guidelines on Perioperative Cardiovascular Evaluation for Noncardiac Surgery). Circulation 2002;105:1257-1267.
188. Goldman L, Caldera DL, Nussbaum SR, et al. Multifactorial index of cardiac risk in noncardiac surgical procedures. N Engl J Med 1977;297:845-850.
189. Golden SH, Peart-Vigilance C, Kao WH, Brancati FL. Perioperative glycemic control and the risk of infectious complications in a cohort of adults with diabetes. Diabetes Care 1999;22:1408-1414.

190. Guvener M, Pasaoglu I, Demircin M, Oc M. Perioperative hyperglycemia is a strong correlate of postoperative infection in type II diabetic patients after coronary artery bypass grafting. Endocr J 2002;49:531-537.
191. Gandhi GY, Nuttall GA, Abel MD, et al. Intraoperative hyperglycemia and perioperative outcomes in cardiac surgery patients. Mayo Clin Proc 2005;80:862-866.
192. Bochicchio GV, Salzano L, Joshi M, et al. Admission preoperative glucose is predictive of morbidity and mortality in trauma patients who require immediate operative intervention. Am Surg 2005;71:171-174.
193. Lazar HL, Philippides G, Fitzgerald C, et al. Glucose-insulin-potassium solutions enhance recovery after urgent coronary artery bypass grafting. J Thorac Cardiovasc Surg 1997;113:354-360; discussion 360-352.
194. Besogul Y, Tunerir B, Aslan R, et al. Clinical, biochemical and histochemical assessment of pretreatment with glucose-insulin-potassium for patients undergoing mitral valve replacement in the third and fourth functional groups of the New York Heart Association. Cardiovasc Surg 1999;7:645-650.
195. Lazar HL, Chipkin S, Philippides G, et al. Glucose-insulin-potassium solutions improve outcomes in diabetics who have coronary artery operations. Ann Thorac Surg 2000;70:145-150.
196. Szabo Z, Arnqvist H, Hakanson E, et al. Effects of high-dose glucose-insulin-potassium on myocardial metabolism after coronary surgery in patients with Type II diabetes. Clin Sci (Lond) 2001;101:37-43.
197. Ulgen MS, Alan S, Akdemir O, Toprak N. The effect of glucose-insulin-potassium solution on ventricular late potentials and heart rate variability in acute myocardial infarction. Coron Artery Dis 2001;12:507-512.
198. Groban L, Butterworth J, Legault C, et al. Intraoperative insulin therapy does not reduce the need for inotropic or antiarrhythmic therapy after cardiopulmonary bypass. J Cardiothorac Vasc Anesth 2002;16:405-412.
199. Lell WA, Nielsen VG, McGiffin DC, et al. Glucose-insulin-potassium infusion for myocardial protection during off-pump coronary artery surgery. Ann Thorac Surg 2002;73:1246-1251; discussion 1251-1242.
200. Rao V, Christakis GT, Weisel RD, et al. The insulin cardioplegia trial: myocardial protection for urgent coronary artery bypass grafting. J Thorac Cardiovasc Surg 2002;123:928-935.
201. Smith A, Grattan A, Harper M, et al. Coronary revascularization: a procedure in transition from on-pump to off-pump? The role of glucose-insulin-potassium revisited in a randomized, placebo-controlled study. J Cardiothorac Vasc Anesth 2002;16:413-420.
202. van den Berghe G, Wouters P, Weekers F, et al. Intensive insulin therapy in the critically ill patients. N Engl J Med 2001;345:1359-1367.
203. Weekers F, Giulietti AP, Michalaki M, et al. Metabolic, endocrine, and immune effects of stress hyperglycemia in a rabbit model of prolonged critical illness. Endocrinology 2003;144:5329-5338.
204. Hansen TK, Thiel S, Wouters PJ, et al. Intensive insulin therapy exerts antiinflammatory effects in critically ill patients and counteracts the adverse effect of low mannose-binding lectin levels. J Clin Endocrinol Metab 2003;88:1082-1088.
205. Mesotten D, Swinnen JV, Vanderhoydonc F, et al. Contribution of circulating lipids to the improved outcome of critical illness by glycemic control with intensive insulin therapy. J Clin Endocrinol Metab 2004;89:219-226.
206. Langouche L, Vanhorebeek I, Vlasselaers D, et al. Intensive insulin therapy protects the endothelium of critically ill patients. J Clin Invest 2005;115:2277-2286.
207. Vanhorebeek I, De Vos R, Mesotten D, et al. Protection of hepatocyte mitochondrial ultrastructure and function by strict blood glucose control with insulin in critically ill patients. Lancet 2005;365:53-59.

208. Finney SJ, Zekveld C, Elia A, Evans TW. Glucose control and mortality in critically ill patients. JAMA 2003;290:2041-2047.
209. van den Berghe G, Wouters PJ, Bouillon R, et al. Outcome benefit of intensive insulin therapy in the critically ill: insulin dose versus glycemic control. Crit Care Med 2003;31:359-366.
210. Kagansky N, Levy S, Rimon E, et al. Hypoglycemia as a predictor of mortality in hospitalized elderly patients. Arch Intern Med 2003;163:1825-1829.
211. Murrary MJ, Brull SJ, Coursin DB. Strict blood glucose control in the ICU: panacea or Pandora's box? J Cardiothorac Vasc Anesth 2004;18:687-689.
212. Norris EJ, Beattie C, Perler BA, et al. Double-masked randomized trial comparing alternate combinations of intraoperative anesthesia and postoperative analgesia in abdominal aortic surgery. Anesthesiology 2001;95:1054-1067.
213. Eckenhoff RG, Johansson JS, Wei H, et al. Inhaled anesthetic enhancement of amyloid-beta oligomerization and cytotoxicity. Anesthesiology 2004;101:703-709.
214. Culley DJ, Baxter MG, Crosby CA, et al. Impaired acquisition of spatial memory 2 weeks after isoflurane and isoflurane-nitrous oxide anesthesia in aged rats. Anesth Analg 2004;99:1393-1397; table of contents.
215. Culley DJ, Baxter MG, Yukhananov R, Crosby G. Long-term impairment of acquisition of a spatial memory task following isoflurane-nitrous oxide anesthesia in rats. Anesthesiology 2004;100:309-314.
216. Culley DJ, Baxter M, Yukhananov R, Crosby G. The memory effects of general anesthesia persist for weeks in young and aged rats. Anesth Analg 2003;96:1004-1009, table of contents.
217. Kehlet H. Modifications of responses to surgery by neural blockade. In Cousins MJ, Bridenbaugh PO (eds): Neural Blockade in Clinical Anesthesia and Management of Pain. Philadelphia, PA: Lippincott-Raven, 1998, pp. 129-175.
218. Rasmussen LS, Johnson T, Kuipers HM, et al. Does anaesthesia cause postoperative cognitive dysfunction? A randomised study of regional versus general anaesthesia in 438 elderly patients. Acta Anaesthesiol Scand 2003;47:260-266.
219. Williams-Russo P, Sharrock NE, Mattis S, et al. Cognitive effects after epidural vs general anesthesia in older adults: a randomized trial. JAMA 1995;274:44-50.
220. Capdevila X, Coimbra C, Choquet O. Approaches to the lumbar plexus: success, risks, and outcome. Reg Anesth Pain Med 2005;30:150-162.

3

GERIATRIC EMERGENCY MEDICINE

*Christopher R. Carpenter, MD, MSc, FACEP; Lowell W. Gerson, PhD**

The American Geriatric Society (AGS) project "Increasing Geriatric Expertise in Surgical and Related Medical Specialties" sponsored an effort to summarize the existing evidence and to identify priorities for future research in geriatrics aspects of several surgical and related medical fields. Ultimately, each specialty's research agenda was disseminated in a book (hereinafter referred to as *New Frontiers*) [1] and a Web site (http://www.frycomm.com/ags/rasp), and many were also disseminated in professional journals, as was, for example, the agenda for emergency medicine. [2] In 2005, the AGS initiated a review of each specialty's recommendations to analyze any progress made and evaluate whether any agenda items should be discarded or new ones added.

This chapter summarizes the findings of our follow-up review for the field of emergency medicine. Overall, little progress has been made on most of the research questions in the time since publication of *New Frontiers*. Therefore, we did not change any of the agenda items. However, new developments have prompted us to add four new topics to the agenda—models of care, driving safety, stroke, and elder abuse and neglect—and to add new agenda items under some of the topics covered in the original agenda. (For discussions of the new topics and all the new agenda items, see the New Horizons in Geriatric Emergency Medicine section at the end of the chapter.)

The Key Questions for geriatrics-oriented research in emergency medicine remain the same, as specified in *New Frontiers*:

EmergMed KQ1: **Can alterations in the process of emergency department care, such as those found to be beneficial elsewhere (ie, geriatric specialty inpatient units), improve the outcomes of older emergency department patients?**

EmergMed KQ2: **What diagnostic and therapeutic interventions can improve outcomes in older emergency department patients with high-risk common complaints, such as abdominal pain and acute coronary syndromes?**

EmergMed KQ3: **In older blunt multiple trauma patients, does early invasive monitoring and aggressive resuscitation result in improved outcomes?**

METHODS

The methods used to locate the evidence in the current review differ somewhat from those used for *New Frontiers*. RAND librarians conducted a PubMed search in July 2005 using the MeSH headings *emergency medicine*, *emergency treatment*, and *emergency service*,

* Carpenter: Assistant Professor, Division of Emergency Medicine, Washington University School of Medicine, St. Louis, MO; Gerson: Professor Emeritus of Epidemiology, Northeastern Ohio Universities College of Medicine, Senior Scientist, Emergency Medicine Research Center, Summa Health System, Akron, OH.

hospital. These headings were combined with the following MeSH terms: *age*, *geriatric assessment*, *aged*, *aged 80 and over*, *frail elderly*, *longevity*, and *geriatrics*. The following limits were placed on all searches: over age 65, English language, humans, years 2000–2005. This PubMed search was repeated in December 2005. Additionally, relevant journals (published between January 2004 and December 2005) were hand searched for topics specific to the overlap between geriatrics and emergency medicine. The hand-searched journals were the following: *Journal of the American Geriatrics Society, Journal of Gerontological Sciences, Age Ageing, Journal of Emergency Medicine, Annals of Emergency Medicine, Academic Emergency Medicine, American Journal of Emergency Medicine, Annals of Internal Medicine, New England Journal of Medicine,* and *JAMA*. Bibliographies of selected studies were also reviewed. Finally, a cited reference search using the Web of Science was conducted for each of those studies referenced in the chapter on geriatric emergency medicine in *New Frontiers*.

The content expert (CRC) reviewed the titles and abstracts derived from the search to identify those that were germane to the goals of research in the emergency care of older patients. These goals were to improve patient care through optimum medical management, disease and injury prevention, and maintenance of well-functioning individuals. The content expert and the senior writing group member (LWG) drafted a paper that synthesized the current literature and suggested areas for further research. This paper was reviewed by a panel consisting of experienced investigators who were AGS members and emergency physicians with expertise in geriatrics. Each new research question was assigned a level, using the rating system developed for *New Frontiers* (see pp. 6–7 for definitions of levels A through D).

The search of PubMed yielded 69 articles using *emergency medicine*, 1276 articles using *emergency treatment*, and 825 articles using *emergency service, hospital*. The search of PubMed and Web of Science, with the addition of the hand search of selected journals, resulted in a list of 2223 articles. Following review of titles and abstracts, 221 articles were obtained for inspection.

PROGRESS IN GERIATRIC EMERGENCY MEDICINE

General Geriatric Emergency Care

Patterns of Emergency Department Use

See *New Frontiers,* p. 54.

EmergMed 1 (Level D): **Observational and analytic studies on emergency department use should continue to come from large databases or national samples (such as the National Hospital Ambulatory Medical Care Survey database) so that the results can be generalized.**

New Research Addressing This Question: The patterns of emergency department (ED) use among older adults have been well described by single-hospital and multicenter studies. Elder ED patients have distinct patterns of use and disease presentation. Recent studies demonstrated that older patients represent 12% to 21% of all ED encounters. Older adults are consistently over-represented in the ED in comparison with their proportions in the general population in their geographic vicinity, and the numbers of older patients are steadily increasing. [3] One third to one half of elder ED presentations result in a hospital admission. The atypical presentations and time-consuming evaluation of older patients often result in under-triage, delayed dispositions, and inaccurate diagnoses. [4,5] Several systematic reviews have evaluated predictors of ED use by older patients, intervention effectiveness, and outcomes. [6–8]

Modification of This Question in Light of New Research: Since the publication of *New Frontiers* no evidence has emerged to prompt a modification of the original question. (For new agenda items on this topic, see the subsection on patterns of ED use in New Horizons in Geriatric Emergency Medicine, at the end of the chapter.)

Physician Training and Comfort

See *New Frontiers,* p. 55.

> *EmergMed 2 (Level A)*: **Randomized controlled trials are needed to assess the effectiveness of interventions (eg, educational models, standardized protocols) for improving quality of care of older emergency department patients.**

New Research Addressing This Question: On the basis of narrowly focused research questions posed to emergency medicine residency directors over a decade ago, the majority of emergency physicians believe that insufficient time is spent on geriatrics issues in residency and that ongoing research is lacking. [9] More recent efforts to describe baseline knowledge and integrate geriatrics principles into medical student educational programs during elective rotations have met with moderate success, [10,11] but no research has evaluated residency or postresidency training in evolving concepts of emergency care for older adults. [12–14] Another survey over 10 years ago of 971 practicing emergency physicians with a 44% response rate reported that these clinicians said they had more difficulty in managing abdominal pain, altered mental status, dizziness, and trauma in older than in younger patients. [15] Although textbooks in general medical geriatrics have incorporated principles of evidence-based medicine in devising clinically relevant questions, assessing the quantity and quality of available evidence to answer these questions, incorporating patient differences and preferences to the available data, and moving from evidence to action, the available textbooks and other learning tools in emergency medicine have not yet incorporated this 21st-century extension of clinical epidemiology. [16,17]

Modification of This Question in Light of New Research: Since the publication of *New Frontiers* no evidence has emerged to prompt a modification of the original question. (For new agenda items on this topic, see the subsection on physician training and comfort in New Horizons in Geriatric Emergency Medicine, at the end of the chapter.)

Environment

See *New Frontiers,* p. 55.

> *EmergMed 3 (Level B)*: **Large studies are needed to confirm the results of patient surveys and focus group interviews. Studies to identify characteristics of the micro-environment that affect outcomes in**

elderly patients (communication, emergency department environment) are needed to identify target areas for improvement.

EmergMed 4 (Level A): **Following evidence-based identification of target areas for improvement, controlled studies of the effect of alterations in the micro-environment on outcomes for older emergency department patients should be performed. Such studies likely cannot be based on random assignments of individuals to interventions; rather, whole micro-environments will have to be compared.**

New Research Addressing These Questions: One prospective study of urban older ED patients identified three variables which ED staff can influence: the patient's perception of time spent in the ED, how well physicians and nurses shared information with the patient and included the patient in decision making, and pain management. [18] Recent reviews have summarized the available patient satisfaction literature [19] and the Institute of Medicine's six quality domains: effective, timely, efficient, safe, patient-centered, and equitable care. [20] One randomized trial of replacing uncomfortable gurneys with reclining chairs found that doing so improved pain and satisfaction scores. [21]

Modification of These Questions in Light of New Research: Since the publication of *New Frontiers* no evidence has emerged to prompt a modification of the original questions. (For new agenda items on this topic, see the subsection on ED environment in New Horizons in Geriatric Emergency Medicine, at the end of the chapter.)

Prehospital Care

See *New Frontiers,* p. 56.

EmergMed 5 (Level B): **Cohort studies should be performed to describe the ability of prehospital care providers to assess older patients in their home environments. Areas where this may be particularly beneficial include the assessment of the home environment of patients with falls and functional decline, and the assessment of potential abuse. This research should focus on whether information about home environment provided by prehospital care providers affects patient outcomes.**

New Research Addressing This Question: The AGS and the National Council of State Emergency Medical Services Training Coordinators developed a textbook and instructional program to train prehospital professionals to deliver state-of-the-art care to older adults (online at http://www.gemssite.com/). No reports of educational or outcomes-based results of these ongoing courses have yet been published. One survey noted that 70% of out-of-hospital providers believe that primary injury prevention should be a routine part of their professional mission, yet only 33% routinely educated their patients on injury prevention behaviors. [22]

Modification of This Question in Light of New Research: Since the publication of *New Frontiers* no evidence has emerged to prompt a modification of the original question. (For new agenda items relevant to aspects of this question, see the subsection on abuse and neglect under Trauma in New Horizons in Geriatric Emergency Medicine, at the end of the chapter.)

Cognitive Impairment

See *New Frontiers,* pp. 57–58.

EmergMed 6 (Level B): **Screening tests for cognitive dysfunction for use in the emergency department should be validated against gold-standard assessment, and efforts should be made to determine if new, shorter screening approaches would be effective.**

EmergMed 7 (Level B): **Prospective cohort studies such as larger-scale longitudinal outcome studies of older patients with impaired cognition are necessary to confirm the finding that patients with undiagnosed delirium have worse outcomes than do those without delirium or with diagnosed and treated delirium.**

EmergMed 8 (Level A): **If research (EmergMed 7) confirms that older patients with delirium that is not diagnosed in the emergency department ultimately have worse outcomes than do those either without delirium or with recognized and treated delirium, interventional trials should be designed to determine the effect on outcomes of better screening and management of cognitive impairment in older emergency department patients.**

New Research Addressing These Questions: Cognitive impairment, including delirium and dementia, is prevalent among older ED patients.[23,24] A recent prospective observational study demonstrated that although 26% of patients at one tertiary care ED had impairment, less than one third of them had documentation of the delirium or cognitive deficit by the emergency physician.[25] Furthermore, when the treating emergency physicians were notified of the impairment, the knowledge did not affect their management decisions on a single patient.[26] Multiple studies have since demonstrated an association between delirium with increased mortality[27–29] and diminished functional outcomes.[30] Other ED-based prospective studies have verified the poor recognition of cognitive impairments among senior patients.[24,31] Several rapid, ED-accessible screening tests for dementia and delirium have been developed.[32–37] Delirium intervention models have not been initiated from the ED in current study settings,[38,39] even though emergency medicine has been called upon to take a more active role in the evaluation and disposition of these patients.[40,41]

Modification of These Questions in Light of New Research: Since the publication of *New Frontiers* no evidence has emerged to prompt a modification of the original questions.

Functional Assessment

See *New Frontiers,* pp. 58–59.

EmergMed 9 (Level B): **Development and testing of measures for functional assessment that are feasible and valid in elderly emergency department patients are needed.**

EmergMed 10 (Level B): **Case-control or cohort studies are needed to determine whether older emergency department patients with func-**

tional impairments have worse outcomes than do those without impairment.

EmergMed 11 (Level A): **Controlled intervention trials are needed to determine whether the detection and management of functional impairment in older emergency department patients have an effect on these outcomes.**

New Research Addressing These Questions: No new research addressing these questions was found.

Modification of These Questions in Light of New Research: Since the publication of *New Frontiers* no evidence has emerged to prompt a modification of the original questions.

Medication Use

See *New Frontiers*, pp. 59–60.

EmergMed 12 (Level B): **Large, long-term studies of the outcomes when older patients are prescribed potentially inappropriate medications are needed.**

EmergMed 13 (Level A): **Interventional trials (randomized or by comparison of micro-environments) are needed of methods to reduce prescription of potentially inappropriate medications for older patients, such as educational sessions or computer-assisted decision support systems integrated into emergency department discharge instructions.**

New Research Addressing These Questions: The Beers criteria for potentially inappropriate medication use in older adults was updated in 2003. [42] Although these criteria have not been validated for use in ED settings, they have been used to characterize medication use problems. Using the older 1997 Beers criteria, a review of the 2000 National Hospital Ambulatory Medical Care Survey demonstrated "inappropriate" medication administration in 12.6% of ED visits by elderly persons from 1992 to 2000. The number of ED medications was found to be the strongest predictor of inappropriate prescribing. [43] Additionally, 25% of patients aged 60 or over at one institution were noted to have pre-existing drug interactions before any medications were prescribed by the emergency physician. [44] Another retrospective study noted that recognized adverse drug-related events were the reason for over 10% of all ED visits. [45] Older ED patients are able to correctly identify only 43% of their prescription medications, [46] and only 39% of community-dwelling older adults bring a medication list with them to the ED, and 34% of those lists are inaccurate. [47]

Modification of These Questions in Light of New Research: Since the publication of *New Frontiers* no evidence has emerged to prompt a modification of the original questions. (For new agenda items relevant to this topic, see the subsection on medication use in New Horizons in Geriatric Emergency Medicine, at the end of the chapter.)

Screening and Comprehensive Geriatric Assessment in the ED

General Geriatric Assessment Tools

See *New Frontiers,* pp. 60–62.

EmergMed 14 (Level B): **Comprehensive emergency department screening of older patients is feasible and inexpensive; however, outcomes have not been affected, possibly because of low compliance with recommendations and follow-up. Potential interventions to improve compliance with recommendations and follow-up, including direct referral to geriatrics teams, should be prospectively evaluated.**

EmergMed 15 (Level B): **The Identification of Seniors at Risk tool should be employed at independent sites to determine its value in selecting high-risk elderly patients for interventional trials of geriatric assessment.**

New Research Addressing These Questions: The deficiencies in the care of older ED patients include a failure to identify high-risk conditions or refer to available community resources. Multiple brief ED screening tools and multidisciplinary interventional teams have been evaluated: Triage Risk Screening Tool,[48] Identification of Seniors at Risk,[49] and the Domain Management Model.[50] Questions of time and resource availability may limit the widespread implementation of these systems in the majority of EDs. The Discharge of Elderly from the Emergency Department (DEED II) study was a prospective randomized controlled trial of a comprehensive geriatric assessment, which was found to lower in-hospital resource consumption without affecting nursing home admission or mortality.[51] Like the DEED II trial, all successful ED interventional trials have included a home assessment component. Most interventional studies used a specialized nurse practitioner to identify and follow elderly patients.[38,51–55]

Modification of These Questions in Light of New Research: Since the publication of *New Frontiers* no evidence has emerged to prompt a modification of the original questions. (For new agenda items relevant to this topic, see the subsection on general geriatric assessment tools in New Horizons in Geriatric Emergency Medicine, at the end of the chapter.)

Screening for Specific Conditions

See *New Frontiers,* pp. 63–64.

EmergMed 16 (Level B): **Studies are needed to develop brief screening instruments for specific conditions for use with older patients in the emergency department.**

EmergMed 17 (Level A): **Screening for asymptomatic conditions in older patients in the emergency department should be done only if detection of the abnormality results in treatment of the disorder and this treatment results in improvement in outcomes. Randomized interventional trials are needed to assess short- and long-term out-**

comes of patients who have screening and treatment for these conditions.

New Research Addressing These Questions: Conditions such as correctable undetected visual acuity deficit, hearing deficit, malnutrition, depression, dementia, delirium, substance abuse, and elder mistreatment have high ED prevalence, validated screening tools, and effective interventions. Nevertheless, case-finding for these conditions is not commonly done in the ED. Depression, for example, affects up to one third of elderly ED patients and one half of hospitalized and homebound elderly patients. Depressed patients use the ED more often than those who are not depressed and have longer lengths of stay when admitted. Brief screening tools, such as a three-question instrument, have been developed to replace the cumbersome Geriatric Depression Scale and the modified Koenig Scale, but they have yet to undergo multicenter validation.[56,57]

No study has addressed the optimal screening test for alcohol abuse in ED older persons, although several relatively brief screens exist: CAGE, Alcohol Use Disorders Identification Test (AUDIT), Michigan Alcoholism Screening Test (MAST-Geriatric Version), and the Alcohol-Related Problems Survey (ARPS). A systematic review of self-reported alcohol screening instruments assessed the CAGE, MAST, and AUDIT screening tools, but did not assess the ARPS.[58] Another study of 574 patients aged 65 or over found the ARPS to be more sensitive than the CAGE, AUDIT, or MAST.[59] The ARPS was specifically designed to assess older adults who are at risk of experiencing problems because of their alcohol consumption alone or in conjunction with their underlying comorbidities, functional status, and medication use. The ARPS is much longer than the AUDIT or CAGE screening tools, though.[60–62]

Brief screening tools for malnutrition (DETERMINE[63] and Subjective Global Assessment[64]), visual acuity,[65] and hearing loss exist, but they are probably underused and have not been evaluated in ED settings.[66] Screening tools for elder mistreatment and cognitive deficiencies are discussed elsewhere in this article.

Modification of These Questions in Light of New Research: Since the publication of *New Frontiers* no evidence has emerged to prompt a modification of the original questions.

Specific Clinical Syndromes

Abdominal Pain

See *New Frontiers,* p. 65.

EmergMed 18 (Level B): **Prospective longitudinal cohort or case-control studies of elderly emergency department patients with abdominal pain are necessary to adequately define which patients with abdominal pain have serious disease and which have benign disease.**

EmergMed 19 (Level B): **The value of history and physical examination findings, laboratory examination, and imaging studies in older emergency department patients should be prospectively evaluated.**

New Research Addressing These Questions: One prospective multicenter study demonstrated a 58% admission rate for adults aged 60 or over who were evaluated for acute, nontraumatic abdominal pain; 18% subsequently required surgery or an invasive procedure and 11% returned to the ED within 2 weeks. [67] In another study EM physicians were found to have used computerized tomography (CT) imaging in 37% of patients, with a diagnostic accuracy of 57% for all patients and 75% for surgical patients. [68] A third study found that EM physicians relied heavily on CT to alter admission decisions in 26% of cases and improve diagnostic certainty. [69]

Modification of These Questions in Light of New Research: Since the publication of *New Frontiers* no evidence has emerged to prompt a modification of the original questions. (For a new agenda item for this topic, see the subsection on abdominal pain in New Horizons in Geriatric Emergency Medicine, at the end of the chapter.)

Falls

See *New Frontiers,* p. 66.

> *EmergMed 20 (Level A)*: **Randomized controlled trials are necessary to assess the value of a falls prevention program in reducing subsequent falls by elderly patients presenting to the emergency department with a fall.**

New Research Addressing This Question: Older adults who present to the ED with a fall often do not receive current guideline care, [70] although ED-initiated home modifications, [71] vestibular assessment, [72] and multidisciplinary falls prevention programs [73] have identified some high-risk fall populations, and subsequent preventive measures have been found to reduce the incidence of subsequent falls. [74,75] A meta–analysis of 40 randomized controlled trials to prevent falls in older adults, mostly outpatient, demonstrated effectiveness in reducing the rate of falling; the most efficacious intervention consisted of multifactorial falls risk assessment and management. [76] The cost-effectiveness of multidisciplinary interventional programs is being assessed in a randomized controlled trial. [77]

Modification of This Question in Light of New Research: Since the publication of *New Frontiers* no evidence has emerged to prompt a modification of the original question. (For new agenda items on this topic, see the subsection on falls in New Horizons in Geriatric Emergency Medicine, at the end of the chapter.)

Infectious Disease

See *New Frontiers,* pp. 66–67.

> *EmergMed 21 (Level B)*: **Up to now, studies of fever and infectious disease in older emergency department patients have been observational and analytic retrospective studies. Prospective observational cohort studies, including longitudinal studies of outcomes and predictors of outcomes, are needed.**

> *EmergMed 22 (Level A)*: **Descriptive studies of emergency-department based immunization programs have found them to be feasible. Intervention trials for older persons are necessary to determine if such programs are beneficial (because they access an underserved**

population) and whether they provide more cost-effective care and reduce adverse outcomes in comparison with usual care.

New Research Addressing These Questions: Fever remains a common and ominous presenting complaint among older ED patients. Identification of afebrile septic patients or febrile patients at increased risk of adverse outcome remains challenging. ED and non-ED studies have been limited to retrospective analyses with often contradictory findings. [78–80] In the United States, 58% of sepsis occurs among patients aged 65 or over. [81] The Surviving Sepsis Campaign guidelines include source control and rapid reduction of broad-spectrum antimicrobial coverage to monotherapy active against the causative organism, particularly among elderly patients with increased likelihood of repeat antibiotic exposures resulting in the accumulation of multi-drug–resistant microbes. [82,83] In an initial trial, early goal-directed therapy was randomized to patients with a mean age of 67,with a 16% absolute reduction in mortality without significantly increased adverse events associated with increasing age. [84]

A review of the National Hospital Ambulatory Medical Care Survey (NHAMCS) for all ED vaccinations between 1992 and 2000 described over 27 million ED vaccinations, although 93% were against tetanus. [85] ED patients are rarely vaccinated against influenza or pneumococcus, despite the increased frequency with which EM physicians manage the complications associated with these infections. [85,86] One single-center ED study noted that only 9% of adults aged 65 or over received an appropriate pneumococcal vaccination, despite the 90% goal set by Healthy People 2010. [87,88] When ED patients are referred to their primary care physician for pneumococcal vaccination, only 10% compliance is observed. [89] Tetanus immunity wanes to 59% in persons aged 70 or over, and 8.3% lack an appropriate rise in antitoxin titers in response to a tetanus booster. [90]

Modification of These Questions in Light of New Research: Since the publication of *New Frontiers* no evidence has emerged to prompt a modification of the original questions. (For new agenda items on this topic, see the subsection on infectious disease in New Horizons in Geriatric Emergency Medicine, at the end of the chapter.)

Acute Coronary Syndromes

See *New Frontiers,* pp. 67–69.

EmergMed 23 (Level B): **Studies of techniques to improve recognition and appropriate treatment of acute coronary syndromes in older emergency department patients should be performed.**

EmergMed 24 (Level A): **Older patients should be included in randomized controlled trials of acute coronary syndromes treatment.**

New Research Addressing These Questions: Older patients, especially the oldest old (aged 85 and over) and women, present atypically with acute coronary syndromes. Although older patients represent 37% of acute myocardial infarctions (AMIs), they consisted of only 2% of study populations from 1960 to 1992 and only 9% from 1992 to 2000. [91] Regardless of the under-representation of seniors in these studies, several large randomized controlled trials have consistently demonstrated the efficacy of thrombolytic therapy in older AMI patients, with diminished relative risk countered by substantial absolute mortality reductions, although several recent observational studies have questioned these results.[92–96] Additionally, several studies have indicated that the older patients most likely to receive the greatest benefit from guideline-based therapy (aspirin, β-blockers, angiotensin-converting enzyme inhibitors) are the least likely to receive them.[97–101] Older age is consistently associated with symptom-to-treatment time delays exceeding 12 hours, with reperfusion therapy efficacy diminished beyond this therapeutic window.[102,103] Although discrepant data exist, randomized trials of percutaneous intervention versus thrombolytics in the elderly patient generally favor percutaneous intervention.[104–112]

Modification of These Questions in Light of New Research: Since the publication of *New Frontiers* no evidence has emerged to prompt a modification of the original questions.

Cardiopulmonary Arrest

See *New Frontiers,* pp. 69–70.

EmergMed 25 (Level B): **Cohort or case-control studies are necessary to determine in which patients resuscitation for out-of-hospital arrest is futile. However, it appears that age alone should not be used to make this decision.**

EmergMed 26 (Level B): **Prospective multicenter longitudinal studies on the clinical course of older emergency department patients with important conditions (abdominal pain, fever, acute coronary syndromes) are needed. (See also the Key Questions, at the beginning of the chapter.)**

New Research Addressing These Questions: Multiple prospective and retrospective studies on the outcome of cardiopulmonary arrest in older patients have recently been the subject of a systematic review.[113] Although the results vary, the majority of studies indicate that age is not an independent predictor of cardiac arrest mortality.[114–116] Instead, premorbid health, performance status, duration of cardiopulmonary arrest, delayed defibrillation, and initial rhythm are predictors of outcome. Patients with unwitnessed arrests and those with asystole have poorer outcomes at any age. Increased availability of cardiopulmonary resuscitation[117,118] and rapid access to automated external defibrillators[114] may improve survival of elderly cardiac arrest victims.

Modification of These Questions in Light of New Research: Since the publication of *New Frontiers* no evidence has emerged to prompt a modification of the original questions. (For a new agenda item on this topic, see the subsection on cardiopulmonary arrest in New Horizons in Geriatric Emergency Medicine, at the end of the chapter.)

TRAUMA

See *New Frontiers,* pp. 70–74.

Triage and Mortality

EmergMed 27 (Level B): **Research on older trauma patients would benefit from standardization of outcomes, including short- and long-term survival and also functional outcome.**

EmergMed 28 (Level B): **Valid and accurate ways to predict outcomes in older trauma patients must be developed on the basis of cohort or case-control studies that can identify risk factors for bad outcomes.**

New Research Addressing These Questions: Increasing age is associated with increased morbidity and mortality in geriatric trauma patients,[119–123] but good outcomes can be achieved when appropriate trauma care is provided to those individuals with survivable injuries.[124–128] Guidelines have sought to summarize the available data and provide a basis for standardization of care while outlining future research initiatives, though existing evidence is of varying quality and heterogeneous design.[129] Therefore, most of the recommendations are based upon Level III evidence. Among the guideline assertions are that all other factors being equal, age alone is not predictive of poor outcomes after trauma and patients aged 55 or over are under-triaged to trauma centers. Some have agreed and called for early trauma team activation using age as a criterion,[130] although others have noted increasing volumes at Level I trauma centers and suggested consideration of the mechanism of injury and comorbidities before deciding to transfer to a tertiary medical center.[131] The EAST guidelines also note extremely high mortality rates for patients aged 55 or over, with base deficits < -6 and for those aged 65 or over with a presenting Glasgow Coma Scale < 8, trauma score < 7, or a respiratory rate < 10. Pre-existing comorbidities independently affect outcomes for older trauma patients adversely.[132,133] Mild traumatic brain injury, either in isolation or in combination with multisystem trauma, is associated with increased mortality and worse functional outcomes.[134–137]

Modification of These Questions in Light of New Research: Since the publication of *New Frontiers* no evidence has emerged to prompt a modification of the original questions. (For new agenda items on this topic, see the subsection on triage and mortality in New Horizons in Geriatric Emergency Medicine, at the end of the chapter.)

Resuscitation

See *New Frontiers*, pp. 74–75.

EmergMed 29 (Level B): **Cohort or case-control studies are needed to determine which older patients are at risk for multiple-organ failure and death after blunt trauma and to construct a predictive model.**

EmergMed 30 (Level B): **Exploratory studies are needed to identify new noninvasive ways of determining which older trauma patients might benefit from invasive monitoring and aggressive resuscitation.**

EmergMed 31 (Level A): **To determine whether early invasive monitoring and aggressive resuscitation of high-risk older trauma patients result in improved outcomes, large-scale randomized controlled trials should be performed, and outcomes that include not only short-term mortality but also long-term mortality and function should be used. (See also the Key Questions, at the beginning of the chapter.)**

New Research Addressing These Questions: The EAST guidelines generated recommendations based only upon Level II or Level III evidence for management of older trauma patients. Pulmonary artery catheter hemodynamic monitoring on any geriatric patient with a high-risk mechanism, chronic cardiovascular disease, or physiologic compromise was one of their recommendations. Additionally, they recommended maintaining cardiac index above 4 L/min/m^2 and oxygen consumption above 170 mL/min/m^2.[129]

Modification of These Questions in Light of New Research: Since the publication of *New Frontiers* no evidence has emerged to prompt a modification of the original questions.

NEW HORIZONS IN GERIATRIC EMERGENCY MEDICINE

Advancements in other specialties with potential impact upon ED care of older adults have prompted the addition of four new topics for the research agenda in emergency care for older patients: models of care, driving safety, stroke, and abuse or neglect. In addition, several questions have been added to the original topics in *New Frontiers* to address the need for alternative study designs or additional information.

GENERAL GERIATRIC EMERGENCY CARE

Patterns of ED Use

ED professionals have identified problems associated with the transfer of patients from long-term-care facilities. These include transfers that are deemed inappropriate and failure to provide information in a timely and useful manner. This is an area in which quality of patient care can be improved. The following questions should be answered.

EmergMed 32 (Level D): **Prospective studies are needed that identify patterns of emergency department use, risk factors, and interventions among older people living in residential and long-term-care facilities, given their exclusion from most emergency department studies of older adults.**

EmergMed 33 (Level C): **Prospective studies are needed to evaluate communication between the emergency department and primary physician and assess the relation of outcomes to the exchange of information, follow-up interval, and patient satisfaction toward services rendered.**

EmergMed 34 (Level A): **Randomized controlled trials with blinded outcome assessors and controlled interventions are needed to study whether measures to improve clinical outcomes in the emergency department can simultaneously reduce service utilization rates of older adults.**

Physician Training and Comfort

Existing initiatives to improve residency training in the care of elderly patients provide models that could be used in the field of emergency medicine. For example, the AGS, as part of its program to increase expertise in surgical and related medical specialties, established the Geriatrics for Specialty Residents (GSR) program. GSR, through a competitive process, identified and supported training projects.

EmergMed 35 (Level C): **Systematic evaluation of training effectiveness on clinically important outcomes is needed. This evaluation should begin with an assessment of the attitudes, knowledge, and skills of residents who participate in any program to improve emergency care for older adults.**

EmergMed 36 (Level B): **Prospective studies are needed to assess the effectiveness of interventions (eg, educational models, standardized protocols) for improving the quality of care of older emergency department patients.**

EmergMed 37 (Level B): **Systematic reviews and, when possible, meta-analyses are needed to summarize the best available diagnostic, prognostic, and therapeutic evidence with regard to care for older adults presenting to the emergency department. These reviews should follow established protocols, such as the Cochrane review methodology, including planned periodic updates.**

Environment

There is discussion, but no evidence, about the effect of the environment on the older patient's care and well-being. The ED environment includes the physical and social environment. Elements such as architecture, physical configuration, equipment, furnishings, décor, and communication are topics that have been discussed. Studies are needed to quantify the environmental effect on the outcomes of care, to identify areas for improvement, and to evaluate the changes. Evidence from individual studies could be synthesized into guidelines for improving processes of care of older ED patients.

EmergMed 38 (Level C): **Large prospective studies, including surveys of patients, caregivers, and staff, and observational studies of emergency department facilities and procedures should be performed to identify areas for improvement of the emergency department micro-environment. These could assess elements such as physical plant and communication during evaluation and pre-discharge, follow-up phone interviews by ancillary personnel, and assistance with social priorities (transportation, follow-up appointment scheduling, and medication procurement).**

EmergMed 39 (Level B): **Prospective studies, including surveys of patients, caregivers, and staff, should be conducted to describe the effect of changes in the micro-environment on processes of care for older emergency department patients.**

EmergMed 40 (Level A): **Randomized trials of the effects of specific modifications of the micro-environment on outcomes for older emergency department patients should be conducted.**

Models of Care

We examined alternative models to hospital care with regard to the decision in the ED to admit the older patient or discharge him or her for care at home. A Cochrane review of "hospital at home" care as an alternative to inpatient management of common admitting diagnoses reviewed 22 trials, with early hospital discharge demonstrating a nonsignificant trend toward decreased mortality for stroke and chronic obstructive pulmonary disease subsets.[138] In the United States, a quasi-randomized trial of community-dwelling elderly patients who required hospital-at-home care for pneumonia, heart failure, cellulitis, or chronic obstructive pulmonary disease demonstrated improved satisfaction scores from patients and family members without a difference in functional status or mortality at 2 weeks.[139] Other researchers have assessed home hospitalization or early hospital discharge after an uncomplicated first ischemic stroke, demonstrating a similar improvement in patient satisfaction in addition to lower rates of depression and nursing home admissions.[140,141]

EmergMed 41 (Level B): **Randomized trials are needed to assess alternatives to inpatient management of selected conditions in appropriate subsets of acutely ill older adults and to assess optimal candidate selection, patient and caregiver satisfaction scores, cost-effectiveness, mortality, and functional outcomes in varying health care settings.**

EmergMed 42 (Level A): **Randomized trials based on results of studies in EmergMed 41 should be conducted to evaluate the effectiveness of home care in selected older patients.**

Driving Safety

Motor vehicle crashes are the leading cause of injury-related mortality in the 65-to-74-year age group and are the second leading cause of death for all adults aged 65 or over. Older drivers are more likely to experience medication- and disease-related functional decline. Because current projections indicate increasing numbers of elderly drivers who are driving more miles per year at older ages than ever before, some have predicted a doubling of the number of automobile-related fatalities in the elderly age group by 2030.[142] Though a number of state motor vehicle policies have proven effective with regard to teenaged drivers, with the exception of mandatory seatbelt laws, these results have not been replicated with older drivers.[143] Because assessments of individual patients, family members, and clinicians are poor predictors of potentially hazardous drivers,[144,145] the American Medical Association and the National Highway Safety Administration have published the Physician's Guide to Assessing and Counseling Older Drivers to facilitate physicians' assessment of the older person's driving skills and guidance to change dangerous behaviors to avoid future accidents.[146] No single finding or combination of deficits has been demonstrated to identify individuals at high risk for future motor vehicle accidents, and no validated tool exists with which to screen elderly patients who use the ED.[147,148]

EmergMed 43 (Level B): **Prospective validation studies of brief, low-cost screening tools for use in the emergency department to identify impaired older drivers are needed; such tools must be acceptable to patients and staff.**

EmergMed 44 (Level A): **Randomized trials are needed to demonstrate that the emergency department identification of chronically impaired elderly drivers can reduce motor vehicle accident mortality and morbidity rates.**

Medication Use

The cross-cutting issues chapter of *New Frontiers* (see pp. 369–419) identified medication misuse, overuse, and underuse as an area of concern. These remain issues for emergency physicians and researchers.

EmergMed 45 (Level B): **Prospective studies are needed to validate the use of Beers' criteria to assess medication use by older emergency department patients.**

EmergMed 46 (Level A): **Prospective studies are needed to determine the prevalence of clinically meaningful adverse drug events among older emergency department patients.**

EmergMed 47 (Level A): **Randomized trials are needed to demonstrate that improved recognition in the emergency department of potential adverse drug events in older patients can reduce the incidence rates of adverse events.**

SCREENING AND COMPREHENSIVE GERIATRIC ASSESSMENT IN THE ED

General Geriatric Assessment Tools

Screening and assessment studies conducted in the ED (see discussion of the Identification of Seniors at Risk[49] and Triage Risk Screening Tool[48] projects in the subsection on general geriatric assessment tools in Progress in Geriatric Emergency Medicine) have primarily been conducted by research personnel and have not been part of normal ED procedures. There has been discussion, but no research, about alternate ways of implementing screening programs.

EmergMed 48 (Level C): **Prospective studies are needed to evaluate the cost-effectiveness of interventions by non-nursing, non-physician specialists such as trained "geriatrics technicians."**

EmergMed 49 (Level B): **All studies of emergency department interventions should include quality-of-life measures and indicators of health care service delivery quality among the outcomes assessed.**

EmergMed 50 (Level A): **Randomized controlled trials of emergency department case-finding interventions should be conducted with**

blinded outcome assessors to measure the effect of these interventions on outcomes of care.

SPECIFIC CLINICAL SYNDROMES

Abdominal Pain

Research published since *New Frontiers* (see descriptions in the subsection on abdominal pain in Progress in Geriatric Emergency Medicine) has cast light on the value of diagnostic testing and imaging in the evaluation of older patients presenting with abdominal pain. However, they do not address the question of whether there is a benefit to the patient with earlier detection.

EmergMed 51 (Level A): **Prospective cohort studies are needed to determine whether the rapid identification of older emergency department abdominal pain patients at high risk for adverse outcomes or need for timely surgical intervention can improve outcomes while lowering overall costs.**

Falls

ED-based and outpatient research published since *New Frontiers* (see descriptions in the subsection on falls in Progress in Geriatric Emergency Medicine) identified successful falls reduction programs. These studies have not created a cost-effective falls prevention strategy for use in the ED.

EmergMed 52 (Level B): **Prospective cohort studies to develop a brief, effective screen are needed to identify patients that are most likely to benefit from falls prevention programs.**

EmergMed 53 (Level A): **Randomized controlled trials are needed to assess the efficacy and cost-effectiveness of emergency department–initiated falls prevention interventions for elderly patients at high risk for falls to reduce repeat falls, injurious falls, and subsequent use of health care resources.**

Infectious Disease

Research published since *New Frontiers* identified lack of tetanus immunity and less-than-optimal rates of pneumococcal and influenza vaccination as continuing issues in prevention of infectious disease in older patients. It is not known whether the less-than-optimal rate of tetanus immunity is due to a delayed amnestic response or lack of prior immunization. Pneumococcal and influenza vaccinations are recommended for older adults. The ED is one venue for administering these vaccinations, but it is not clear whether the ED is a cost-effective location for an immunization program.

EmergMed 54 (Level B): **Prospective cohort studies are needed to determine whether older adults' less-than-optimal tetanus immunity is the consequence of a delayed amnestic response to tetanus immunization or a lack of previous immunizations or immunosenescence.**

EmergMed 55 (Level B): **Randomized controlled trials of emergency department–based immunization programs for pneumococcus and influenza are needed to determine whether such programs are cost-effective and whether they reduce pneumonia and influenza incidence and death rates.**

Stroke

A Cochrane review of thrombolytics in acute ischemic stroke treated within 3 hours of symptom onset noted a significant decrease in the odds of dependency or death, [149] but with the exception of the National Institute of Neurological Disorders and Stroke trial, all studies specifically excluded those over 80 years of age. [150–152] Therefore, little information is available to confidently assess the safety or efficacy of thrombolysis in this stroke population. A retrospective review of acute ischemic stroke patients aged 80 or over demonstrated an intracranial hemorrhage rate of 10%, with no improvement in overall mortality when compared with historical cohorts. [153] A multicenter retrospective review of those aged 80 or over demonstrated no differences in favorable or poor outcomes, though a nonsignificant tendency for higher in-hospital mortality was noted. [154] Some have proposed stroke-specific Acute Care for Elders (ACE) units, [155] and others have established home care models for managing uncomplicated acute stroke patients. [140,141] Model systems for stroke care begin in the ED and require integration between the ED and other hospital departments.

EmergMed 56 (Level B): **Randomized controlled trials evaluating models of care for uncomplicated elderly ischemic stroke patients presenting to the emergency department, including Acute Care for Elders (ACE) units and early discharge to home with supportive care, should be conducted. These trials should assess cost-effectiveness, patient satisfaction, and long-term outcomes, including death and disability.**

EmergMed 57 (Level A): **Randomized controlled trials of older acute ischemic stroke patients presenting within 3 hours of symptom onset should be conducted with intravenous tissue plasminogen activator to assess bleeding risk and functional outcomes.**

Cardiopulmonary Arrest

Research published since *New Frontiers* demonstrated the value of automated external defibrillators (see descriptions in the section on cardiopulmonary arrest in Progress in Geriatric Emergency Medicine). The value for aged populations specifically has not been demonstrated.

EmergMed 58 (Level A): **Prospective community trials of cardiopulmonary resuscitation training for seniors and rapid access to automated external defibrillators are needed to evaluate the effect of early resuscitation and defibrillation on age-, gender-, and**

disease-matched controls for important outcomes such as death and return to baseline function.

TRAUMA

Triage and Mortality

Research published since *New Frontiers* (see descriptions in the section on triage and mortality in Progress in Geriatric Emergency Medicine) indicates the need for the following additions to the research agenda.

EmergMed 59 (Level B): **All research concerning the older trauma patient should use similar functional outcomes and standardized definitions of what constitutes "elderly" and "pre-existing medical condition."**

EmergMed 60 (Level A): **Prospective trials are needed to evaluate the diagnostic and prognostic value of injury mechanism, age, traumatic brain injury, and injury severity scores in improving outcomes in older emergency department patients with blunt and penetrating trauma.**

Abuse and Neglect

Elder mistreatment includes abuse, neglect, exploitation, and abandonment of an older person. Recognized as a significant problem since the 1970s, elder mistreatment affects an estimated 1.3% to 10% of the elderly age group, with differing results likely related to widely varying definitions of abuse. Although several causative theories have provided the basis upon which screening tools have been developed, little research has tested these competing theories, even though they form the foundation of assessment instruments being used. A variety of screening and intervention tools exist, though some are too time-consuming for routine use in the ED , and many require input from the caregiver, who may or may not be present during the ED evaluation. Few have been validated in ED settings, and the prevalence of elder mistreatment among different demographic subsets of those utilizing the ED has not been studied.[156–161]

EmergMed 61 (Level B): **Screening tests for elder mistreatment suitable for use in the emergency department should be developed and validated against the tests developed for other settings.**

EmergMed 62 (Level B): **Cross-sectional studies are needed to estimate the prevalence of elder mistreatment among older emergency department patients.**

EmergMed 63 (Level A): **If a high prevalence of elder mistreatment is found (see EmergMed 62) and a rapid identification tool is validated (see EmergMed 61), interventional trials of elder mistreatment detection and management in the emergency department should be performed.**

REFERENCES

1. Solomon DH, LoCicero J, 3rd, Rosenthal RA (eds): New Frontiers in Geriatrics Research: An Agenda for Surgical and Related Medical Specialties. New York: American Geriatrics Society, 2004 (online at http://www.frycomm.com/ags/rasp).
2. Wilber ST, Gerson LW. A research agenda for geriatric emergency medicine. Acad Emerg Med 2003;10:251-260.
3. Downing A, Wilson R. Older people's use of accident and emergency services. Age Ageing 2005;34:24-30.
4. Rutschmann OT, Chevalley T, Zumwald C, et al. Pitfalls in the emergency department triage of frail elderly patients without specific complaints. Swiss Med Wkly 2005;135:145-150.
5. Schumacher JG. Emergency medicine and older adults: continuing challenges and opportunities. Am J Emerg Med 2005;23:556-560.
6. Aminzadeh F, Dalziel WB. Older adults in the emergency department: a systematic review of patterns of use, adverse outcomes, and effectiveness of interventions. Ann Emerg Med 2002;39:238-247.
7. Hastings SN, Heflin MT. A systematic review of interventions to improve outcomes for elders discharged from the emergency department. Acad Emerg Med 2005;12:978-986.
8. McCusker J, Karp I, Cardin S, et al. Determinants of emergency department visits by older adults: a systematic review. Acad Emerg Med 2003;10:1362-1370.
9. Jones JS, Rousseau EW, Schropp MA, Sanders AB. Geriatric training in emergency medicine residency programs. Ann Emerg Med 1992;21:825-829.
10. Lee M, Wilkerson L, Reuben DB, Ferrell BA. Development and validation of a geriatric knowledge test for medical students. J Am Geriatr Soc 2004;52:983-988.
11. Shah MN, Heppard B, Medina-Walpole A, et al. Emergency medicine management of the geriatric patient: an educational program for medical students. J Am Geriatr Soc 2005;53:141-145.
12. LaMascus AM, Bernard MA, Barry P, et al. Bridging the workforce gap for our aging society: how to increase and improve knowledge and training. Report of an expert panel. J Am Geriatr Soc 2005;53:343-347.
13. Levine SA, Caruso LB, Vanderschmidt H, et al. Faculty development in geriatrics for clinician educators: a unique model for skills acquisition and academic achievement. J Am Geriatr Soc 2005;53:516-521.
14. Potter JF, Burton JR, Drach GW, et al. Geriatrics for residents in the surgical and medical specialties: implementation of curricula and training experiences. J Am Geriatr Soc 2005;53:511-515.
15. McNamara RM, Rousseau E, Sanders AB. Geriatric emergency medicine: a survey of practicing emergency physicians. Ann Emerg Med 1992;21:796-801.
16. Leipzig RM. Evidence-based medicine in geriatrics. In Cassel CK, Leipzig RM, Cohen HJ, et al. (eds): Geriatric Medicine: An Evidence-Based Approach. New York, NY: Springer-Verlag, 2003, pp. 3-14.
17. Meldon S, Ma OJ, Woolard R (eds): Geriatric Emergency Medicine. New York, NY: McGraw-Hill, 2004,
18. Nerney MP, Chin MH, Jin L, et al. Factors associated with older patients' satisfaction with care in an inner-city emergency department. Ann Emerg Med 2001;38:140-145.
19. Boudreaux ED, O'Hea EL. Patient satisfaction in the emergency department: a review of the literature and implications for practice. J Emerg Med 2004;26:13-26.
20. Magid DJ, Rhodes KV, Asplin BR, et al. Designing a research agenda to improve the quality of emergency care. Acad Emerg Med 2002;9:1124-1130.

21. Wilber ST, Burger B, Gerson LW, Blanda M. Reclining chairs reduce pain from gurneys in older emergency department patients: a randomized controlled trial. Acad Emerg Med 2005;12:119-123.
22. Jaslow D, Ufberg J, Marsh R. Primary injury prevention in an urban EMS system. J Emerg Med 2003;25:167-170.
23. Fick DM, Kolanowski AM, Waller JL, Inouye SK. Delirium superimposed on dementia in a community-dwelling managed care population: a 3-year retrospective study of occurrence, costs, and utilization. J Gerontol A Biol Sci Med Sci 2005;60:748-753.
24. Elie M, Rousseau F, Cole M, et al. Prevalence and detection of delirium in elderly emergency department patients. CMAJ 2000;163:977-981.
25. Hustey FM, Meldon SW. The prevalence and documentation of impaired mental status in elderly emergency department patients. Ann Emerg Med 2002;39:248-253.
26. Hustey FM, Meldon SW, Smith MD, Lex CK. The effect of mental status screening on the care of elderly emergency department patients. Ann Emerg Med 2003;41:678-684.
27. Kakuma R, du Fort GG, Arsenault L, et al. Delirium in older emergency department patients discharged home: effect on survival. J Am Geriatr Soc 2003;51:443-450.
28. McCusker J, Cole M, Abrahamowicz M, et al. Delirium predicts 12-month mortality. Arch Intern Med 2002;162:457-463.
29. Tierney MC, Charles J, Naglie G, et al. Risk factors for harm in cognitively impaired seniors who live alone: a prospective study. J Am Geriatr Soc 2004;52:1435-1441.
30. McCusker J, Cole M, Dendukuri N, et al. The course of delirium in older medical inpatients: a prospective study. J Gen Intern Med 2003;18:696-704.
31. Chiovenda P, Vincentelli GM, Alegiani F. Cognitive impairment in elderly ED patients: need for multidimensional assessment for better management after discharge. Am J Emerg Med 2002;20:332-335.
32. Irons MJ, Farace E, Brady WJ, Huff JS. Mental status screening of emergency department patients: normative study of the quick confusion scale. Acad Emerg Med 2002;9:989-994.
33. Laurila JV, Pitkala KH, Strandberg TE, Tilvis RS. Confusion assessment method in the diagnostics of delirium among aged hospital patients: would it serve better in screening than as a diagnostic instrument? Int J Geriatr Psychiatry 2002;17:1112-1119.
34. McCusker J, Cole MG, Dendukuri N, Belzile E. The delirium index, a measure of the severity of delirium: new findings on reliability, validity, and responsiveness. J Am Geriatr Soc 2004;52:1744-1749.
35. Monette J, Galbaud du Fort G, Fung SH, et al. Evaluation of the Confusion Assessment Method (CAM) as a screening tool for delirium in the emergency room. Gen Hosp Psychiatry 2001;23:20-25.
36. Nishiwaki Y, Breeze E, Smeeth L, et al. Validity of the Clock-Drawing Test as a screening tool for cognitive impairment in the elderly. Am J Epidemiol 2004;160:797-807.
37. Wilber ST, Lofgren SD, Mager TG, et al. An evaluation of two screening tools for cognitive impairment in older emergency department patients. Acad Emerg Med 2005;12:612-616.
38. Milisen K, Foreman MD, Abraham IL, et al. A nurse-led interdisciplinary intervention program for delirium in elderly hip-fracture patients. J Am Geriatr Soc 2001;49:523-532.
39. Flaherty JH, Tariq SH, Raghavan S, et al. A model for managing delirious older inpatients. J Am Geriatr Soc 2003;51:1031-1035.
40. Christensen RC. Assessing new-onset mental status changes in patients with dementia. Am J Emerg Med 2004;22:228-229.
41. Modawal A. Model and systems of geriatric care: "delirium rooms"—but where and at what cost? J Am Geriatr Soc 2004;52:1023; author reply 1024.

42. Fick DM, Cooper JW, Wade WE, et al. Updating the Beers criteria for potentially inappropriate medication use in older adults: results of a US consensus panel of experts. Arch Intern Med 2003;163:2716-2724.
43. Caterino JM, Emond JA, Camargo CA, Jr. Inappropriate medication administration to the acutely ill elderly: a nationwide emergency department study, 1992-2000. J Am Geriatr Soc 2004;52:1847-1855.
44. Gaddis GM, Holt TR, Woods M. Drug interactions in at-risk emergency department patients. Acad Emerg Med 2002;9:1162-1167.
45. Hohl CM, Dankoff J, Colacone A, Afilalo M. Polypharmacy, adverse drug-related events, and potential adverse drug interactions in elderly patients presenting to an emergency department. Ann Emerg Med 2001;38:666-671.
46. Chung MK, Bartfield JM. Knowledge of prescription medications among elderly emergency department patients. Ann Emerg Med 2002;39:605-608.
47. Stromski C, Popavetsky G, Defranco B, Reed J. The prevalence and accuracy of medication lists in an elderly ED population. Am J Emerg Med 2004;22:497-498.
48. Meldon SW, Mion LC, Palmer RM, et al. A brief risk-stratification tool to predict repeat emergency department visits and hospitalizations in older patients discharged from the emergency department. Acad Emerg Med 2003;10:224-232.
49. Dendukuri N, McCusker J, Belzile E. The Identification of Seniors at Risk screening tool: further evidence of concurrent and predictive validity. J Am Geriatr Soc 2004;52:290-296.
50. Siebens H. The Domain Management Model—a tool for teaching and management of older adults in emergency departments. Acad Emerg Med 2005;12:162-168.
51. Caplan GA, Williams AJ, Daly B, Abraham K. A randomized, controlled trial of comprehensive geriatric assessment and multidisciplinary intervention after discharge of elderly from the emergency department—the DEED II study. J Am Geriatr Soc 2004;52:1417-1423.
52. Guttman A, Afilalo M, Guttman R, et al. An emergency department-based nurse discharge coordinator for elder patients: does it make a difference? Acad Emerg Med 2004;11:1318-1327.
53. McCusker J, Dendukuri N, Tousignant P, et al. Rapid two-stage emergency department intervention for seniors: impact on continuity of care. Acad Emerg Med 2003;10:233-243.
54. McCusker J, Jacobs P, Dendukuri N, et al. Cost-effectiveness of a brief two-stage emergency department intervention for high-risk elders: results of a quasi-randomized controlled trial. Ann Emerg Med 2003;41:45-56.
55. Mion LC, Palmer RM, Meldon SW, et al. Case finding and referral model for emergency department elders: a randomized clinical trial. Ann Emerg Med 2003;41:57-68.
56. Fabacher DA, Raccio-Robak N, McErlean MA, et al. Validation of a brief screening tool to detect depression in elderly ED patients. Am J Emerg Med 2002;20:99-102.
57. Raccio-Robak N, McErlean MA, Fabacher DA, et al. Socioeconomic and health status differences between depressed and nondepressed ED elders. Am J Emerg Med 2002;20:71-73.
58. O'Connell H, Chin AV, Hamilton F, et al. A systematic review of the utility of self-report alcohol screening instruments in the elderly. Int J Geriatr Psychiatry 2004;19:1074-1086.
59. Fink A, Tsai MC, Hays RD, et al. Comparing the alcohol-related problems survey (ARPS) to traditional alcohol screening measures in elderly outpatients. Arch Gerontol Geriatr 2002;34:55-78.
60. Fink A, Morton SC, Beck JC, et al. The alcohol-related problems survey: identifying hazardous and harmful drinking in older primary care patients. J Am Geriatr Soc 2002;50:1717-1722.
61. Girard DD, Partridge RA, Becker B, Bock B. Alcohol and tobacco use in the elder emergency department patient: assessment of rates and medical care utilization. Acad Emerg Med 2004;11:378-382.

62. Onen SH, Onen F, Mangeon JP, et al. Alcohol abuse and dependence in elderly emergency department patients. Arch Gerontol Geriatr 2005;41:191-200.
63. Incorporating nutrition screening and interventions into medical practice: a monograph for physicians. The Nutritional Screening Initiative. American Academy of Family Physicians, American Dietetic Association, National Council on Aging, 1994.
64. Detsky AS, Smalley PS, Chang J. The rational clinical examination: is this patient malnourished? JAMA 1994;271:54-58.
65. Watson GR. Low vision in the geriatric population: rehabilitation and management. J Am Geriatr Soc 2001;49:317-330.
66. Hastings OM, Zenko MM. Malnutrition and dehydration in the geriatric adult. Geriatr Emerg Med Rep 2000;1:41-50.
67. Lewis LM, Banet GA, Blanda M, et al. Etiology and clinical course of abdominal pain in senior patients: a prospective, multicenter study. J Gerontol A Biol Sci Med Sci 2005;60:1071-1076.
68. Hustey FM, Meldon SW, Banet GA, et al. The use of abdominal computed tomography in older ED patients with acute abdominal pain. Am J Emerg Med 2005;23:259-265.
69. Esses D, Birnbaum A, Bijur P, et al. Ability of CT to alter decision making in elderly patients with acute abdominal pain. Am J Emerg Med 2004;22:270-272.
70. Donaldson MG, Khan KM, Davis JC, et al. Emergency department fall-related presentations do not trigger fall risk assessment: a gap in care of high-risk outpatient fallers. Arch Gerontol Geriatr 2005;41:311-317.
71. Gerson LW, Camargo CA, Jr., Wilber ST. Home modification to prevent falls by older ED patients. Am J Emerg Med 2005;23:295-298.
72. Murray KJ, Hill K, Phillips B, Waterston J. A pilot study of falls risk and vestibular dysfunction in older fallers presenting to hospital emergency departments. Disabil Rehabil 2005;27:499-506.
73. Close JC, Hooper R, Glucksman E, et al. Predictors of falls in a high risk population: results from the prevention of falls in the elderly trial (PROFET). Emerg Med J 2003;20:421-425.
74. Haines TP, Bennell KL, Osborne RH, Hill KD. Effectiveness of targeted falls prevention programme in subacute hospital setting: randomised controlled trial. BMJ 2004;328:676.
75. Lord SR, Tiedemann A, Chapman K, et al. The effect of an individualized fall prevention program on fall risk and falls in older people: a randomized, controlled trial. J Am Geriatr Soc 2005;53:1296-1304.
76. Chang JT, Morton SC, Rubenstein LZ, et al. Interventions for the prevention of falls in older adults: systematic review and meta-analysis of randomised clinical trials. BMJ 2004;328:680.
77. Hendriks MR, van Haastregt JC, Diederiks JP, et al. Effectiveness and cost-effectiveness of a multidisciplinary intervention programme to prevent new falls and functional decline among elderly persons at risk: design of a replicated randomised controlled trial [ISRCTN64716113]. BMC Public Health 2005;5:6.
78. Fontanarosa PB, Kaeberlein FJ, Gerson LW, Thomson RB. Difficulty in predicting bacteremia in elderly emergency patients. Ann Emerg Med 1992;21:842-848.
79. Marco CA, Schoenfeld CN, Hansen KN, et al. Fever in geriatric emergency patients: clinical features associated with serious illness. Ann Emerg Med 1995;26:18-24.
80. Mellors JW, Horwitz RI, Harvey MR, Horwitz SM. A simple index to identify occult bacterial infection in adults with acute unexplained fever. Arch Intern Med 1987;147:666-671.
81. Angus DC, Linde-Zwirble WT, Lidicker J, et al. Epidemiology of severe sepsis in the United States: analysis of incidence, outcome, and associated costs of care. Crit Care Med 2001;29:1303-1310.
82. Dellinger RP, Carlet JM, Masur H, et al. Surviving Sepsis Campaign guidelines for management of severe sepsis and septic shock. Crit Care Med 2004;32:858-873.

83. Girard TD, Opal SM, Ely EW. Insights into severe sepsis in older patients: from epidemiology to evidence-based management. Clin Infect Dis 2005;40:719-727.
84. Rivers E, Nguyen B, Havstad S, et al. Early goal-directed therapy in the treatment of severe sepsis and septic shock. N Engl J Med 2001;345:1368-1377.
85. Pallin DJ, Muennig PA, Emond JA, et al. Vaccination practices in U.S. emergency departments, 1992-2000. Vaccine 2005;23:1048-1052.
86. Greci LS, Katz DL, Jekel J. Vaccinations in pneumonia (VIP): pneumococcal and influenza vaccination patterns among patients hospitalized for pneumonia. Prev Med 2005;40:384-388.
87. Rudis MI, Stone SC, Goad JA, et al. Pneumococcal vaccination in the emergency department: an assessment of need. Ann Emerg Med 2004;44:386-392.
88. Healthy People 2010: Understanding and Improving Health. 2nd ed. Washington DC: U.S. Department of Health and Human Services. U.S. Government Printing Office, 2000.
89. Manthey DE, Stopyra J, Askew K. Referral of emergency department patients for pneumococcal vaccination. Acad Emerg Med 2004;11:271-275.
90. Talan DA, Abrahamian FM, Moran GJ, et al. Tetanus immunity and physician compliance with tetanus prophylaxis practices among emergency department patients presenting with wounds. Ann Emerg Med 2004;43:305-314.
91. Lee PY, Alexander KP, Hammill BG, et al. Representation of elderly persons and women in published randomized trials of acute coronary syndromes. JAMA 2001;286:708-713.
92. Ball SG. Thrombolysis: too old and too young. Heart 2002;87:312-313.
93. Estess JM, Topol EJ. Fibrinolytic treatment for elderly patients with acute myocardial infarction. Heart 2002;87:308-311.
94. Soumerai SB, McLaughlin TJ, Ross-Degnan D, et al. Effectiveness of thrombolytic therapy for acute myocardial infarction in the elderly: cause for concern in the old-old. Arch Intern Med 2002;162:561-568.
95. Stenestrand U, Wallentin L. Fibrinolytic therapy in patients 75 years and older with ST-segment-elevation myocardial infarction: one-year follow-up of a large prospective cohort. Arch Intern Med 2003;163:965-971.
96. Thiemann DR, Coresh J, Schulman SP, et al. Lack of benefit for intravenous thrombolysis in patients with myocardial infarction who are older than 75 years. Circulation 2000; 101:2239-2246.
97. Barchielli A, Buiatti E, Balzi D, et al. Age-related changes in treatment strategies for acute myocardial infarction: a population-based study. J Am Geriatr Soc 2004;52:1355-1360.
98. Alter DA, Manuel DG, Gunraj N, et al. Age, risk-benefit trade-offs, and the projected effects of evidence-based therapies. Am J Med 2004;116:540-545.
99. Magid DJ, Masoudi FA, Vinson DR, et al. Older emergency department patients with acute myocardial infarction receive lower quality of care than younger patients. Ann Emerg Med 2005;46:14-21.
100. Rathore SS, Mehta RH, Wang Y, et al. Effects of age on the quality of care provided to older patients with acute myocardial infarction. Am J Med 2003;114:307-315.
101. Rathore SS, Wang Y, Radford MJ, et al. Quality of care of Medicare beneficiaries with acute myocardial infarction: who is included in quality improvement measurement? J Am Geriatr Soc 2003;51:466-475.
102. Grossman SA, Brown DF, Chang Y, et al. Predictors of delay in presentation to the ED in patients with suspected acute coronary syndromes. Am J Emerg Med 2003;21:425-428.
103. Lee DC, Pancu DM, Rudolph GS, Sama AE. Age-associated time delays in the treatment of acute myocardial infarction with primary percutaneous transluminal coronary angioplasty. Am J Emerg Med 2005;23:20-23.

104. Bach RG, Cannon CP, Weintraub WS, et al. The effect of routine, early invasive management on outcome for elderly patients with non-ST-segment elevation acute coronary syndromes. Ann Intern Med 2004;141:186-195.
105. Cohen M, Gensini GF, Maritz F, et al. Prospective evaluation of clinical outcomes after acute ST-elevation myocardial infarction in patients who are ineligible for reperfusion therapy: preliminary results from the TETAMI registry and randomized trial. Circulation 2003;108:III14-III21.
106. de Boer MJ, Ottervanger JP, van't Hof AW, et al. Reperfusion therapy in elderly patients with acute myocardial infarction: a randomized comparison of primary angioplasty and thrombolytic therapy. J Am Coll Cardiol 2002;39:1723-1728.
107. Goldenberg I, Matetzky S, Halkin A, et al. Primary angioplasty with routine stenting compared with thrombolytic therapy in elderly patients with acute myocardial infarction. Am Heart J 2003;145:862-867.
108. Kotamaki M, Strandberg TE, Nieminen MS. Clinical findings, outcome and treatment in patients > or = 75 years with acute myocardial infarction. Eur J Epidemiol 2003;18:781-786.
109. Minai K, Horie H, Takahashi M, et al. Long-term outcome of primary percutaneous transluminal coronary angioplasty for low-risk acute myocardial infarction in patients older than 80 years: a single-center, open, randomized trial. Am Heart J 2002;143:497-505.
110. Moriel M, Behar S, Tzivoni D, et al. Management and outcomes of elderly women and men with acute coronary syndromes in 2000 and 2002. Arch Intern Med 2005;165:1521-1526.
111. Niebauer J, Sixt S, Zhang F, et al. Contemporary outcome of cardiac catheterizations in 1085 consecutive octogenarians. Int J Cardiol 2004;93:225-230.
112. Yagi M, Nakao K, Honda T, et al. Clinical characteristics and early outcomes of very elderly patients in the reperfusion era. Int J Cardiol 2004;94:41-46.
113. Kaye P. Early prediction of individual outcome following cardiopulmonary resuscitation: systematic review. Emerg Med J 2005;22:700-705.
114. Bunch TJ, White RD, Khan AH, Packer DL. Impact of age on long-term survival and quality of life following out-of-hospital cardiac arrest. Crit Care Med 2004;32:963-967.
115. Herlitz J, Eek M, Engdahl J, et al. Factors at resuscitation and outcome among patients suffering from out of hospital cardiac arrest in relation to age. Resuscitation 2003;58:309-317.
116. Herlitz J, Engdahl J, Svensson L, et al. Can we define patients with no chance of survival after out-of-hospital cardiac arrest? Heart 2004;90:1114-1118.
117. Swor R, Compton S, Farr L, et al. Perceived self-efficacy in performing and willingness to learn cardiopulmonary resuscitation in an elderly population in a suburban community. Am J Crit Care 2003;12:65-70.
118. Swor R, Fahoome G, Compton S. Potential impact of a targeted cardiopulmonary resuscitation program for older adults on survival from private-residence cardiac arrest. Acad Emerg Med 2005;12:7-12.
119. Demetriades D, Murray J, Martin M, et al. Pedestrians injured by automobiles: relationship of age to injury type and severity. J Am Coll Surg 2004;199:382-387.
120. Schulman AM, Claridge JA, Young JS. Young versus old: factors affecting mortality after blunt traumatic injury. Am Surg 2002;68:942-947; discussion 947-948.
121. Clark DE, DeLorenzo MA, Lucas FL, Wennberg DE. Epidemiology and short-term outcomes of injured Medicare patients. J Am Geriatr Soc 2004;52:2023-2030.
122. Hannan EL, Waller CH, Farrell LS, Rosati C. Elderly trauma inpatients in New York state: 1994-1998. J Trauma 2004;56:1297-1304.
123. Nirula R, Gentilello LM. Futility of resuscitation criteria for the "young" old and the "old" old trauma patient: a national trauma data bank analysis. J Trauma 2004;57:37-41.
124. Grossman M, Scaff DW, Miller D, et al. Functional outcomes in octogenarian trauma. J Trauma 2003;55:26-32.

125. Inaba K, Goecke M, Sharkey P, Brenneman F. Long-term outcomes after injury in the elderly. J Trauma 2003;54:486-491.
126. McKevitt EC, Calvert E, Ng A, et al. Geriatric trauma: resource use and patient outcomes. Can J Surg 2003;46:211-215.
127. Richmond TS, Kauder D, Strumpf N, Meredith T. Characteristics and outcomes of serious traumatic injury in older adults. J Am Geriatr Soc 2002;50:215-222.
128. Sieling BA, Beem K, Hoffman MT, et al. Trauma in nonagenarians and centenarians: review of 137 consecutive patients. Am Surg 2004;70:793-796.
129. Jacobs DG, Plaisier BR, Barie PS, et al. Practice management guidelines for geriatric trauma: the EAST Practice Management Guidelines Work Group. J Trauma 2003;54:391-416.
130. Demetriades D, Karaiskakis M, Velmahos G, et al. Effect on outcome of early intensive management of geriatric trauma patients. Br J Surg 2002;89:1319-1322.
131. Liberman M, Mulder DS, Sampalis JS. Increasing volume of patients at level I trauma centres: is there a need for triage modification in elderly patients with injuries of low severity? Can J Surg 2003;46:446-452.
132. Grossman MD, Miller D, Scaff DW, Arcona S. When is an elder old? Effect of preexisting conditions on mortality in geriatric trauma. J Trauma 2002;52:242-246.
133. McGwin G, Jr., MacLennan PA, Fife JB, et al. Preexisting conditions and mortality in older trauma patients. J Trauma 2004;56:1291-1296.
134. Coronado VG, Thomas KE, Sattin RW, Johnson RL. The CDC traumatic brain injury surveillance system: characteristics of persons aged 65 years and older hospitalized with a TBI. J Head Trauma Rehabil 2005;20:215-228.
135. Mosenthal AC, Lavery RF, Addis M, et al. Isolated traumatic brain injury: age is an independent predictor of mortality and early outcome. J Trauma 2002;52:907-911.
136. Reynolds FD, Dietz PA, Higgins D, Whitaker TS. Time to deterioration of the elderly, anticoagulated, minor head injury patient who presents without evidence of neurologic abnormality. J Trauma 2003;54:492-496.
137. Susman M, DiRusso SM, Sullivan T, et al. Traumatic brain injury in the elderly: increased mortality and worse functional outcome at discharge despite lower injury severity. J Trauma 2002;53:219-223; discussion 223-214.
138. Shepperd S, Iliffe S. Hospital at home versus in-patient hospital care. Cochrane Database Syst Rev 2005:CD000356.
139. Leff B, Burton L, Mader SL, et al. Hospital at home: feasibility and outcomes of a program to provide hospital-level care at home for acutely ill older patients. Ann Intern Med 2005;143:798-808.
140. Ricauda NA, Bo M, Molaschi M, et al. Home hospitalization service for acute uncomplicated first ischemic stroke in elderly patients: a randomized trial. J Am Geriatr Soc 2004;52:278-283.
141. Thorsen AM, Holmqvist LW, de Pedro-Cuesta J, von Koch L. A randomized controlled trial of early supported discharge and continued rehabilitation at home after stroke: five-year follow-up of patient outcome. Stroke 2005;36:297-303.
142. Lyman S, Ferguson SA, Braver ER, Williams AF. Older driver involvements in police reported crashes and fatal crashes: trends and projections. Inj Prev 2002;8:116-120.
143. Morrisey MA, Grabowski DC. State motor vehicle laws and older drivers. Health Econ 2005;14:407-419.
144. Brown LB, Ott BR, Papandonatos GD, et al. Prediction of on-road driving performance in patients with early Alzheimer's disease. J Am Geriatr Soc 2005;53:94-98.
145. Ott BR, Anthony D, Papandonatos GD, et al. Clinician assessment of the driving competence of patients with dementia. J Am Geriatr Soc 2005;53:829-833.

146. Physician's guide to assessing and counseling older drivers. Washington, DC: National Highway Traffic Safety Administration, 2003.
147. Fitten LJ. Driver screening for older adults. Arch Intern Med 2003;163:2129-2131; discussion 2131.
148. Li I, Smith RV. Driving and the elderly. Clin Geriatr 2003;11:40-46.
149. Wardlaw JM, Zoppo G, Yamaguchi T, Berge E. Thrombolysis for acute ischaemic stroke. Cochrane Database Syst Rev 2003:CD000213.
150. Tissue plasminogen activator for acute ischemic stroke. The National Institute of Neurological Disorders and Stroke rt-PA Stroke Study Group. N Engl J Med 1995;333:1581-1587.
151. Clark WM, Wissman S, Albers GW, et al. Recombinant tissue-type plasminogen activator (Alteplase) for ischemic stroke 3 to 5 hours after symptom onset. The ATLANTIS Study: a randomized controlled trial. Alteplase Thrombolysis for Acute Noninterventional Therapy in Ischemic Stroke. JAMA 1999;282:2019-2026.
152. Hacke W, Kaste M, Fieschi C, et al. Randomised double-blind placebo-controlled trial of thrombolytic therapy with intravenous alteplase in acute ischaemic stroke (ECASS II). Second European-Australasian Acute Stroke Study Investigators. Lancet 1998;352:1245-1251.
153. Simon JE, Sandler DL, Pexman JH, et al. Is intravenous recombinant tissue plasminogen activator (rt-PA) safe for use in patients over 80 years old with acute ischaemic stroke?—the Calgary experience. Age Ageing 2004;33:143-149.
154. Tanne D, Gorman MJ, Bates VE, et al. Intravenous tissue plasminogen activator for acute ischemic stroke in patients aged 80 years and older: the tPA stroke survey experience. Stroke 2000;31:370-375.
155. Allen KR, Hazelett SE, Palmer RR, et al. Developing a stroke unit using the acute care for elders intervention and model of care. J Am Geriatr Soc 2003;51:1660-1667.
156. Anetzberger GJ. Elder abuse identification and referral: the importance of screening tools and referral protocols. J Elder Abuse Neglect 2001;13:3-22.
157. Dong X. Medical implications of elder abuse and neglect. Clin Geriatr Med 2005;21:293-313.
158. Fulmer T, Guadagno L, Bitondo Dyer C, Connolly MT. Progress in elder abuse screening and assessment instruments. J Am Geriatr Soc 2004;52:297-304.
159. Gorbien MJ, Eisenstein AR. Elder abuse and neglect: an overview. Clin Geriatr Med 2005;21:279-292.
160. Harrell R, Toronjo CH, McLaughlin J, et al. How geriatricians identify elder abuse and neglect. Am J Med Sci 2002;323:34-38.
161. Lachs MS, Pillemer K. Elder abuse. Lancet 2004;364:1263-1272.

4

GERIATRIC GENERAL SURGERY

*Sandhya Lagoo-Deenadayalan, MD, PhD; Walter J. Pories, MD, FACS**

The elderly age group is a fast-growing part of the American population. The proportion of the population aged 85 years and older is projected to increase from 4 million to 19 million by 2050. [1] The growing demands of this elderly population include the increasing need for surgical intervention. [2,3] In the United States the number of patients aged 65 years and older who undergo one or more of five common operations exceeds 1 million per year. Data from the National Cancer Institute Surveillance, Epidemiology and End Results Program show that 56% of newly diagnosed cancer and 71% of cancer deaths are in the age group 65 years or older. [4]

Over the past decade increasing numbers of elderly persons have been found to be more fit and active than ever before. Aging is associated with an increase in the incidence of cancer, gastrointestinal disorders, and vascular disorders, and larger numbers of older adults now desire timely surgical intervention so that they can return to their regular activities with the least possible delay. Many retrospective and prospective studies have shown that age alone is not a contraindication to most surgical procedures when adequate attention is paid to peri-operative care. The advent of minimally invasive surgery, both laparoscopic and endoluminal techniques, have resulted in early recovery following surgical intervention. Advantages include decreased length of stay in hospitals, early ambulation, decreased postoperative pain, and earlier return to preoperative levels of functioning.

The present overview updates the discussion of needed research in geriatric general surgery that was published in *New Frontiers in Geriatrics Research* [5] by describing subsequent contributions to the literature. It also includes relevant information on research conducted in younger patients that are indicative of critical issues that need to be addressed specifically in an older population. New findings that address agenda items from *New Frontiers* are described in the section Progress in Geriatric General Surgery. Research that suggests the need for additions to the research agenda is discussed in the section New Horizons in Geriatric General Surgery at the end of the chapter.

We suggest no changes in the Key Questions in geriatric general surgery that were proposed in *New Frontiers:*

> ***GenSurg KQ1*: How can elderly patients at high risk for emergency procedures be identified?**
>
> ***GenSurg KQ2*: What are the differences in pathophysiology of the disease processes in the older patient leading to surgical emergencies?**
>
> ***GenSurg KQ3*: What factors impact on procedure-specific risk-benefit projections in elderly patients?**

* Lagoo-Deenadayalan: Department of Surgery, Duke University Medical Center, Durham, NC; Pories: Professor of Surgery and Biochemistry, Department of Surgery, Brody School of Medicine, East Carolina University, Greenville, NC.

METHODS

The MEDLINE database was searched via the DIALOG Information Service. The period covered was from January 2000 to November 2006. The search strategy combined the MeSH terms for specific surgical procedures with terms denoting old age and also with the various terms for risk factors, postoperative care, postoperative complications, comorbidity, mortality, quality of life, prognosis, recovery, outcome, length of stay, and functional status. An additional requirement was that the term *age* or *aged* be present in the title or that the term *age factors* be present in the MeSH heading. The search resulted in 722 references. A final selection from these was made on the basis of a review of titles and abstracts.

PROGRESS IN GERIATRIC GENERAL SURGERY

Procedures and Outcomes

See *New Frontiers,* pp. 85–86.

> ***GenSurg 1 (Level B)*: Prospective cohort studies of specific surgical procedures are needed to identify the risk factors in the geriatric population for specific negative and positive outcomes.**

New Research Addressing This Question: Our literature search identified relevant research in three areas: abdominal, biliary, and colorectal surgery.

A retrospective review of 125 octogenarians who over a 6-year period underwent major abdominal surgery showed emergency surgical procedures to be associated with increased morbidity in the elderly age group. The mean age of the patients was 84.6 years. Outcomes measured were whether complications developed, 30-day mortality, and whether there was return to premorbid function. Nearly half were emergency cases. Most operations were on the stomach, small bowel, or large bowel. Multivariate analysis revealed emergency operations to be associated with significantly increased odds of morbidity. Likewise, a poor American Society of Anesthesiologists (ASA) classification, a comorbidity index greater than 5, development of acute coronary syndrome, and anastomotic leakage were also found to significantly increase the odds of morbidity. Low serum albumin and hemoglobin and renal impairment were also predictors of adverse outcome. For elective cases, 82.8% of patients were able to return to their premorbid functional status. The study suggests that efforts to improve outcome in geriatric surgery patients should emphasize a shift toward elective surgery and away from emergency surgery and should also target the optimization of predictors of adverse outcome. [6]

Fifty percent of women and 16% of men in their 70s have been shown to have gallbladder disease, and 20% of the abdominal procedures performed in those older than 80 years are hepatobiliary. In a retrospective study of 5884 patients undergoing laparoscopic cholecystectomy, it was demonstrated that patients aged 70 years and older have a twofold increase in complicated biliary tract disease and conversion rates over those seen in younger patients. Pulmonary and cardiac complications were common in the elderly patients. Complicated biliary disease resulted in a nearly tenfold increase in conversion rate for patients aged 65 years and older, with an increase in morbidity to 27% for patients undergoing conversion. [7] The rate of conversion from a laparoscopic procedure to an open procedure is higher in emergency cases. This was evaluated in a series of 117 patients aged 80 years and older (median age 83 years) undergoing laparoscopic cholecystectomy. The conversion rate was 3% in elective cases and 10% in emergency cases.[8]

A study of bile duct injuries during cholecystectomy reported that the adjusted hazard ratio for death during the follow-up is significantly higher for patients with a common bile duct injury than for those without injury, and the hazard significantly increases with advancing age and comorbidities and decreases with the experience of the surgeon. Complicated gallstone or bile duct disease might necessitate referral to an experienced hepatobiliary surgeon for improvement in the outcomes of elderly patients undergoing laparoscopic cholecystectomy. The risk of bile duct injuries increases with age, male sex, and a low annual hospital volume of cholecystectomies.[9]

In a prospective study comparing presenting findings and outcomes in patients younger than 50 years and 50 years or older (N = 519) with appendicitis, the presence of symptoms for longer than 24 hours was found to be significantly more common in the older group. Complication rates were also significantly higher (20% versus 8%) in the older group, as were mortality rates (2.9% versus 0.24%) and perforation rates (35% versus 13%).[10] Increasing time between appendicitis symptom onset and treatment may be a risk factor for a ruptured appendix, but little is known about how the risk changes with passing time. A retrospective chart review revealed that the risk of rupture is greater in patients with 36 hours or more of untreated symptoms and age of 65 years and older. This study suggests that, especially in the elderly population, delaying surgery beyond 36 hours from symptom onset results in higher risk of rupture and increased morbidity.[11]

Colorectal emergency requiring radical surgery is becoming more common in the older age group, and problems remain as regards the best management policy. A retrospective study evaluated 105 elderly patients, aged 65 years and older, with colorectal disease who underwent an emergency operation. Forty-five patients had benign disease, with a predominance of diverticulitis, and 60 patients had colorectal carcinoma. A resection operation either with primary anastomosis or Hartmann's procedure was performed in 75% of cases; in the rest, only palliation was achieved. Forty-three percent of the patients with colorectal cancer emergency were aged 80 years or older. The mortality rate was higher for patients with perforation than for those with obstruction. Advanced age was found not to be a contraindication to radical surgery for colorectal emergency. In the majority, a resection operation was feasible. In high-risk patients, colostomy was found to be a life-saving alternative.[12]

Modification of This Question in Light of New Research: Further studies are indicated in the elderly population to assess whether postoperative outcomes and quality of life are improved when older adults are offered elective surgery for chronic conditions such as chronic cholecystitis, recurrent gallstone pancreatitis, or chronic diverticulitis. Elderly patients often have multiple comorbidities that can increase the risk of poor outcomes when surgery is performed for acute and complicated biliary disease or complicated diverticulitis following two or more episodes of diverticulitis. These studies will help to re-evaluate the practice of elective resection as a strategy for reducing the mortality and morbidity from complicated intra-abdominal pathology.

GenSurg 2 (Level B): **Prospective studies are needed to compare outcomes in younger and older patients for specific surgical procedures in outpatient settings or with short hospital stays. For example, is it**

possible to safely perform laparoscopic antireflux surgery in older patients with a 23-hour hospital stay?

New Research Addressing This Question: Ultra-short anesthetic agents and advances in the ability to monitor the depth of anesthesia have helped to improve anesthetic recovery in elderly patients following outpatient surgery. This has resulted in quicker recovery from anesthesia, with decreased nausea and vomiting. Postoperative cognitive dysfunction still remains a problem in a small proportion of elderly patients. [13]

While the success of outpatient and short-term inpatient laparoscopy still can be assured only by surgeons' high experience and minimal complications, several other factors contribute to good outcomes. These include meticulous attention to detail in the preoperative assessments, efficient postoperative management, a reliable social setting, and collaboration with local physicians involved in primary care of the patient. [14] Several studies have shown that laparoscopic cholecystectomy, hernia repairs, and fundoplication can be performed safely in a hospital-affiliated outpatient setting, resulting in a significant reduction in procedure costs. Most patients studied were ASA grade I or II. [15–17]

Modification of This Question in Light of New Research: These studies included but were not limited to elderly patients. Prospective studies are still needed to stratify elderly patients according to their suitability for outpatient surgery.

***GenSurg 3 (Level B)*: Case-control studies are needed to identify factors that place elderly patients at high risk for requiring emergency surgical procedures.**

New Research Addressing This Question: Elderly patients with longstanding symptomatic cholelithiasis and chronic cholecystitis are at increased risk for developing gallstone pancreatitis, acute gangrenous cholecystitis, and possible gallbladder perforation. These conditions are associated with significant morbidity and occasionally are difficult to diagnose, as can be the case with gallbladder perforation. In the study detailed here, data were collected prospectively over a 10-year period of patients undergoing laparoscopic cholecystectomy. Two hundred eight of 11,360 patients who underwent cholecystectomy were diagnosed with gangrenous cholecystitis, and 30 were diagnosed with gallbladder perforation. In comparison with patients with gangrenous cholecystitis, patients with gallbladder perforation presented at an older age (53 versus 60 years; $P < .05$), had more cardiovascular comorbidity (29% versus 50%; $P < .05$) and postoperative complications (19% versus 37%; $P < .05$), required more intensive care unit admissions (9% versus 33%; $P < .001$), and had longer hospital stays (8 versus 13 days; $P < .001$). Early cholecystectomy within 24 hours was found to improve outcome ($P < .05$). [18] An additional risk factor for elderly patients is the increased risk of biliary tract disease in postmenopausal women using estrogen therapy. [19]

Retrospective studies have been conducted to evaluate outcomes in patients presenting with acute cholecystitis, mild acute pancreatitis, or cholangitis who were treated conservatively. In one such study, 42% of the patients who did not receive cholecystectomy at the time of the first admission subsequently presented again to the emergency department, and 70% of all the patients studied required further inpatient admission related to gallstone-associated pathology within the study period; 61% underwent cholecystectomy at a median range of 70 days from index admission. [20] Similar studies are needed in the elderly population, as the morbidity associated with repeat presentation with symptoms is high in this patient population. This is critical in patients with gallstone pancreatitis, in whom delay of laparoscopic cholecystectomy for more than 4 weeks after gallstone pancreatitis is associated with a high unplanned readmission rate, even with liberal use of preoperative cholangiography.[21]

Three factors have been shown in one study to predict a high mortality rate in elderly patients, aged 70 and over, who undergo emergency surgery for complicated colorectal carcinoma. These are peri-operative transfusion, a high Acute Physiology and Chronic Health Evaluation (APACHE II) score, and the presence of perforation proximal to the tumor. This study suggests that the presence of these factors and the knowledge that they can independently predict mortality can help determine the operative plan and the need for more intensive postoperative care.[22]

Modification of This Question in Light of New Research: Better understanding of predictors of the need for emergency surgery in the elderly population is still needed. Prospective studies comparing outcome measures following elective or emergent surgery are also needed.

> ***GenSurg 4 (Level B)*: Basic studies are needed to elucidate the differences in pathophysiology of the diseases and disorders in the elderly patient that lead to a high risk of requiring emergency surgical procedures.**

New Research Addressing This Question: The age-associated decline in liver function may be caused by mechanisms operating on the cellular level, such as age-associated mitochondrial damage in hepatocytes, functional decline of Kupffer cells, and defects of the respiratory chain in the liver during aging. One study found advanced age to be associated with a higher incidence of choledocholithiasis ($P = .01$) and an increased incidence of complications probably secondary to increased incidence of inflamed or scarred gallbladder or the presence of choledocholithiasis.[23] The presentation of peptic ulcer disease in the elderly patient is more subtle and atypical than in younger patients. With the increase in prevalence of *Helicobacter pylori* infection in the elderly age group, there has been a concomitant increase in the incidence of peptic ulcer disease in this population.[24] *H. pylori* infection and the use of nonsteroidal anti-inflammatory drugs (NSAIDs) are independent risk factors for peptic ulcer disease. NSAIDs and selective serotonin-reuptake inhibitors together can increase the risk of gastrointestinal bleeding.[25]

Modification of This Question in Light of New Research: The risk factors in elderly patients for emergency surgery still need to be determined tô help prospectively identify those who should receive early elective intervention.

> ***GenSurg 5 (Level A)*: Guidelines for educating physicians to recognize diseases and risk factors that might predict an older patient's need for emergency surgical procedure should be developed; the guidelines would be based on findings of the research recommended in GenSurg 3 and GenSurg 4.**

New Research Addressing This Question: With the steady increase in the aging population, there has been a rise in both elective and emergent surgical procedures in patients aged 70 years or older. A retrospective study of 469 such patients assessed the effect of sex, type of admission, main surgical diagnosis, benign or malignant nature, site of disease, concomitant disease, and preoperative ASA grade on postoperative outcomes. The incidence of various procedures for specific indications was as follows: Hepatopancreatic biliary conditions, 39.6%; colorectal, 19.4%; hernia, 18.8%; upper gastrointestinal, 15.3%; and endocrine disease, 6.9%. The study concluded that factors that increased the risk of postoperative death were the emergency nature of the surgery, the presence of comorbidities, an ASA score of III-V, and upper gastrointestinal surgery.[26]

Scoring systems for the enumeration of morbidity and mortality are useful predictors of postoperative outcomes, but they have to be validated within individual practices. Studies comparing the observed morbidity and mortality in patient populations following a given procedure need to be compared with values predicted by specific scoring systems to check for concordance. A study examined the validity of a physiology and operative severity score for enumeration of mortality and morbidity (POSSUM)[27] in predicting morbidity and mortality in 76 patients aged 80 and older undergoing laparoscopic cholecystectomy. Patients were identified from the surgical operations database of one hospital. Information on clinical and operative factors as described in POSSUM was collected. The ratios of observed to POSSUM-estimated morbidity and 30-day mortality were calculated. Observed and POSSUM scores were similar in predicting morbidity. However, POSSUM scoring overpredicted mortality in this patient population.[28]

Modification of This Question in Light of New Research: Scoring systems should be used to modify peri-operative care for elderly patients undergoing emergent procedures, and observational studies should be carried out to evaluate the effect of such interventions on outcomes following surgery.

ENDOCRINE DISEASE

Parathyroid Disease

See *New Frontiers,* p. 87.

> ***GenSurg 6 (Level B)*: Research is needed to determine the effect of hyperparathyroidism on quality of life, longevity, functional status, and cognitive status of older patients.**

New Research Addressing This Question: Evaluation of the quality of life following parathyroidectomy is critical. A study conducted over 16 months evaluated the health-related quality of life of 61 patients following parathyroidectomy for hyperparathyroidism. The mean age of patients in the study was 61 years. The patients filled out health status questionnaires preoperatively and during two subsequent postoperative visits, and the results were evaluated. During the postoperative visits, patients' perception of their general health, muscle strength, energy level, and mood showed significant improvement ($P < .05$), suggesting that parathyroidectomy for hyperparathyroidism is associated with marked improvement in a patient's quality of life.[29,30] These and other studies were not targeted solely on the study of elderly patients. However, a retrospective analysis of 54 patients aged 80 years or older with symptomatic primary hyperparathyroidism showed similar improvement in symptoms of fatigue, weight loss, bone pain, depression, and constipation following parathyroidectomy.[31]

Primary hyperparathyroidism is one of the risk factors for bone loss, osteoporosis, and fractures in elderly people. A cohort study of 3213 patients with a mean age of 61 years and a diagnosis of primary hyperparathyroidism compared the effects of surgery (60%)

with nonsurgical management (40%). Patients who underwent surgery were found to have a lower incidence of fractures (hazards ratio 0.69, 0.56 to 0.84) and gastric ulcers (0.59, 0.41 to 0.84). Mortality was lower in the patients who were treated surgically. There was no difference in the occurrence of cardiovascular events following surgical intervention or following nonsurgical treatment. [32]

Improvement of cognitive impairment following parathyroidectomy is one of the expected benefits of the procedure. It has not been proven conclusively that cognitive impairment caused by hyperparathyroidism can be reversed by parathyroidectomy. However, case studies of three patients, two women aged 79 and 80 and a man aged 84, revealed cognitive impairment caused by primary hyperparathyroidism. In these three patients, parathyroidectomy led to a marked improvement in the symptoms. [33]

Modification of This Question in Light of New Research: Further studies are needed to evaluate improvement in symptoms, progression of osteoporosis, and cognitive function in elderly patients following parathyroidectomy.

GenSurg 7 (Level B): **Observational comparison of older and younger patients is needed to suggest whether hyperparathyroidism is recognized and treated surgically in the same percentage of older and younger patients.**

New Research Addressing This Question: Although primary hyperparathyroidism is common in elderly patients, referral for parathyroidectomy may be delayed because of concerns regarding the fitness for surgery of older persons and the perceived risk of increased morbidity and mortality in this age group. A retrospective analysis of 54 patients aged 80 years and older with primary hyperparathyroidism was conducted. Twenty-two percent of these patients had a mean delay of 5 years before a surgical referral was requested. [31] The concern regarding the morbidity associated with anesthesia and surgical stress of parathyroidectomy has decreased with the advent of minimally invasive parathyroidectomy. [34]

Modification of This Question in Light of New Research: Further studies are needed to evaluate the benefit of early referral of elderly patients with symptomatic hyperparathyroidism. Studies are also needed to determine whether minimally invasive parathyroidectomy can offer a reliable and safe alternative for the elderly patient with multiple comorbidities. Comparisons of treatment modalities and outcomes between younger and older patients are also needed.

Thyroid Disease

See *New Frontiers,* p. 87. For a new agenda item, see the subsection on thyroid disease in New Horizons in Geriatric General Surgery at the end of the chapter.

BREAST CANCER

See *New Frontiers,* pp. 88–90. For new agenda items, see the subsection on breast cancer in New Horizons in Geriatric General Surgery at the end of the chapter.

GenSurg 8 (Level A): **Randomized controlled trials should be performed to determine the effect of screening mammography on survival,**

treatment morbidity, functional outcomes, and costs as a function of age.

New Research Addressing This Question: The annual breast cancer mortality rate declined between 1987 and 1997. However, this decline was only 9% for women aged 70 to 79 years, much lower than the 19% for women aged 20 to 49 and the 18% for women aged 50 to 69. The difference may be due to the fact that older women are not screened as vigorously as younger women or that they receive less aggressive treatment. [35,36]

Breast cancer—specific mortality has been found to be higher in the younger woman (aged 55 to 64 years). In this group, 75% of deaths are a result of breast cancer, but this is true in only 27.6% of women aged 85 and older. The majority of elderly breast cancer patients present with stage I and II disease. However, despite this stage distribution, most elderly patients undergo modified radical mastectomy instead of breast conservation surgery. [36]

The screening studies available for detecting breast cancer are self-examination, physical examination by a health care professional, and mammography. Other avenues being explored are digital mammography and magnetic resonance imaging. The use of mammography in older women does affect survival. Women undergoing at least two mammograms between age 70 and 79 have shown a 2.5-fold reduction in cancer-related mortality. [37] Mammography has also shown reduced mortality in women up to the age of 85 in spite of the presence of moderate comorbidities. [38]

The value of obtaining routine mammograms in women aged 65 years and older has not been documented. The American Geriatrics Society position statement recommends annual or at least biennial mammography until age 75 and biennially or at least every 3 years thereafter, with no upper age limit for women with an estimated life expectancy of 4 or more years. [39] Previous studies had suggested that screening mammography could reduce the mortality rates from breast cancer between the ages of 50 and 69 and that this advantage could extend to patients aged 70 to 74 years. A retrospective cohort study evaluated the relationship between the use of screening mammography and the size and stage of breast cancer at the time of diagnosis in 12,038 older women who received a diagnosis of breast cancer over a 2-year period. The results indicated that women aged 75 years and older are less likely to have undergone a screening mammogram than women aged 69 to 74 years. More importantly, an increase in the use of mammography was found to be associated with smaller tumor size and a lesser stage of cancer at the time of diagnosis. This finding is more significant in older women than in younger women. [40]

A retrospective cohort study conducted in women aged 67 years and older sought to establish the relationship between the use of mammography, stage of the breast cancer at the time of diagnosis, and breast cancer mortality. The 11,399 women in the study were divided into three age groups: 67 to 74 years, 75 to 85, and 85 or older. Lack of use of mammography was found to be associated with a higher incidence of presentation with stage II or higher advanced breast cancer in all age groups. For all women, but especially for women between the ages of 67 and 85, lack of mammography is significantly associated with an increase in the risk of dying from breast cancer. [37]

Modification of This Question in Light of New Research: Questions that remain to be answered are whether physical breast examination is as effective as mammography in older women and whether mammograms should be performed at intervals longer than 1 year in women over 70 years age. Such research will lead to the establishment of evidence-based guidelines for the use of routine mammography in older women. Studies are also needed to evaluate differences in outcomes when older women are screened as vigorously as their younger counterparts and receive similarly aggressive treatment.

GenSurg 9 (Level A): **Randomized controlled trials of breast cancer therapy in older women should be performed to compare the use of tamoxifen alone with the use of tamoxifen plus surgery in subgroups of ages ranging from 50 to 90 years. Outcomes measured would include survival, treatment morbidity, function, and cost. Subgroup analyses would identify which patients are likely to respond well to tamoxifen alone.**

New Research Addressing This Question: The 2001 St. Gallen Seventh International Consensus Panel recommends that postmenopausal women with breast cancer (with the exception of those who are low-risk node-negative patients and those who are estrogen-receptor negative) should receive 5 years of tamoxifen therapy.[41] However, several studies show that older women are less likely than younger women to receive tamoxifen. A study of patterns of adjuvant tamoxifen prescription and patterns of discussion regarding such therapy between patients and physicians revealed that older patients (those aged 80 years and older, those with multiple comorbidities, and those with estrogen receptor–negative status) were less likely to report discussion regarding tamoxifen therapy with their physicians.[42]

In a cohort study of 5464 women diagnosed with node-positive operable breast cancer, adjuvant chemotherapy was found to result in improved survival only in patients aged 65 to 69. No benefit was seen in patients aged 70 years and older,[43] similar to what had been seen in previously published randomized clinical trials. Collaborative meta-analyses of 194 unconfounded randomized trials of adjuvant chemotherapy and hormonal therapy started in 1995 have yielded interesting results. Six-month treatment with anthracycline-based polychemotherapy with FAC (fluorouracil/Adriamycin/cyclophosphamide) or FEC (fluorouracil/epirubicin/cyclophosphamide) reduced the annual breast cancer death rate by 38% in women younger than 50 years and by 20% in women aged 50 to 69. These results were found to occur regardless of estrogen-receptor status, nodal status, tumor characteristics, and use of tamoxifen. Unfortunately, women aged 70 or older were not included in the study. More interestingly, the use of tamoxifen for estrogen receptor–positive disease reduced the annual death rate by 31% regardless of the use of chemotherapy, age, progesterone-receptor status, and other tumor characteristics. This included patients aged 70 years and older.[44]

The European Organization for Research and Treatment of Cancer 10851 trial randomized women aged 70 years and older to modified radical mastectomy or to tamoxifen 20 mg daily for life. Median follow-up was 11.7 years in the mastectomy group and 10.2 years in the tamoxifen group.[45] This trial was preceded by two earlier trials—the Nottingham City trial comparing wedge resection with tamoxifen (20 mg twice daily) and the St. George's trial comparing total mastectomy or wide local excision versus tamoxifen alone (20 mg daily for 2 years).[46] All three trials showed that overall survival and breast cancer-specific survival were equivalent with operation or tamoxifen.

Surgery as a primary treatment modality offers the best chance for local control. Progression of disease while on tamoxifen therapy requires subsequent surgical intervention in a large number of patients. The optimal treatment for breast cancer in a woman who is physically fit is surgery, not endocrine therapy.[47] It has been suggested, therefore, that primary endocrine therapy should be reserved for selected patients with multiple comorbidities, those with limited life expectancy, and those who refuse surgical treatment.

Modification of This Question in Light of New Research: Further studies are needed to evaluate the outcomes of adjuvant tamoxifen therapy in older postmenopausal women with breast cancer (with the exception of those with low-risk node-negative status and estrogen receptor–negative status).

GenSurg 10 (Level A): **Randomized controlled trials are needed to determine the minimum duration of tamoxifen therapy that is required for optimal effect in older breast cancer patients.**

New Research Addressing This Question: Although tamoxifen therapy is the gold standard adjuvant treatment in estrogen receptor–positive early breast cancer, it does have several disadvantages. Patients undergoing tamoxifen therapy are at increased risk of endometrial cancer and other life-threatening events. They may also develop resistance to tamoxifen. This has led to a keen interest in developing alternatives to tamoxifen. A prospective randomized trial was planned in which, following 2 to 3 years of tamoxifen treatment, patients were randomly assigned either to receive anastrozole (aromatase inhibitor) 1 mg per day or to continue receiving tamoxifen 20 mg per day, for a period of 5 years. A total of 448 patients with node-positive, estrogen receptor–positive tumors were enrolled, and disease-free survival was measured over a period of 36 months. Disease-free survival and local recurrence–free survival were significantly longer in the anastrozole group ($P = .0002$).[48]

Overall survival was assessed in a randomized prospective study of women between the ages of 50 and 70 years with T1-3, N0-3 breast carcinoma. They were randomized to 2 years versus 5 years of adjuvant tamoxifen, and studies were performed after 12 years of follow-up. In studying the entire population and patients who were estrogen-receptor positive, the researchers concluded that tamoxifen usage did not affect overall survival. However, in younger patients (aged 55 or younger) with estrogen receptor–positive disease, the 5-year treatment was found to be associated with a 44% decrease in the risk of death. This advantage was not present in the older age group.[49]

One study conducted a 10-year follow up of 18,000 women with breast cancer in 47 randomized trials of chemotherapy. The study showed that younger women, those aged under 50 years, who were treated with chemotherapy gained a significantly increased relapse-free survival (average of 10.3 months) and an overall survival (average of 5.4 months) in comparison with patients in the no-treatment group. The same benefit was seen in older women, aged 50 to 69 years, who received chemotherapy, also in comparison with older women in the no-treatment group. When the older and younger women in the chemotherapy group were compared, the size of the benefit for the older women was found to be less. Even within this group, however, there was a smaller subgroup of patients who had estrogen receptor–negative tumors and therefore did not receive tamoxifen. In this subgroup, the benefits of polychemotherapy were comparable to those seen in the younger patients.[50]

Modification of This Question in Light of New Research: Further studies are needed to evaluate the impact of switching to anastrozole after the first 2 to 3 years of treatment with tamoxifen in patients with early breast cancer who are aged 70 years and older. Discussions are warranted as to whether the overall benefit of a treatment modality should be determined by comparison with younger patients undergoing similar treatment or with older patients who do not undergo the treatment.

GenSurg 11 (Level A): **Randomized controlled trials are needed to compare rates of recurrence and survival in groups of older breast cancer patients who are treated with and without axillary dissection.**

New Research Addressing This Question: The presence of multiple comorbidities in the older patient can limit interventions such as an axillary node dissection and can affect decisions regarding the type of surgery and subsequent adjuvant therapy.

A cohort study of 464 women aged 64 years or older who were newly diagnosed with breast cancer (stage I or II) and undergoing breast-conservation surgery yielded interesting results. Most of the women studied, 63.4%, also underwent axillary node dissection. Although increasing age was associated with decreasing odds of node dissection, it was found that irrespective of age, women in the lowest quartile of physical functioning were less likely to undergo axillary node dissection than those with excellent functioning. Also, patients cared for by surgeons with special training in oncology were less likely to undergo node dissection. Age, therefore, does not seem to be the only determinant in the decision regarding whether or not to proceed with axillary node dissection in older women with stage I or II breast cancer.[51]

The utility of sentinal lymph node (SLN) dissection in determining subsequent therapy was evaluated in a prospectively collected breast cancer SLN mapping database. A total of 730 breast cancer SLN mapping patients were studied; 261 (35.8%) were aged 70 years or older. Axillary lymph node dissection was performed in 88.9% of patients with metastases detected by hematoxylin and eosin stain, and 84.65% of patients with metastases documented by immunohistochemistry. Hormonal and cytotoxic chemotherapy were administered more frequently (86.9% and 24%) in SLN-positive patients than in SLN-negative patients (54.3% and 2.8%). In the patients studied, SLN status affected treatment algorithms. With a mean follow-up of 15.4 months, 8.2% of patients with positive SLN developed distant metastases, as compared with no patients with negative SLN.[52]

Another retrospective study evaluated SLN biopsy using smaller-sized tin colloid in 122 patients; 40 patients were over 60 years of age and 82 patients were 60 years or younger. The 95% confidence intervals (CI) for successful mapping rate, false negative rate, and accuracy of the two groups overlapped. It was concluded that SLN biopsy can therefore be feasible and useful in elderly patients.[53]

Modification of This Question in Light of New Research: The results of SLN mapping and biopsy in elderly patients significantly influences subsequent therapy decisions, including axillary lymph node dissection, hormonal therapy, and cytotoxic chemotherapy. The effect of regularly recommending SLN mapping and biopsy and axillary lymph node dissection in elderly women should be evaluated.

STOMACH DISORDERS

See *New Frontiers,* pp. 91–93. For new agenda items on gastroesophageal reflux disease (GERD) and achalasia, see the subsections on these conditions in New Horizons in Geriatric General Surgery at the end of the chapter.

Ulcer Disease

See *New Frontiers,* p. 92.

GenSurg 12 (Level B): **Observational cohort studies are needed to determine if presentation and pathophysiology of peptic ulcer disease are different in older people.**

New Research Addressing This Question: Elderly persons are known to be at higher risk for GERD, pill-induced esophagitis, peptic ulcer disease, and complications of NSAID use.[54] Retrospective studies of patients who underwent surgery for treatment of peptic ulcer disease over a 15-year period showed that for elderly patients the percentage requiring emergency surgical intervention is significantly higher than for their younger counterparts. The older patients are also more likely to present with hemodynamic instability and require a longer hospital stay. NSAID use was also found to be higher in the elderly age group.[55]

Modification of This Question in Light of New Research: Future studies should evaluate the effects of endoscopic surveillance of elderly patients presenting with new-onset symptoms of ulcer disease.

GenSurg 13 (Level B): **Prospective cohort studies are needed to seek clues as to how complications of peptic ulcer disease in older patients can be prevented.**

New Research Addressing This Question: One of the ways in which it may be possible to reduce the incidence of acute presentations would be to recommend endoscopy for identification of mucosal disease in patients who are older than 45 years and who present with new-onset weight loss, vomiting, anemia, dysphagia, or gastrointestinal bleeding.[54]

Modification of This Question in Light of New Research: Future studies should evaluate the effects of follow-up and possible endoscopic surveillance of elderly patients who have previously undergone surgery for peptic ulcer disease and who present with recurrent symptoms.

GenSurg 14 (Level B): **Cohort studies on older patients are needed to identify risk factors for peptic ulcer disease.**

New Research Addressing This Question: Presentation of peptic ulcer disease in the elderly patient is more subtle and atypical than in the younger patient. With the increase in prevalence of *H. pylori* infection in the elderly age group, there has been a concomitant increase in the incidence of peptic ulcer disease in these patients.[24] *H. pylori* infection and NSAIDs use are independent risk factors for peptic ulcer disease. NSAIDs with selective serotonin-reuptake inhibitors together can increase the risk of gastrointestinal bleeding.[25]

Modification of This Question in Light of New Research: Future studies are needed to evaluate the ability of gastroprotective agents to cause a decrease in the rate of gastrointestinal bleeding in patients on NSAIDs and selective serotonin-reuptake inhibitors. Observational studies are needed to evaluate the effect of substituting alternatives to NSAIDs in the elderly population.

***GenSurg 15 (Level B)*: Observational cohort studies are needed of putative methods to reduce the morbidity and mortality of emergency operations for peptic ulcer disease in older patients.**

New Research Addressing This Question: Management of peptic ulcer disease in the elderly patient is a challenging task. There is an increase in the number of elderly patients presenting with complications of peptic ulcer disease such as perforation and bleeding. Observational studies evaluating 13 patients older than 70 years of age and presenting with perforated gastric ulcer were carried out in a tertiary hospital from 1995 to 2003. Surgical procedures performed were simple closure with an omental patch in 11 patients and antrectomy in 2 patients. Three patients died in the postoperative period. Of these, 2 were transferred from an outside hospital. The study also included 28 elderly patients with a mean age of 79.6 years with bleeding gastric ulcer who were admitted during the same period. All patients were managed with medical therapy and endoscopic intervention. The study concluded that early diagnosis and treatment were the two main factors that resulted in favorable outcomes in elderly patients presenting with perforated gastric ulcers. Medical management and endoscopic intervention were successful in controlling gastric ulcer bleeding in elderly patients. The need for surgery in these cases was found to arise only after two failed endoscopic interventions.[56]

A prospective cohort study was carried out in 96 patients presenting with perforated peptic ulcer in order to assess the predictors of the risk, rate, and number of postoperative complications. Patients underwent either a Graham patch closure or a gastrojejunostomy with total truncal vagotomy. The results showed that comorbidities, abdominal distension, and the need for blood transfusion were risk factors for postoperative complications and for the higher number of such complications. The rate of development of complications was influenced by a history suggestive of shock and A− blood group. This study documents the need for early recognition of the above-mentioned risk factors so that postoperative management can be optimized, resulting in improved outcomes.[57]

Modification of This Question in Light of New Research: GenSurg 15 has been answered and can be dropped from the research agenda.

***GenSurg 16 (Level A)*: Randomized controlled trials of the most promising method for reducing the morbidity and mortality of emergency surgery for peptic ulcer disease in older patients are needed.**

New Research Addressing This Question: One study enrolled 72 consecutive patients to evaluate the role of intensive resuscitation in the outcome of patients with upper gastrointestinal bleeding. The factors thought to be associated with increased morbidity and mortality are age, associated comorbidities, and hemodynamic stability. To prevent bias in comparing improperly balanced patient groups, the groups were designed to be similar with respect to variables such as age, shock, comorbid conditions, cause of bleeding, and major stigmata of recent hemorrhage. Both groups had 36 patients, with 22/36 in the observational group with peptic ulcer disease and 24/36 patients in the intensive resuscitation group with peptic ulcer disease. Other causes of bleeding included esophageal varices, esophageal ulcers, and malignancy. Irrespective of age, timely correction of hemodynamic instability, correction of hematocrit, and coagulopathy resulted in decreased morbidity and mortality ($P = .04$).[58]

Modification of This Question in Light of New Research: Similar studies are needed focusing solely on elderly patients with stratification based on their comorbidities and specifically on patients with ulcer disease.

> ***GenSurg 17 (Level B)*: Cohort studies are needed to seek alternatives to nonsteroidal anti-inflammatory drugs for use by older patients.**

New Research Addressing This Question: No research of the type recommended has been done.

Modification of This Question in Light of New Research: Alternatives to NSAIDs that may be beneficial for use by older patients are needed. This item should remain on the research agenda.

> ***GenSurg 18 (Level A)*: As possibly safer nonsteroidal anti-inflammatory drugs are developed, they should be tested in randomized controlled trials for safe use by older patients.**

New Research Addressing This Question: No research of the type recommended has been done.

Modification of This Question in Light of New Research: This item should remain on the research agenda.

Gastric Cancer

See *New Frontiers,* pp. 92–93.

> ***GenSurg 19 (Level B)*: Outcome studies and prospective cohort studies are needed to build evidence as to optimum treatment for each stage of gastric cancer, including ways to palliate the near-terminal and terminal phases.**

New Research Addressing This Question: The incidence of gastric cancer is increasing in elderly patients, though not in younger patients. The higher mortality observed in the elderly patients and the poor survival rate leads to a surgical approach that mostly tends to palliate symptoms rather than obtain a curative resection.[59]

One study analyzed outcomes for 3431 patients treated for gastric cancer between 1977 and 1998. Patients in group 1 were aged 70 years or older and in group 2 were younger than 70 years. The incidence of intestinal type (Lauren classification) and distally located cancers were higher in the older age group. Total gastrectomies and extended lymph node dissection were performed more commonly in the younger group. There was a significant difference between the groups in 5-year survival: 24% for group 1 and 35% for group 2. Following more radical procedures, the 5-year survival increased: 35% in group 1 and 53% in group 2. The researchers concluded that surgical resection is therefore the treatment of choice for gastric cancer and that advancing age is not a contraindication.[60]

One study found postoperative complications and mortality rates to be higher in elderly patients undergoing resection for gastric cancer. However, in this patient population it may be beneficial to use biological markers to determine if they will benefit from preoperative high-dose chemotherapy. Positive p53 immunostaining and positive p53 mutation status before chemotherapy and histologic regression following high-dose chemotherapy followed by surgical resection has been shown to be associated with prolonged overall survival. These studies were conducted in 25 patients, 3 of whom were aged 60 years or older.[61] The use of a Comprehensive Geriatric Assessment tool that takes into account the individual operative risk can help optimize the choice of treatment.[62]

A study of 135 elderly patients (aged 75 years or older), and 665 middle-aged patients (45 to 65 years old) with gastric cancer undergoing surgery noted distinct characteristics in the elderly patients. These included a predominance of males and advanced-stage disease; also, deaths from other cancers and comorbid disease were more common in the elderly group. The authors concluded that follow-up and management of their other diseases would improve survival of elderly gastric cancer patients.[63]

Laparoscopic hand-assisted surgery for early gastric cancer in young and elderly patients has been evaluated to test the feasibility of the procedure and to compare outcomes. The controls were patients undergoing standard open gastrectomy. Blood loss was found to be less in elderly patients undergoing laparoscopic surgery than in younger patients and control patients. The overall 5-year survival rates were not significantly different in the elderly and younger groups.[64]

The utility of gastrojejunostomy for the palliation of gastric outlet obstruction in irresectable or incurable gastric carcinoma was investigated in a retrospective review of 67 patients who underwent a gastrojejunostomy for gastric outlet obstruction caused by gastric carcinoma. Sixty patients were discharged from hospital once they had resumed normal eating. Their median survival after surgery was 9 months, which suggests that gastrojejunostomy offers worthwhile palliation and possibly prolongs survival for this significant group of patients.[65]

Palliative procedures are often indicated in patients with advanced biliary and pancreatic tumors. Placement of self-expandable metal stents inserted either endoscopically or under fluoroscopic control has shown encouraging results. A retrospective study of 33 patients who had a metal stent positioned was conducted. They ranged in age from 45 to 94 years, with a mean age of 75. Indications were a pancreatic adenocarcinoma (27 patients), a stricture of a gastrojejunal anastomosis due to recurrent pancreatic tumor (4), and a stricture of a gastrojejunal anastomosis secondary to gastric cancer surgery (2). There were no immediate complications. Improvement in the quality of life was obtained in all patients, with a median duration of hospitalization of 8 days and mean survival rate of 12 weeks. Such palliative procedures have therefore been shown to be safe and well tolerated, and to demonstrate improved quality of life.[66]

Modification of This Question in Light of New Research: Future studies can be conducted prospectively in elderly patients presenting with gastric cancer at various stages to determine which stage and which biological marker profile can help determine the treatment that carries the least morbidity and mortality with overall good outcomes.

GenSurg 20 (Level B): **Cohort or outcome studies are needed to gain information about the effectiveness of using newer treatment methods, such as photodynamic therapy, for treating elderly patients with stomach disorders.**

New Research Addressing This Question: The therapeutic efficacy of endoscopic photodynamic therapy for advanced gastric cancer is limited. In one small study, immunotherapy combined with photodynamic therapy was evaluated in two elderly (aged 92 and 89 years) men with complicated advanced gastric cancer. Two or three courses of the combined therapy safely stopped tumor bleeding, and the initial poor prognoses of a few months of survival seemed to be improved (patient 1, over 32 months; patient 2, 14 months).[67]

Modification of This Question in Light of New Research: Cohort or outcome studies are still needed to prove the efficacy of this multimodal treatment for elderly patients with gastric cancer.

COLORECTAL DISEASE

See *New Frontiers,* pp. 94–96.

Diverticular Disease

See *New Frontiers,* pp. 94–95.

> ***GenSurg 21 (Levels B and A)*: Nonrandomized or randomized trials comparing appropriate management options for complications of diverticular disease in older patients are needed.**

New Research Addressing This Question: An elderly patient presenting with acute perforated diverticulitis presents a serious challenge, especially in the presence of multiple comorbidities. It is therefore critical to evaluate prognostic factors that can serve as indicators of outcomes following surgical intervention. A retrospective study of 172 patients with perforated diverticulitis admitted over a 19-year period was conducted. Of these, 71 patients were aged 70 years or older. The Mannheim Peritonitis Index Score was found to be useful in predicting mortality in this patient population. The score includes purulent peritonitis (6 points), fecal peritonitis (12 points), age over 50 years (5 points), female gender (5 points), preoperative duration of peritonitis for more than 24 hours (4 points), and organ failure—ie, kidney or lung failure, shock, or intestinal obstruction (7 points). Patients with scores greater than 21 were considered to have a poor prognosis. Although mortality was found to be related to age, age alone was not considered to be an independent predictor.[68]

Patients presenting with acute perforated diverticulitis can undergo either a primary resection and anastomosis or a Hartmann procedure that involves resection of the diseased segment with a proximal end colostomy.[69] Evaluation of postoperative outcomes following Hartmann's reversal showed a higher incidence of prolonged ileus, respiratory infections, and the need for reoperation in comparison with outcomes following a primary resection and anastomosis. There was no difference in the readmission rates or early postoperative mortality.[70]

Alternatively, primary resection and anastomosis with a diverting ileostomy may also be considered. Although a diverting ileostomy may not decrease the incidence of postoperative leak, it can reduce the associated morbidity. In two groups of 20 patients who were studied retrospectively over a 5-year period, complications were found to be more common after Hartmann's reversal than after loop ileostomy reversal. The mean age for the Hartmann's reversal group was 56 years (range 40 to 74) and for the loop ileostomy reversal group was 55 years (range 28 to 76). This finding suggests that segmental colonic excision with anastomosis and loop ileostomy may be an attractive alternative to minimize morbidity with stoma reversal.[71]

Age is a risk factor in acute lower gastrointestinal hemorrhage. Diverticular disease is an important cause. In contrast to elective resection for diverticulosis, emergent management of lower gastrointestinal bleeding can have significant death and complication rates. Preoperative condition and functioning are key predictors of peri-operative complications in the elderly patient. Although the risk of surgical complications increases only slightly with age for elective surgery, it increases dramatically for emergent surgery.[72] Every effort must therefore be made to avoid urgent operations by attending to pre-existing symptoms. These may be neglected in the elderly age group.

A retrospective study of 43 patients older than 80 years with acute lower gastrointestinal hemorrhage revealed that the cause is more likely to be diverticular disease, as opposed to benign ano-rectal and small intestinal pathology in the younger population. Older patients have a higher incidence of comorbidities, such as prior colorectal surgery seen in 9% of patients, or indications for anticoagulant and anti-aggregant medication in 26% of patients. Endoscopy provided a diagnosis in 59% (N = 23) of cases, while arteriography provided a diagnosis in two of the four cases. Urgent surgical intervention was required in 16% of cases. Though conservative management of acute lower gastrointestinal hemorrhage in elderly patients is usually successful, increasing age is associated with high morbidity and mortality, and with relapse of hemorrhage.[73] In patients who present with rebleeding, prolonged observation may be more dangerous than intervention. This and similar studies highlight the role of meticulous peri-operative care in improving overall outcomes in elderly patients.

Modification of This Question in the Light of New Research: Prospective randomized trials are needed to determine the usefulness of early definitive surgery in patients aged 70 years or older who have presented with one or two episodes of acute diverticulitis. Patients in such a study should be divided into groups on the basis of whether they are at low, intermediate, or high risk for any surgical procedure. This will enable identification of patients most likely to benefit from early intervention.

Prospective randomized trials are needed to evaluate outcomes in elderly patients following primary resection and anastomosis in comparison with Hartmann's takedown.

Colorectal Cancer

See *New Frontiers,* pp. 95–96. For new agenda items, see the subsection on colorectal cancer in New Horizons in Geriatric General Surgery at the end of the chapter.

GenSurg 22 (Level A): **Randomized controlled trials are needed to compare the various colorectal cancer screening methods now in use for their efficacy in elderly patients.**

New Research Addressing This Question: Two randomized controlled studies have demonstrated decreased mortality from colorectal cancer in asymptomatic patients between the ages of 50 and 80 undergoing yearly fecal occult blood tests.[74] Serial screening endoscopy is particularly advantageous, as it leads to the identification and removal of adenomatous polyps. The progression model for colorectal neoplasia is now well established, and it is now accepted that progression from normal colonic epithelium to adenomatous polyps and finally to infiltrating adenocarcinoma is associated with activation of oncogenes and inactivation of tumor-suppressor genes.

In a cross-sectional study of 15,406 asymptomatic persons aged 50 years or older, 18% were found to have had an inadequate examination. The screening method used was a sigmoidoscopy. In men, inadequate examinations increased from 10% in men aged 50 to 59 years to 22% in those aged 80 and older. In women, the inadequacy was even more marked, with inadequate examinations in 19% of women aged 50 to 59 years and in 32% of women aged 80 and older.[75] Prospective randomized studies are needed to evaluate and compare the adequacy of colonoscopy and sigmoidoscopy in these patient populations so that recommendations can be made with regard to screening protocols.

Full colonoscopy is more advantageous, as polyps can occur exclusively in the proximal colon. It is also more cost-effective if performed once every 10 years, as compared with yearly fecal occult blood testing or more frequent sigmoidoscopies, because compliance with the latter is low.[76]

There are no guidelines for screening and surveillance colonoscopy in the elderly patient. In a study of 1112 patients with an average age of 83.1 years, the diagnostic yield in asymptomatic patients undergoing routine screening and surveillance colonoscopy was low. The procedure could be safely performed, with major complications in only 0.6% of the patients. Indications for the procedure were as follows: polyp surveillance, 227 (19%); altered bowel habits, 168 (14%); iron-deficiency anemia, 132 (11%); and cancer follow-up, 108 (9%). Eighty-six examinations (7%) were performed solely for an indication of colorectal cancer screening; 22% of patients had more than one indication for colonoscopy. The screening group did not have any malignancies. Overall, 45 malignancies were found (3.7%), and 2 malignancies (0.7%) were found in patients undergoing colonoscopy for polyp surveillance. The study concluded that colonoscopy should be limited to elderly patients with symptoms or specific clinical findings.[77]

Modification of This Question in the Light of New Research: Questions that remain to be answered are the determination of the upper age limit after which screening is not beneficial and the efficacy of virtual colonoscopy in the elderly patient in avoiding the 3% risk of perforation that currently exists as a complication of colonoscopy. Research might also be focused on screening that targets elderly individuals with known higher risk for colorectal cancer.

> ***GenSurg 23 (Level B)*: Exploratory studies are needed to elucidate the roles of emerging technologies in the management of colorectal cancer in elderly patients.**

New Research Addressing This Question: Several studies now confirm that laparoscopic resection for colon cancer is not inferior to open surgery in terms of oncologic outcomes. One randomized multicenter study of patients with a mean age of 70 years showed that recurrence rates at 3 years were the same in both open and laparoscopic groups. Postoperative mortality and morbidity rates were also similar. Length of stay and use of parenteral narcotics were shorter in the laparoscopic group.[78]

Robotic assistance has facilitated laparoscopy by offering magnified, three-dimensional visualization and articulating instruments that better simulate the movements of the human hand. Data on the use of this technology in colon surgery is just beginning to emerge.

Transanal endoscopic microsurgery, which uses specialized instruments to resect rectal tumors, has also recently been introduced. The role for this modality in the treatment of rectal tumors in the elderly patient is not yet defined.

Modification of This Question in Light of New Research: Prospective studies are needed to determine whether newer technologies, such as robotic techniques for low anterior resection or transanal endoscopic microsurgery for rectal tumors, will improve the overall results of surgical treatment of colorectal cancer in older patients.

LIVER RESECTION

See *New Frontiers,* pp. 96–97. For a new agenda item, see also the subsection on liver resection in New Horizons in Geriatric General Surgery at the end of the chapter.

> *GenSurg 24 (Level B)*: **Cohort studies are needed to determine the role, safety, and efficacy of newer liver-directed therapies in older patients, for example, cryoablation, radiofrequency ablation, and hepatic artery infusion.**

New Research Addressing This Question: Although several studies have evaluated the role of cryoablation, radiofrequency ablation, and hepatic artery infusion, there are no studies that have evaluated these modalities in the elderly patient.

Modification of This Question in the Light of New Research: The role of these different modalities still needs to be evaluated in elderly patients. This item should remain on the research agenda.

BILIARY DISEASE

See *New Frontiers,* pp. 97–98.

> *GenSurg 25 (Level A)*: **Randomized controlled trials are needed to compare the safety and effectiveness for older patients of outpatient or short-stay cholecystectomy with the safety and effectiveness of longer hospital stays.**

New Research Addressing This Question: Elderly patients with gallbladder disease tend to present with complications of cholelithiasis such as acute cholecystitis, choledocholithiasis, or gallstone pancreatitis and require more urgent intervention. Early referral in this group for an elective operation can minimize the morbidity and mortality secondary to complicated gallbladder disease.[79] Cholecystectomy is one of the most commonly performed general surgical procedures in elderly patients. Laparoscopic cholecystectomy continues to be the procedure of choice for the management of gallstone disease. It has been shown that elective laparoscopic cholecystectomy for uncomplicated disease in the elderly age group has comparable safety and efficacy to that seen in younger populations.[80]

A retrospective chart review of 47 patients with a median age of 71 undergoing laparoscopic cholecystectomy was undertaken to evaluate the outcomes of the procedure. The mean postoperative stay for the patients aged 70 years or older was significantly longer than for the younger group, although 30% of the older patients had only a one-night postoperative stay.[81] Patients undergoing surgery for symptomatic cholelithiasis require a shorter postoperative hospital stay than those undergoing surgery for acute cholecystitis or gallstone pancreatitis.

A retrospective review of 70 patients aged 80 or older who underwent cholecystectomy for biliary disease showed that 17 patients presented for elective surgery and 54 presented with complications of cholelithiasis. The conversion rate was 12.5% in the elective group and 37% in the emergent group. The average length of stay was 3.7 days in those who underwent elective laparoscopic surgery but 11.7 days for patients who underwent emergent laparoscopic surgery. Morbidity and mortality did not differ significantly between laparoscopic and open procedures performed for acute disease.[80] A prospective study evaluated 421 patients aged 65 or older undergoing laparoscopic cholecystectomy. The patients were divided into two groups: those 65 to 79 years old and those 80 to 95 years old. A study database was analyzed. Advanced age was found to be associated with higher mean ASA scores (P = .001) and a higher incidence of choledocholithiasis (P = .01). There was an increased incidence of grade 1 and 2 complications (ie, those requiring either bedside intervention or invasive procedures including surgery) in the older patients (P = .05), probably secondary to increased incidence of inflamed or scarred gallbladder or the presence of choledocholithiasis.[23]

Modification of This Question in the Light of New Research: Randomized controlled trials may be difficult to perform, as the safety and effectiveness of outpatient or short-stay cholecystectomy for the elderly patient has already been established. Therefore, this question can be dropped from the research agenda.

***GenSurg 26 (Level B)*: Basic physiologic and biochemical studies are needed to learn why older patients are more likely than younger patients to present with complicated biliary disease.**

See the discussion of research relating to GenSurg 3 and GenSurg 4.

PANCREATIC DISEASE

See *New Frontiers,* p. 98.

***GenSurg 27 (Level B)*: Cohort or case-control studies are needed to determine what are the most appropriate selection criteria for pancreatic resection in older patients.**

New Research Addressing This Question: Pancreatic cancer is the fourth leading cause of death in both men and women, and each year approximately 28,000 Americans die of the disease. The mean age for local-stage adenocarcinoma of the pancreas in a group of 1331 patients was found to be 71.2 years, indicating that it is an important cause of morbidity and mortality in an aging population.[82] Data extracted from the Surveillance, Epidemiology and End Results (SEER) Program of the National Cancer Institute for the period 1997 to 2001 also revealed an incidence of ~60% of pancreatic cancers diagnosed between ages of 65 and 84.[83] The growth in the older population and the increasing incidence associated with age results in a greater number of elderly patients in need of surgery for management of pancreatic cancer. Although the appropriateness of extensive surgery, such as a pancreatic duodenectomy, in elderly patients has been questioned, several studies have shown that long-term survival after pancreatic resection is similar in elderly and younger patients. Therefore, the decision to proceed with curative pancreatic resection should be made independently of the patient's age, taking into consideration instead factors that can affect long-term outcomes.[84] The rate of cancer-directed surgery has been found to be 26.2% for adenocarcinoma of the pancreas. However, the rate of cancer-directed surgery was significantly lower for patients older than 70 years than in patients 40 to 50 years of age (20% versus 55% to 56%, respectively).[82] This pattern is probably due to concern that an elderly patient may not be able to tolerate the stress of surgery because of decreased physiologic reserve. A tool such as Comprehensive Geriatric Assessment to define the individual's operative risk would help to optimize the surgical management of elderly patients with resectable pancreatic cancer. [85]

The overall response to surgical resection in pancreatic cancer is still suboptimal, with survival times being less than 12 months. The addition of chemotherapy in these patients has increased the mean survival to about 24 months. Advances in chemotherapy such as those discussed below are possible only in patients with resected disease. Postoperative adjuvant treatment and expected changes in outcomes following such treatment therefore become important factors that should be considered while deciding selection criteria regarding surgical resection for pancreatic cancer in the elderly patient.

The European Study Group for Pancreatic Cancer 1 trial is the largest study of adjuvant treatment. It is a multicenter randomized trial of adjuvant chemoradiotherapy and chemotherapy (5FU) in patients with resected pancreatic cancer. After a median follow-up of 47 months, a highly significant difference in median survival in favor of chemotherapy was reported. The 2- and 5-year survival rates for chemotherapy were 40% and 21%, while the 2- and 5-year survival rates without chemotherapy were 30% and 8%. No benefit was seen in patients who received chemoradiotherapy. [86] Adjuvant chemotherapy has also been shown to be effective in treating pancreatic cancer in a randomized controlled trial in Japan. [87]

A meta-analysis of the randomized adjuvant therapy trials for pancreatic cancer concluded that chemotherapy is more effective than chemoradiotherapy in the treatment of resected pancreatic cancer. Patients younger than 60 years formed 45% of the patient population in these studies, while those 60 years and older formed 55%. Adjuvant chemoradiation did not lead to a significant difference in the risk of death and did not significantly change 2-year and 5-year survival rates in patients with pancreatic cancer. However, a subgroup analysis found that adjuvant chemoradiation was more effective in patients with positive resection margins. [88]

There have been significant advances in imaging, staging, surgical techniques, and peri-operative care of the patient with pancreatic cancer. This has now resulted in operative mortality of $< 5\%$ in high-volume centers. However, the 5-year survival rate of patients diagnosed with pancreatic cancer has not changed from what it has been over the past two decades and is still only a dismal 5%. One of the most recent studies evaluated clinical and demographic factors to test their effect on outcomes of pancreatico-duodenectomy in two groups of patients, one group aged 70 years and older, and the other group younger than 70 years. Significantly higher morbidity and mortality was observed in the older age group (morbidity of 49.1% versus 45.8%, and mortality of 10.5% versus 3.7%). These were attributed to increased comorbidities, reduced functional reserve, decreased tolerance to stress, and the texture of the pancreatic remnant. A soft pancreatic remnant has been found to increase the rate of leak from the pancreatico-jejunal anastomoses. [89] Even though there is no documented correlation between age and the texture of the pancreatic remnant, modification of the procedure in older patients with a soft pancreatic remnant may yield better outcomes. [90]

Pancreatic duct lesions are now thought most likely to be the precursors of infiltrating duct adenocarcinomas. This is associated with multiple genetic alterations that include activating point mutations in the K-ras gene, overexpression of HER-2/neu, and the inactivation of several tumor suppressor genes.[91] Early detection and resection of intraductal pancreatic neoplasms and the use of chemoprevention in patients with intraductal papillary mucinous neoplasms and those at increased inherited susceptibility to pancreatic cancer may be important areas of future research. Additionally, evaluation of genetic alterations in samples of pancreatic secretions may prove to be an important screening tool for patients with increased susceptibility to pancreatic cancer.[92]

Modification of This Question in Light of New Research: Future studies evaluating the use of ligation of the duct of Wirsung or use of temporary fibrin glue for occlusion of the main duct in elderly patients with a soft pancreatic remnant may show a reduced peri-operative morbidity and mortality in this patient population. Future studies to identify genetic markers for susceptibility to pancreatic cancer should be performed to help select the group of older patients who would most benefit from resection for pancreatic duct lesions.

***GenSurg 28 (Level A)*: Exploratory prospective cohort studies are needed to suggest how elderly patients with pancreatic cancer are best palliated.**

New Research Addressing This Question: A retrospective review was conducted of the notes of all patients (mean age 64.5 years) who underwent gastroduodenal stent insertion for malignant gastroduodenal obstruction. The primary tumor was gastric in 20 patients, pancreatico-biliary in 15, and metastatic in 5. A stent was successfully placed in all cases. The researchers conclude that the use of enteral stents achieves good palliation and allows discharge from the hospital and reintroduction of an enteral diet.[93]

Patients with pyloroduodenal obstruction secondary to malignancy generally undergo an open gastrojejunostomy (OGJ) to bypass the obstruction. Other methods now available for palliation include laparoscopic gastrojejunostomy (LGJ) and endoscopic stenting (ES). In one study, 181 patients with malignant pyloroduodenal obstruction, of whom 56 patients had OGJ, 14 had LGJ, and 16 had ES, were evaluated to study differences in outcomes, with particular emphasis on time to starting free oral fluids and light diet, length of stay, and survival. No significant differences in age, sex, ASA grade, and level of obstruction were found between the matched OGJ (n = 16), LGJ (n = 14), and ES (n = 16) groups. Patients who underwent ES were able to tolerate free oral fluids and light diet earlier, and had a decreased length of stay after the procedure than the surgical group, with values showing a significant difference. The incidence of complications was significantly higher in the surgical group than in the stenting group. In spite of the fact that survival was shortest in the ES group, there were significant benefits following ES as compared with OGJ and LGJ.[94] Combined biliary and duodenal stenting for the palliation of pancreatic cancer can also be performed safely and successfully. Stents allowed effective recanalization of the biliary tract and duodenum, relieving both jaundice and vomiting. This procedure should be considered as an alternative to palliative surgery, especially in critically ill patients.[95]

Modification of This Question in Light of New Research: Future studies should be directed at evaluating the proper timing for palliative intervention with reference to use of chemotherapy and chemoradiotherapy in patients with unresectable disease. Randomized prospective trials are indicated in elderly patients with positive resection margins to compare adjuvant chemotherapy and adjuvant chemoradiotherapy. Future studies should evaluate the efficacy of gemcitabine in patients with advanced metastatic adenocarcinoma of the pancreas. Studies also need to be performed with advanced radiation techniques that are now available and can be used without delaying the chemotherapy schedules for these patients.

Cerebrovascular Disease

See *New Frontiers,* pp. 99–100.

GenSurg 29 (Level B, then A): **Cohort studies followed possibly by randomized controlled trials are needed to determine beyond what age carotid endarterectomy is minimally or not beneficial.**

New Research Addressing This Question: The use of antihypertensive medications, particularly the successful treatment of systolic hypertension, has resulted in the primary prevention of fatal or nonfatal strokes in hypertensive and high-risk patients aged 60 years and older. In addition to antihypertensives, antiplatelet agents are also indicated in elderly patients with nonembolic strokes. Additionally, the use of statins has been shown to prevent strokes in high-risk elderly persons aged up to 82 years. Although surgical intervention with carotid endarterectomy is indicated in carotid artery stenosis of 70% or more and outcomes are even better in elderly than in younger patients, medical treatment is still the first-line treatment in asymptomatic elderly patients with less than 70% stenosis. Thus, prevention of cardiovascular disease should be addressed aggressively in the elderly age group, especially in patients aged 75 and older.[96]

A retrospective review of all primary carotid endarterectomies (CEAs) performed by a single surgeon from 1990 to 2003 for severe symptomatic or asymptomatic carotid disease was conducted. Outcomes in patients younger than 80 years and in those aged 80 years and older were compared. Descriptive demographic data, risk factors, surgical details, peri-operative strokes and deaths, and other complications were recorded, as well as the 30-day stroke risk and death rates. In the period studied, 1260 CEAs were performed in 1099 patients; 1145 were performed in 987 patients younger 80 years, and 115 were performed in 112 patients aged 80 and older. In the younger group, 11 peri-operative strokes occurred in the 1145 procedures (0.8%), and in the older group, no strokes occurred in the 115 procedures. The death rates were 0% for the octogenarians and 0.3% for the younger group. This study demonstrates that patients aged 80 and older can undergo CEA with no more peri-operative risks than younger patients.[97]

Carotid angioplasty and stenting is often the preferred treatment for severe carotid occlusive disease in patients labeled as high risk, including those aged 80 or older. A retrospective review evaluated the records and imaging studies of patients aged 80 years or older who underwent attempted carotid angioplasty and stenting, both with and without distal embolic protection. Study results suggest that elderly patients undergoing this procedure with adjunctive distal embolic protection are at a lower risk of peri-procedure adverse events. The researchers concluded that routine clopidogrel use, smaller hardware profile, careful patient selection, and increased experience of the surgeon probably contributed to these results.[98] Another similar study of carotid endarterectomy showed that peri-operative and postoperative mortality and morbidity as well as the long-term stroke-free rate do not differ significantly in patients 80 years or older and those younger than 80.[99] More importantly, it suggests that increasing age need not be a barrier to surgery and that the patient can benefit from having the procedure most suited to the pathology.

Surgery for carotid artery occlusive disease can be safely performed under local anesthesia in selected patients aged 75 years and older. One study evaluated 262 carotid operations that were performed under local anesthesia between 1998 and 2004. Of these operations, 34% were carotid reconstructions in 70 patients older than 75 years. Indications for surgery included asymptomatic critical stenosis in 26% of patients, transient ischemic symptoms in 46%, and stroke with persisting neurologic deficit in 25%. Comorbidities included coronary artery disease in 38% and arterial hypertension in 72%. Eighty-four percent were ASA class 3 patients. In spite of this, in-hospital mortality was not significantly different from that of the younger patients.[100]

Patients with carotid artery disease can undergo either CEA or CAS. High-risk patients in need of these procedures are those with multiple comorbidities and those who have undergone previous neck irradiation or previous CEA. One study evaluated 545 high-risk patients who underwent CEA and 148 patients who underwent CAS to compare outcomes following these procedures. The incidence of death, stroke, or myocardial infarction was evaluated during the follow-up, with follow-up times of 18 months for CAS and 23 months for CEA. Significant differences were present in patient age (CAS, 75 ± 11.0 years versus CEA, 71 ± 9 years, $P = .012$), but there were no differences in gender or smoking history. The incidence of per procedural complications did not vary significantly between patients treated with CAS and those treated with CEA. CAS is therefore believed to be similar to CEA in safety and efficacy, even in high-risk patients.[101]

Complete occlusion of the contralateral carotid artery has been thought to increase the risk of CEA. Two groups of patients were evaluated in a retrospective study of 221 CEAs: those with contralateral occlusion and those with contralateral patency. Data regarding preoperative demographic features, indications for surgery, operative techniques, and follow-up results were available for 170 of the 221 procedures performed, with 16 of these patients having complete occlusion. Parameters evaluated did not vary between study groups except for the fact that there was increased use of general anesthesia ($P = .05$) in the group with complete occlusion. There were no deaths, and peri-operative stroke rates were not statistically different between groups (complete occlusion group, 6.3%; contralateral patency group, 2.6%; $P = .39$). Long-term patency and stroke-free survival rates at 5 years exceeded 90% and did not vary significantly between groups. This study therefore suggests that contralateral carotid artery occlusion need not be a contraindication for CEA and does not affect outcomes.[102]

Modification of This Question in Light of New Research: Prospective randomized trials are still needed to evaluate the effects of surgery versus medical therapy on the risk of stroke and long-term outcomes in elderly patients with complete occlusion of the contralateral carotid artery. Further trials are needed to demonstrate the long-term efficacy of carotid angioplasty and stenting in comparison with carotid endarterectomy. Studies are also needed to evaluate the use of cerebral protection devices and self-expanding stents to minimize peri-operative morbidity.

GenSurg 30 (Level B): **Prospective studies are needed to determine the incidence and prevalence of cerebrovascular disease in older patients. As with screening for other conditions, prospective studies**

are needed to evaluate the impact of screening for carotid disease on longevity, quality of life, stroke rate, and financial implications. Cohort studies are needed to determine if there is a subset of older patients (eg, smokers, those with hypertension) who benefit from screening for carotid disease.

New Research Addressing This Question: Stroke is the third leading cause of death and a foremost cause of serious, long-term disability in the United States. Older people are more susceptible to cerebrovascular accidents; however, with educated intervention the incidence of debilitating strokes can be markedly reduced. Several risk factors contribute to the increased incidence of strokes in the elderly age group and to the associated morbidity and mortality. These include hypertension, dyslipidemia, diabetes mellitus, and atrial fibrillation. Institution of appropriate treatment and behavioral modifications such as adherence to a healthy diet, regular exercise, and cessation of cigarette smoking can decrease the incidence of strokes among older adults. Other factors that can affect outcomes following a stroke include early recognition of stroke symptoms, quick access to evaluation and treatment, and an intensive rehabilitation program geared to the needs and capabilities of the elderly patient. [103] Diabetes and obesity are two important modifiable risk factors for stroke. [104] Studies have supported a causal role of inflammation in carotid atherosclerosis and emphasize the importance of gene-gene and gene-environment interactions in this pathogenic pathway. [105]

Patients who are at risk for developing a stroke due to significant narrowing of the internal carotid artery are known to benefit from CEA. Diagnosis of the narrowing of the internal carotid artery is usually made by duplex scanning. In a study of 64 patients, angiography was performed in addition to duplex scanning prior to the decision to proceed with CEA. Of these, 14% did not qualify for CEA on the basis of angiographic findings. In 17% of the patients, the angiographic studies showed details of the distal vasculature that were not evident on duplex scanning, and three of these patients were excluded from surgery because of extensive distal disease. The risk of angiography is low, with only one patient experiencing a transient ischemic attack at the time of angiography. The study shows that there are limitations to using duplex scanning alone and that angiographic evaluation has its merits in helping to determine the appropriate candidate for surgery. [106]

Modification of This Question in Light of New Research: Future studies should identify stroke risk factors and primary and secondary prevention strategies in the context of aging, with special consideration of the identification and management of acute stroke, recovery, and rehabilitation for older adults who survive stroke. There is also the need to evaluate the role of additional noninvasive carotid imaging such as magnetic resonance angiography or computed tomographic angiography in addition to conventional duplex scanning in the assessment of elderly patients with carotid artery disease.

PERIPHERAL OCCLUSIVE DISEASE

See *New Frontiers,* pp. 101–102.

***GenSurg 31 (Level B)*: Cohort studies comparing the results of endovascular therapy, thrombolytic therapy, and interventional vascular radiology in older patients are needed.**

New Research Addressing This Question: In one study angiographic and clinical results of popliteal, infrapopliteal, and multilevel disease treated with percutaneous transluminal angioplasty (PTA) were evaluated retrospectively in 37 patients aged over 80 years with chronic critical leg ischemia. All patients were at high surgical risk; 81.5% had chronic nonhealing wounds, and 37% had multilevel disease. One hundred and two lesions were treated by angioplasty. Angiographic results obtained at the end of the procedure and clinical outcomes at 1-year follow-up were studied. Patency following angioplasty was present in only 14.8% of the patients. However, overall limb salvage was seen in 74% of patients, and symptomatic relief of rest pain was present in 57%. The temporary vascular patency achieved by angioplasty resulted in complete and partial wound healing in 80% of patients. These outcomes justify the use of endovascular interventions in the elderly population with chronic critical leg ischemia.[107]

A prospective database of patients undergoing endovascular treatment for superficial femoral artery disease was maintained to evaluate the consequences of early failure (30 days or less) after endovascular treatment. The database was maintained from 1986 to 2004. Intention-to-treat analysis was performed, and angiograms of the lesion, with run-offs before and after the procedure, were evaluated. Results were standardized to current Transatlantic Intersociety Consensus and Society for Vascular Surgery criteria. A total of 360 patients with an average age of 65 years underwent 441 procedures. There was no mortality within 90 days of the procedure, and the morbidity was 4%. The failure of the endoluminal procedure did not affect the level of amputation or the level of the distal anastomosis of a bypass graft subsequently performed. The study showed that there is no disadvantage to performing an endoluminal procedure and that it is justifiable to offer aggressive endoluminal approaches to superficial femoral artery disease as a first-line therapy in all patients.[108]

Although patients who present with rest pain are offered operative bypass procedures, patients with claudication are not offered operative bypass unless the claudication interferes significantly with their lifestyle or ability to work. The hesitation to offer operative bypass procedures is due to the fact that the procedure is invasive. Endovascular treatment of atherosclerotic disease below the inguinal ligament has been shown to yield good short-term results. The procedure itself has a low morbidity. More important, it does not interfere with the success of surgical alternatives in the future. These advantages make it difficult to deny this intervention to patients with claudication. The option of endovascular treatment for infrainguinal atherosclerotic disease therefore needs to be offered to patients with significant claudication. More important, outcomes following these procedures should be compared with results of nonsurgical interventions and not with results following operative bypass procedures.[109]

Modification of This Question in Light of New Research: Prospective randomized studies are still needed comparing results of endovascular therapy, thrombolytic therapy, and interventional vascular radiology in older patients. This item should remain on the research agenda.

GenSurg 32 (Level B): **Cohort studies are needed to determine selection criteria for lower-extremity bypass in older patients.**

New Research Addressing This Question: No research addressing this question was found.

Modification of This Question in Light of New Research: This question should remain unchanged on the research agenda.

GenSurg 33 (Level B): **Exploratory studies (eg, case series, cohort studies, outcomes studies) are needed to learn how best to improve limb salvage rates in peripheral vascular disease in older patients.**

New Research Addressing This Question: Aggressive arterial reconstruction in patients with critical lower limb ischemia improves the chances of limb salvage and patient survival. In one study, 114 patients who were admitted for assessment of an ischemic leg underwent preoperative angiography and subsequent definitive treatment: either bypass surgery, amputation, or lumbar sympathectomy. Surprisingly, preoperative risk factors, including age, sex, pre-existing diabetes mellitus, presenting symptoms, and ankle systolic pressure, did not have any effect on limb salvage or mortality. Bypass procedures were attempted in 76 limbs, with 61 patients undergoing a femoropopliteal bypass. Peri-operative mortality was 4% in these patients. Graft patency rates were 77.7% at the end of 1 month and 62.5% at the end of 1 year. These results justify attempts at revascularization. [110] Another study of infrainguinal bypass for critical limb ischemia reported that, despite the achievement of the anticipated graft patency and limb salvage results, 25% of patients did not realize wound healing at 1 year of follow-up, 19% had lost ambulatory function, and 5% had lost independent living status. [111]

Alternate modalities have also been found to be effective in treating patients with lower-extremity critical ischemia. Another study reported successful performance of percutaneous transluminal angioplasty in 18 patients with critical ischemia (mean age 72.8 years). The mean stent length was 30.29 mm, and mean stent diameter was 3.23 mm. Mean follow-up was 256 days. The overall 6-month survival rate was 94.4%, and the limb salvage rate was 94%. These results suggest that treatment with sirolimus-eluting stents is effective and safe for patients with critical ischemia. [112]

Modification of This Question in Light of New Research: Studies in elderly patients with critical limb ischemia should address the effect of pursuing an aggressive policy of revascularization on limb salvage and survival rates. Prospective natural history studies are needed to further define the functional outcomes and their predictors after infrainguinal bypass for critical limb ischemia. Treatment with sirolimus-eluting stents can be considered effective and safe for patients with critical ischemia and should be further evaluated in the elderly patient population.

ABDOMINAL AORTIC ANEURYSM

See *New Frontiers,* pp. 102–103.

Outcomes following elective and emergent repair of abdominal aortic aneurysms (AAAs) are significantly different, and this is particularly noticeable in elderly patients with multiple comorbidities. Factors that affect treatment decisions included ASA grade ≥ 4, inoperable malignancy, New York Heart Association class III, $FEV_1 < 35\%$, creatinine > 6.0 mg/dL, and patient and family choice. In one parallel-group observational study, outcomes were evaluated following operative and nonoperative management. Thirty-three percent of the patients were octogenarians. In this patient population, 5-year survival was highest in patients treated electively (83%). Five-year survival was 42% in the nonoperative group and least in those undergoing emergency repair (20%). [113]

***GenSurg 34 (Level B)*: Studies are needed to identify criteria for selecting patients who should be screened for abdominal aortic aneurysm and the screening methods to use.**

New Research Addressing This Question: Ultrasound is the standard imaging tool; if performed by trained personnel, it has a sensitivity and specificity approaching 100% and 96%, respectively, for the detection of infrarenal AAA. The US Preventive Services Task Force has released recommendations for AAA screening. It states that screening benefits patients who have a relatively high risk for dying from an aneurysm; the major risk factors are age 65 years or older, male sex, and smoking at least 100 cigarettes in a lifetime. [114] The guideline recommends one-time screening with ultrasound for AAA in men aged 65 to 75 years who have ever smoked. Patients with abdominal aortic diameter of 3 cm or less do not require further screening. Those with an aneurysm of 3 to 4 cm should be screened every 12 months; those with an aneurysm of 4 to 4.5 cm should be screened every 6 months; and those with an aneurysm larger than 4.5 cm should be referred to a vascular surgeon. No recommendation was made for or against screening in men aged 65 to 75 years who have never smoked, and the task force recommended against screening women. Men with a strong family history of AAA should be counseled about the risks and benefits of screening as they approach 65 years of age. [115]

A study to evaluate the cost-effectiveness of screening for AAAs showed that screening men aged 64 to 73 years is cost-effective. [116] Women are usually not considered for AAA screening because of the lower prevalence of the disease among women. This position may, however, be questioned, given the higher risk of rupture and the longer life expectancy of women. A study evaluating the cost-effectiveness of screening 65-year-old women for AAA showed that the incremental cost-effectiveness ratio is similar to that found for screening men, which reflects the fact that the lower AAA prevalence in women is balanced by a higher rupture rate. Screening women for AAA may be cost-effective, and future evaluations on screening for AAA should include women. [117]

Modification of This Question in Light of New Research: This question has been answered, and GenSurg 34 can be dropped from the research agenda.

***GenSurg 35 (Level A)*: Randomized controlled trials are needed to compare results using newer endovascular repairs in elderly high-risk patients with results in traditional surgical abdominal aortic aneurysm repair.**

New Research Addressing This Question: With the projected increase in the elderly population, an increase in the number of elderly patients presenting with AAA is expected. In addition to conventional open repair of abdominal aneurysms, endoluminal approaches now offer an alternative means of treating these patients. The mortality rates for open repair of AAA vary from 2.7% to 5.8%. No survival benefit is found if the aneurysm is less than 5.5 cm. Elderly patients with cardiac disease, renal insufficiency, and pulmonary insufficiency are at high risk for morbidity and mortality. However, it has been shown in separate studies that if surgery is denied, the mortality from rupture of the AAA is between 35% and 49%, [118] suggesting that factors other than age alone should be taken into account when surgical intervention is considered.

Endovascular aneurysm repair (EVAR) is a new technology to treat patients with AAA when the anatomy is suitable. Uncertainty exists about how endovascular repair compares with conventional open surgery. The EVAR trial 1 comparing these treatments in patients judged fit for open AAA repair randomized 1082 elective patients to receive either EVAR (n = 543) or open AAA repair (n = 539). Patients aged at least 60 years with aneurysms of diameter 5.5 cm or more who were fit enough for open surgical repair were recruited for the study at 41 British hospitals proficient in the EVAR technique. Patients (983 men, 99 women) had a mean age of 74 years and mean AAA diameter of 6.5 cm. Of the total group studied, 1047 (97%) underwent AAA repair and 1008 (93%) received their allocated treatment. [119] The 30-day mortality rate in the EVAR group was 1.7% (9/531) versus 4.7% (24/516) in the open-repair group. By per-protocol analysis, 30-day mortality for EVAR was 1.6% versus 4.6% for open repair. Secondary interventions were more common in patients allocated to EVAR (9.8% versus 5.8%, *P* = .02). [120] In older patients with suitable anatomy, EVAR can be performed with minimal morbidity and short length of stay. Older patients not suitable for EVAR constitute a higher risk group because of increased incidence of coronary artery disease and the need for more complex repairs. However, the mortality rate in this group was only 4.6%. [121]

In the EVAR trial 2, the authors investigated whether EVAR to exclude AAA in patients considered unfit for open surgical repair improves survival in comparison with no intervention. The randomized controlled trial included 338 patients aged 60 years or older with an aneurysm of at least 5.5 cm in diameter, of whom 166 were to receive EVAR and 172 no intervention. The endpoints were all-cause mortality, aneurysm-rated mortality, postoperative complications, health-related quality of life, and hospital costs. The 30-day operative mortality in the EVAR group was 9%, and the no-intervention group had a rupture rate of 9 per 100 person years. No significant difference in aneurysm-related mortality was found between the two groups; the overall mortality rate after 4 years was 64%. The authors concluded that EVAR has considerable 30-day operative mortality in patients already unfit for open AAA repair and that it does not improve survival over no intervention. [122]

Factors that affect outcomes of both open and endovascular repair of AAA include preoperative cardiac status and renal function. Older patient age is independently associated with a higher risk of major postoperative complications after AAA repair. One study found that increasing age correlates with a higher risk of having one or more complications (ages 51 to 60: 18.8%; 61 to 70: 27.3%; 71 to 80: 31.2%; 80 and older: 34.3%; $P < .01$). Comparison of the oldest and youngest age groups revealed higher rates of the following in the oldest patients: pulmonary insufficiency 13.9% versus 6.4%, pneumonia 7.7% versus 3.0%, reintubation 9.5% versus 3.9%, acute renal failure 8.8% versus 2.5%, myocardial infarction 4.3% versus 1.6%, and mortality 7.9% versus 1.1%. [123]

It is interesting to note that glomerular filtration rate (GFR) can help stratify the risk of peri-operative and long-term mortality in patients undergoing EVAR more accurately than serum creatinine alone. Mortality following EVAR is no doubt affected by the need for contrast agents that are nephrotoxic. Patients with GFR of less than 45 exhibit decreased survival after EVAR. Peri-operative mortality in patients with a GFR of 45 to 60 is similar to that seen in patients with a GFR below 45. However, late survival in patients with a GFR between 45 and 60 is similar to that of patients with a GFR higher than 60. This suggests that the use of alternative, better contrast agents that are less likely to be nephrotoxic or the use of renal protection techniques may improve outcomes after EVAR. [124]

Modification of This Question in Light of New Research: Future studies stratifying patients according to their comorbidities are needed to determine the optimal use of cardiac and renal protective agents during EVAR or open repair of AAA.

PRESSURE ULCERS

See *New Frontiers,* p. 103.

***GenSurg 36 (Level B)*: Cohort studies are needed to suggest whether prevention and treatment strategies for pressure ulcers that are applicable to younger patients are also applicable to older patients.**

New Research Addressing This Question: More than two thirds of all pressure ulcers occur in elderly persons. Although the risk factors for and the incidence of pressure ulcers are well documented in younger patients, few studies have addressed the problem in the older patients. A prospective cohort study was designed to estimate the incidence and identify risk factors for lower-extremity pressure ulcers in older adult patients confined to bed. The study enrolled 259 patients who were aged 65 years or older, confined to bed, and without lower-extremity pressure ulcers at the time of enrollment. Cox regression analysis indicated three factors to be independently related to the risk of new lower-extremity pressure ulcer: low ankle-brachial index value (hazards ratio 0.075; 95% CI, 0.023 to 0.242), length of period of confinement to bed (hazards ratio 1.010; 95% CI, 1.004 to 1.015), and male gender (hazards ratio 2.951; 95% CI, 1.450 to 6.009).[125]

Economic studies have shown that the costs of preventing and treating pressure ulcers approach those of treating cancer and cardiovascular disease. Most of these costs are incurred in lengthy hospital stays and the use of antipressure beds. In addition to improper mattresses, poor seating—often in collapsible wheelchairs or in gerichairs—contributes to pressure ulcer formation. Pressure sores may also develop when the head of the bed is continuously elevated at least 30 degrees (for nasogastric tube feeding or as a precaution against aspiration).[126]

A multicenter retrospective cohort study used medical record abstraction to obtain 2425 patients aged 65 years and older who had been discharged from acute care hospitals after treatment for pneumonia, cerebrovascular disease, or congestive heart failure. Six processes of care for preventing pressure ulcers were evaluated: daily skin assessment, the use of a pressure-reducing device, documentation of the patient's being at risk, repositioning at least every 2 hours, nutritional consultation for patients with nutritional risk factors, and pressure ulcer staging. The associations between processes of care and the incidence of pressure ulcer were determined with Kaplan-Meier survival analyses. Estimates of adherence with each process of care were as follows: daily skin assessment, 94%; use of pressure-reducing device, 7.5%; documentation of risk, 22.6%; repositioning, 66.2%; nutritional consultation, 34.3%; stage 1 pressure ulcer staged, 20.2%; and stage 2 or greater ulcer staged, 30.9%. This study suggests that there still remain numerous opportunities to improve care relating to the prediction and prevention of pressure ulcers in older patients.[127]

Malnutrition plays a critical role in the incidence of pressure ulcers in old age. Studies have shown that improved nutritional status helps prevent the development of pressure ulcers in younger patients. In one study of a 15-day nutritional intervention with two oral supplements of 200 kcal added to a 1800 kcal hospital diet in 672 critically ill older inpatients, that patients showed a tendency to have fewer pressure ulcers at days 5, 10, and 14. The study also clearly showed the problems in achieving nutritional goals despite offering adequate quantities.[128] Another study evaluated the effect of supplemental tube feeding (1500 kcal, 60 g protein) during nighttime for two groups of inpatients with hip fractures, one group receiving tube-fed supplementation, the control group receiving no supplementation. All patients received a standard hospital diet in the daytime. Despite a low acceptance of the tube, intakes of energy and protein were 2 to 3 times higher and nutritional status was largely improved in the supplemented group, but without any effect on the development and severity of pressure ulcers.[129]

Severe malnutrition, impaired oral intake, and the risk of pressure ulcer formation appear to be interrelated. Energy and nutrients, such as proteins and vitamins B and C, that are deficient in old age are needed in pressure ulcer healing. Attention should be focused on early recognition of a depleted nutritional status in the older patient and on an adequate and supervised intake of energy (35 kcal/kg) and protein (1.5 g/kg), with provision of the recommended daily allowances of micronutrients and correction of the nutrient deficiencies of old age.[130]

Modification of This Question in Light of New Research: Prospective randomized trials are needed to determine the value of indicators enabling early recognition and intervention to prevent the development of pressure ulcers and to compare outcomes between younger and older patients, especially in the postoperative period.

NEW HORIZONS IN GERIATRIC GENERAL SURGERY

THYROID DISEASE

The average age for patients presenting for surgery for multinodal goiter has steadily increased, from 56.6 years in 1995 to 63.2 years in 2003. Although total thyroidectomy has replaced subtotal thyroidectomy as the treatment of choice for multinodal goiter, this has not been validated for the elderly patient. An analysis of 279 patients who underwent total thyroidectomy for multinodal goiter studied differences in outcome secondary to age. The duration of the operation, intraoperative blood loss, the weight of the resected thyroid gland, and the proportion of retrosternal goiter were found to be significantly higher in the group aged 70 years or older. The incidence of surgically related complications, such as recurrent laryngeal nerve palsy and hypoparathyroidism, were similar in young and elderly patients.[131]

Thyroid nodules are clinically detectable in about 4% to 7% of the general population. However, the incidence of subclinical nodules discovered by thyroid ultrasonography exceeds 50% in women aged over 60 years. Though about 5% of clinical thyroid nodules are cancerous, in surgical specimens not previously submitted for cytologic analysis, the incidence may range from 8% to 20%. Thyroid cancers are usually differentiated carcinomas and have a favorable prognosis. However, undifferentiated carcinoma or anaplastic carcinoma accounts for about 2% to 14% of thyroid cancer and has a dismal prognosis.[132] It may arise from longstanding papillary carcinoma and occurs in the elderly population.

Thyroid cancer in the elderly patient has a poor prognosis because of its aggressiveness. The extreme aggressiveness of anaplastic carcinoma makes it impossible to perform the curative treatment because of direct invasion to trachea and adjacent vital structures. Accordingly, palliative surgery and adjuvant treatment, such as radiation therapy and chemotherapy, could be considered for salvage and quality of life. Thyroid hormone replacement after total thyroidectomy should be undertaken cautiously in the elderly patient to avoid the adverse bone effect (osteoporosis) and cardiac effect (tachycardia, atrial fibrillation, and premature atrial contraction).[133]

Advances in the accurate diagnosis of thyroid tumors may be beneficial in an elderly population. A particular problem is distinguishing between follicular thyroid carcinoma and benign follicular thyroid adenoma. Researchers have found four genes (*DDIT3, ARG2, ITM1,* and *C1orf24*) to differ between the two classes of thyroid tumor and that a linear combination of expression levels distinguishes follicular thyroid carcinoma from follicular thyroid adenoma (estimated predictive accuracy of 0.83). They also found immunohistochemistry for *DDIT3* and *ARG2* to show consistent staining for carcinoma in an independent set of 59 follicular tumors.[134] Tests based on a combination of these markers might improve preoperative diagnosis of thyroid nodules, allowing better treatment decisions and reducing long-term health costs in the elderly age group.

> ***GenSurg 37 (Level B)*: Observational studies are needed to elucidate the differences between older and younger patients with regard to the biological behavior, diagnostic approach, and invasiveness of thyroid malignant nodules as well as to clarify the differences in the safety of surgical intervention, postoperative quality of life, and adverse consequences of longstanding tumor.**

Breast Cancer

The use of postmastectomy radiotherapy in elderly women with high-risk breast cancer has been studied recently. The study analyzed 233 women aged 70 years and over with tumors larger than 5 cm or with four or more axillary nodes. Of these women, 147 were treated with radiotherapy and 86 women were treated without it. Although the tumor size distribution and systemic therapy was the same in both groups, a higher number of women who received radiotherapy had four or more positive lymph nodes and positive surgical margins. Elderly women who had radiotherapy had a lower local recurrence rate than those who did not have radiotherapy. There was no difference between the two groups in the incidence of distant recurrence, disease-free survival, or overall survival.[135]

Trastuzumab is a humanized monoclonal antibody used in the treatment of breast cancer. Cancers that overexpress human epidermal growth-factor receptor 2 (HER2) are associated with a poor prognosis and aggressive disease. Trastuzumab has been approved as an additional first-line chemotherapeutic agent in patients with HER2-positive metastatic breast cancer and has been found to improve the time to disease progression, objective response rate, duration of response, and overall survival in randomized multicenter trials. It has also been approved for monotherapy in women with HER2-positive metastatic breast cancer who had already undergone chemotherapy and as a standard component of adjuvant therapy for patients with HER2-positive early-stage breast cancer.[136]

Concern for the ability of the older woman with breast cancer to tolerate the rigors of chemotherapy may lead to undertreatment and higher mortality in these patients. Older women are still under-represented in clinical trials. These factors can be changed by physician education and by trials designed especially for the older woman with breast cancer. Chemotherapy should be considered for older women with breast cancer who fall into high-risk groups: namely, women with node-positive tumors, those with poorly differentiated tumors even if they are node-negative, and those with hormone receptor–negative tumors. Additionally, if agents such as aromatase inhibitors are more effective than tamoxifen in reducing breast cancer recurrence in postmenopausal women, these agents should be used more widely.[137]

It is critical that elderly patients be included in clinical trials. Older women are as interested in enrollment in clinical trials as younger women. When asked to participate, 56% of younger patients and 50% of older patients chose to participate in clinical trials.[138] However, in the early 1990s, even though 22.8% of newly diagnosed breast cancer patients were aged 75 years or older, only 2.7% of those enrolled in the National Cancer Institute cooperative trials were in this age group. Reasons for this lack of enrollment include the older patients' comorbidities and lower financial and social support. Increasing age has also been found to be associated with deviation from established guidelines. While 6% of patients younger than 65 years did not receive standard treatment, 22.2% of patients aged 65 or older did not receive the treatment. Reasons cited in the younger cohort included prohibitive medical conditions, favorable primary tumor, or patient refusal. No reasons were documented for the older cohort.[139]

A review of tumor biology in two US databases showed that with increasing age, there is a more frequent expression of hormone receptors, lower rates of tumor cell proliferation, greater frequency of diploidy, and lower expression of HER2 and epidermal growth factor. In older women, more tumors express estrogen receptor and progesterone receptors, have lower proliferative rates, are diploid, have normal levels of p53, and do not express epidermal growth-factor receptor or C-erb B_2.[140] Even though these biological characteristics suggest that older women with breast cancer have more indolent disease, this does not translate into the expected clinical outcome, as seen in a study evaluating women with locoregional disease treated with mastectomy without systemic therapy. Women aged 70 years and older had lower distant disease-free survival rates than women aged 40 to 70 years at 10 years, both in node-positive and node-negative groups.[141]

***GenSurg 38 (Level A)*: Randomized controlled trials are needed to compare rates of recurrence and survival in groups of older breast cancer patients who are treated with postmastectomy radiotherapy and with polychemotherapy.**

***GenSurg 39 (Level B)*: Observational studies are needed to evaluate the benefit of adjuvant therapy in elderly women presenting with breast cancer with high-risk indicators.**

***GenSurg 40 (Level B)*: Observational studies are needed to evaluate how age, menopausal status, and estrogen-receptor levels impact benefits from chemotherapy and endocrine therapy.**

***GenSurg 41 (Level A)*: Prospective randomized trials are needed to study short-term and long-term outcomes following the use of aromatase inhibitors in postmenopausal women, and the incorporation of trastuzumab into adjuvant therapy of women with HER2- or neu-positive breast cancer.**

Gastroesophageal Reflux Disease

See *New Frontiers,* pp. 91–92, 93.

The prevalence of GERD has risen in recent years. Some studies report similar prevalence rates for both younger and older people: approximately 20%. [142] Others suggest that the prevalence is higher in the elderly age group. [143] A prospective study of the prevalence of endoscopy-positive GERD showed an incidence of 5.8%, with a higher incidence in men. This study found age to have a minimal effect on prevalence in men but the prevalence rate to rise among women as they age. [144] Elderly persons have also been found to have a higher rate of paraesophageal hernias. [145] In another study, upper gastrointestinal endoscopy was performed on 300 patients who presented for surveillance colonoscopy and had not previously undergone esophagoscopy. Endoscopy revealed that Barrett's esophagus was present in 16.7% of the patients; it was more common in men (21.7%) than in women (10.8%). GERD symptoms were present in 35% of patients. Interestingly, Barrett's esophagus was present in 19.8% of symptomatic and 14.9% of asymptomatic cases; 92% of the patients had Barrett's esophagus of less than 3 cm. [146]

Several factors are responsible for the increased incidence of GERD in the elderly age group. These include changes in esophageal motility and gastric emptying. Other factors are *H. pylori* infection, pill-induced esophagitis, peptic ulcer disease, and complications resulting from use of NSAIDs. [54] The role of *H. pylori* infection in the development of hiatal hernia has been studied. Patients without peptic ulcer disease but with endoscopic evidence of a hiatal hernia were divided into three age groups: those aged 45 years or younger, those aged 46 to 60 years, and those aged 61 years or older. Aging was found to be associated with a higher incidence of hiatal hernias and also an increased incidence of *H. pylori* and corpus-based gastritis. However, there was a 46.8% decrease in GERD symptoms in the oldest patient population (compared with 66.6% and 52.1%). This could be due to the blunting of symptoms of GERD seen with aging. However, *H. pylori* infection was found to be higher in patients without GERD than with GERD (66.4% versus 57.3%, $P < .05$) and higher in patients with nonerosive GERD than with erosive GERD (62.8% versus 48.6%). [147]

Although there are data suggesting decreased salivation with aging, acid clearance is as effective in older adults as in younger adults. [148] The length of upper esophageal sphincter high-pressure zone in the elderly person is significantly less than in young person, as is the upper esophageal sphincter resting pressure. No significant difference between elderly and young persons was found in the same parameters evaluated for the lower esophageal sphincter. [149] The prevalence of hiatal hernia, gastric mucosal atrophy, and reflux esophagitis was studied in a 2788 patients over a 3-year period. Gastric mucosal atrophy was divided into two groups: closed and open. The atrophic border is the boundary between the pyloric and fundic gland territories. Endoscopically, this is recognized by evaluating the color and height of the gastric mucosa. In patients with open gastric mucosal atrophy, the atrophy boundary is in the lateral wall or along the greater curvature; in the closed type, the atrophic border is along the lesser curvature or the antrum. The prevalence of reflux gastritis and hiatal hernia was found to increase with age in women but not in men. [150]

The frequency of complications of GERD is higher in elderly patients. This may be due to differences in symptom thresholds for young and elderly patients. Elderly patients present with more advanced disease and with significant mucosal damage. Older patients with GERD may not present with typical symptoms of heartburn and regurgitation. Instead, they may present with dysphagia, weight loss, vomiting, and anemia. GERD may remain undiagnosed in this patient population. [151] They may also present with atypical symptoms, such as a chronic cough, sleep apnea syndrome, or exacerbation of asthma. [152] Laxity of the esophageal sphincter in older patients makes them more liable to aspiration, especially when they are obese or have a feeding tube. Exacerbation of asthma and chronic obstructive pulmonary disease in the elderly patient are often secondary to chronic aspiration. Once GERD is detected, therapeutic interventions aimed at correction are likely to reduce morbidity and medical expenditure in these patients. [153]

Once esophagitis is diagnosed endoscopically, proton-pump inhibitors relieve symptoms faster than H_2-receptor antagonists. One double blind, randomized, controlled trial found that after resolution of acute esophagitis, treating elderly patients with pantoprazole results in fewer relapses than placebo. [154] Discontinuation of medical therapy for longer than 6 months was found to be responsible for a significant increase in the relapse rate. [155] Another study evaluated the prokinetic and salivary stimulating effects of cisapride in 15 younger and 15 older adults. Both cisapride as well as peppermint lozenges were found to decrease the number of swallows taken to clear the acid infused into the distal esophageal and to return pH to 4. [148] Further studies are needed to evaluate the effect of various drugs such as (5-HT) 4-receptor agonists in the treatment of GERD. [156] Endoscopy should be performed more expeditiously when elderly patients present with symptoms of reflux [143] and medical therapy instituted. Failure to respond to medical management should prompt a surgical referral for an elective antireflux procedure.

Studies have shown that elderly patients have equivalent postoperative results without an increase in postoperative complications following laparoscopic antireflux procedures. [157] In one study, the mean hospital stay following a laparoscopic antireflux procedure was found to be 2.2 ± 1 day in a group of 30 octogenarians and nonagenarians; there was one conversion to a laparotomy, two complications, and no deaths. [145] A retrospective review of 304 consecutive patients who underwent laparoscopic fundoplication for GERD was carried out; 63 of the patients were aged 65 years or older. The older patients more often had regurgitation and respiratory symptoms in addition to heartburn. Hiatal hernias were more common among elderly patients (77% versus 51%). The younger and older groups otherwise proved to be similar in key respects: duration of surgery, a low incidence of intraoperative or postoperative complications, a median hospital stay of 24 hours, and resolution of heartburn in approximately 90% of the patients. The authors therefore concluded that laparoscopic antireflux surgery is as safe in elderly patients as in younger patients and that clinical outcomes are as good. [158]

Surgical intervention has always been indicated for older patients with severe GERD, especially for those who had become refractory to medical management. The advent of laparoscopic antireflux procedure helped to dissipate the hesitation in offering surgery to older patients, probably because it is a minimally invasive procedure. A study comparing outcomes following laparoscopic Nissen fundoplications in 108 patients aged 70 and older with 108 concurrent patients younger than 60 years at similar durations of follow-up found reflux and dysphagia scores to be significantly improved for both older and younger patients. After fundoplication, older patients had lower dysphagia scores and lower reflux scores. A larger number of patients aged 70 or older (91%) as opposed to patients younger than 60 (84%) said that they would undergo laparoscopic Nissen fundoplication again, if necessary. The study concluded that laparoscopic fundoplication safely ameliorates symptoms of GERD in elderly patients, with symptomatic outcomes superior to those seen in younger patients.[159]

Recently, newer minimally invasive methods for the treatment of GERD have begun to appear. Several types of endoscopic therapy are presently under investigation. Whether these techniques will provide additional options for the treatment of GERD in older patients remains to be determined.[160]

GenSurg 42 (Level A): **Randomized prospective studies are needed to compare short-term and long-term outcomes of transendoscopic plication with laparoscopic Nissen fundoplication in elderly patients.**

ACHALASIA

The incidence of achalasia has been increasing over the past decade and may be due to increased incidence of evaluation with esophageal manometry. In one study, 28 consecutive patients were evaluated before and after laparoscopic Heller-Dor myotomy. A gastrointestinal quality-of-life index was used, and a minimum follow-up of 1 year was obtained. Patients were stratified by age: those under 70 years and those 70 years or older. Gastrointestinal symptoms and physical, social, and emotional function were found to be significantly improved in both groups. It was determined, therefore, that the medium-term outcomes of this procedure are not affected by age.[161]

GenSurg 43 (Level B): **Observational studies are needed to evaluate the efficacy of surgical management of achalasia in the elderly patient.**

COLORECTAL CANCER

In one study, 100 patients undergoing surgery for colorectal cancer were screened preoperatively for circulating levels of interleukin (IL)-1β, IL-6, and IL-1 receptor antagonist. Low preoperative levels of IL-1 receptor antagonist were found to be associated with increased incidence of postoperative infection (P = .0001). This finding was observed in elderly patients ($P < .05$) with low body mass index. These findings explain the increased risk of infection in the elderly malnourished patient, possibly as a consequence of a defective adaptive immune system.[162]

Anastomotic leakage following surgery for colorectal cancer is an important cause of increased morbidity and mortality. A prospective study of patients undergoing elective colorectal resection performed by a single surgeon at a university hospital over a 3.5-year period sought to identify risk factors for anastomotic leakage. Preoperative steroid use, longer duration of surgery, and contamination of the operative field were found to be independent risk factors for increased incidence of leakage. Importantly, age did not affect the incidence of anastomotic leakage; the incidence of leakage was 4%, 2.3%, and 2.3% in patients aged 60 years or younger, 61 to 70 years, and over 70 years (P = .610). The study also revealed that a diverting ostomy did not affect the incidence of leakage from the distal anastomotic site.[163]

A retrospective cohort study of 533 patients who over an 8-year period underwent stomal closure was conducted. Univariate analysis showed increasing age to be the only predictor for mortality in patients with stomal closure. Median age of the survivors was 56 years (range 43 to 68); that of nonsurvivors was 61 years (55 to 75), $P = .02$. Sex, type of ostomy, and primary cause were not found to affect mortality rates.[164]

A study of clinical and pathologic parameters comparing rectal cancer patients younger than 65 years with those 65 years or older was carried out in 177 patients accepted consecutively from 1991 to 2002. In the two age groups, postoperative mortality and morbidity were not significantly different. The duration of surgical procedures and the incidence of postoperative complications were variables that were independently associated with 30-day mortality. Patients aged 65 or older demonstrated a significantly worse overall survival ($P = .003$), cancer-specific survival ($P = .02$), and disease-free survival ($P = .03$). In addition to several other factors considered in a multivariate analysis, age of 65 years or older was found to be a risk factor for both overall survival and disease-free interval. While short-term prognosis for elective rectal cancer procedure in patients 65 years or older was similar to that of younger patients, long-term cancer-related survival was found to be statistically lower in older patients.[165]

Researchers have shown that preoperative chemoradiation in elderly rectal cancer patients is feasible and helps to downstage the tumor. A study of 28 rectal cancer patients aged 70 years and older who were treated preoperatively with radiotherapy and 5FU concomitant chemotherapy found no evidence of acute gastrointestinal toxicity, and all the patients underwent surgery without severe peri-operative complications. Complete pathologic response to pT0 (ie, no residual tumor detected in resected specimen by pathologic microscopic examination) was found in 3 patients (11%). Overall T downstaging occurred in 61%. Mean follow-up was 34 months (range 4 to 84). Kaplan Meier Overall Survival at 5 years was 74% (95% CI 54 to 95) and the Disease Free Survival results at 5 years was 65% (95% CI 38 to 93). No treatment-related death was observed.[166]

Treatment of locally advanced or recurrent rectal cancer in elderly patients aged 75 years or older was evaluated in one study of 86 consecutive patients undergoing elective surgery after irradiation with 46–50 Gy for either primary locally advanced rectal cancer (n = 51) or recurrent rectal cancer (n = 35). As seen in younger patients, the study concluded that thorough preoperative evaluation and well-planned and well-executed surgery are critical in achieving potentially curative results in patients with acceptable morbidity. Five-year survival was estimated to be 29% for locally advanced primary cancer without metastases and 32% for locally recurrent rectal cancer. Estimated 5-year local recurrence rates were not significantly different in R0 resections and R1 resections ($P = .434$ ns) and for locally advanced and recurrent rectal cancer ($P = .248$ ns), respectively.[167]

***GenSurg 44 (Level A)*: Prospective randomized trials are needed to evaluate the best management strategies for colorectal cancer in elderly patients.**

***GenSurg 45 (Level B)*: Observational studies are warranted to evaluate the effect of various factors, including tumor grading, preoperative carcinoembryonic antigen level, and gender, on cancer-free survival and overall survival in elderly patients with colorectal cancer.**

***GenSurg 46 (Level A)*: Prospective randomized trials are needed to compare short-term and long-term outcomes in elderly patients who**

undergo total mesorectal excision as opposed to those who undergo transanal excision with adjuvant therapy.

LIVER RESECTION

Liver resection is indicated for colorectal metastases, hepatocellular carcinoma, gallbladder cancer, and hilar bile duct cancer. [84,168]

Hepatic resection is a standard treatment for patients with hepatic metastases secondary to colorectal carcinoma. Colorectal cancer is the third most common cause of cancer deaths worldwide, and approximately 50% to 60% of these patients have hepatic metastases. Several groups have demonstrated that hepatic resection for colorectal metastases is safe and feasible for patients aged 70 years and older. Mortality and morbidity rates have been found to be comparable among younger (< 70 years) and elderly (70 and older) patients. [168,169] A retrospective chart review of 212 consecutive patients with colorectal cancer who underwent potentially curative resection of hepatic metastases between 1992 and 2004 was carried out; 62 patients were 70 years or older and 150 patients were younger than 70 at the time of surgery. There was no significant difference in the rate of postoperative complications or mortality following surgery between the young and older patients. Survival rates in younger patients at 1, 3, and 5 years were significantly better than in the older patients. However, in the older group, survival rates of 79.4%, 46.55%, and 34.1% at 1, 3 and 5 years suggest that age need not be considered a contraindication for hepatic resection. [170] These studies prove that hepatic resection for colorectal metastases is a safe option in elderly patients, provided comorbidities are addressed as they would be in younger patients.

Resection of colorectal liver metastasis involves an anatomic or nonanatomic resection with a 1-cm margin around the tumor. Little is known about the significance of portal vein invasion by colorectal liver metastases; once it is diagnosed, an anatomic major hepatic resection may be necessary for potential curative treatment. [171]

Hepatocellular carcinoma is the fourth most common cause of cancer deaths worldwide, with the peak incidence occurring in the sixth decade of life; 76% of these cases occur in Asia. Mortality rates following hepatic resection for hepatocellular carcinoma are below 10% and do not significantly differ between young and elderly patients. Some groups have reported significantly lower blood loss [172] and lower complication rates in elderly patients. [173] Long-term outcomes have been found to be comparable between young and elderly patients.

Hepatic resection is commonly performed in the United States for resection of metastatic disease and primary hepatocellular malignancies. The prognosis for elderly patients after hepatic resection for hepatocellular carcinoma has been found to be less favorable than that for younger patients, and cirrhosis was found to lead not only to poor survival but also to high mortality in the elderly age group. [174] Hepatic resection in aged patients may have a superimposed surgical risk. An observational study using a nationally representative database showed that in high-volume hospitals and patients older than 65 years, hepatic lobectomy (versus wedge resection), primary hepatic malignancy (versus metastases), and the severity of underlying liver disease were independent risk factors for in-hospital mortality. With regard to age, using a dichotomous age variable with a cut-off point of 65 years, researchers found that patients aged 65 years and older had a 7.8%

in-hospital mortality rate that was significantly greater than the mortality rate of 4.7% for younger patients ($P = .003$).[175]

A retrospective study of 193 patients undergoing hepatic resection showed that elderly patients can undergo the procedure as safely as the control group (younger than 75 years) as long as a careful selection of the patient is performed. Patients excluded were cirrhotic patients with Child-Pugh class B and C, Child-Pugh class A requiring resection of more than two hepatic sectors (trisegmentectomy or extended hepatectomy), patients with thrombosis involving the portal vein trunk or one of the two major branches, noncirrhotic patients with primary disease involving both primary portobiliary branches or the retrohepatic inferior vena cava or the three major hepatic veins. Age was not considered as an isolated exclusion criterion. Importantly, concomitant diseases were found to be more common in the patients older than 75 years, with a statistically significant difference (62.5% of the older group versus 32.9% of the control group, $P = .002$).[176]

GenSurg 47 (Level B): **Cohort studies are needed to determine the efficacy of hepatic resection for colorectal metastases and hepatocellular carcinoma in elderly patients**

SEPSIS

The problem of sepsis is of critical importance in the elderly patient. Incidence rates in the United States for severe sepsis rise sharply with age, from 0.2 cases per 1000 among children aged 5 to 14 years to 26.2 cases per 1000 among elderly adults aged 85 years or older. Sepsis develops in 750,000 people annually, and more than 210,000 of them die.[177,178] It is predicted that the incidence of sepsis will increase by 1.5% per year, resulting in 934,000 cases in the United States in the year 2010 and 1,110,000 cases in 2020. Most of this rise can be attributed to the high incidence of sepsis in the elderly age group and the overall aging of the US population. Mortality from sepsis also increases with increasing age, rising from 10% among children to 38.4% among those aged 85 years or older. Sepsis is the leading cause of death in critically ill patients in the United States.[179] The total annual cost for severe sepsis is estimated to be $16.7 billion. Because sepsis affects the elderly age group disproportionately, more than half of all annual costs—$8.7 billion—is spent on the care of patients aged 65 years or older. Sepsis has been commonly defined as an "uncontrolled inflammatory response." Multiple trials targeted at reducing this inflammatory response have proven unsuccessful.[180–182] More importantly, several patients with sepsis have demonstrated immunosuppression with loss of delayed-type hypersensitivity and an inability to clear the inciting infection.[183] This suggests that in established sepsis, there may be a shift toward an anti-inflammatory or immunosuppressive state. This deactivation of leucocytes from septic patients resembles the phenomenon of endotoxin tolerance. Endotoxin tolerance is defined as a reduced capacity of the host to respond to lipopolysaccharide following a first exposure to this stimulus. Although it may be an adaptive response that tends to limit inflammation during a bacterial infection, it may also favor subsequent infections in survivors of septic shock.

Between 42% and 52% of intensive care unit admissions involve patients aged 65 years or older. These patients also account for approximately 60% of all intensive care unit days. This is because elderly patients have multiple comorbidities, including decreased cardiopulmonary and renal reserve, making them more prone to developing progressive organ failure. Elderly intensive care unit patients are also at a higher risk of developing delirium, another factor that is associated with significant morbidity. Severity of illness and age are the important factors determining intensive care unit survival. It is therefore critical to look for indicators that might dictate the need for more intensive postoperative care in elderly patients undergoing emergent and elective surgery and to continue to maintain a high index of suspicion in the peri-operative period. Our aging society dictates that we must have strict guidelines to optimize care of the older adult who develops critical illness. [184] One study identified several independent predictors of surgical site infection in older people, including comorbid conditions (chronic obstructive pulmonary disease and obesity), peri-operative variables (wound class), and socioeconomic factors (private insurance, which was associated with lower risk). [185]

GenSurg 48: *(Level B)*: **Observational studies are needed to evaluate the physiologic effect of aging on risk factors for sepsis.**

GenSurg 49 (Level B): **Observational and interventional studies are needed to help design and implement interventions to prevent surgical site infections in high-risk older patients.**

REFERENCES

1. Guyer B, Freedman MA, Strobino DM, Sondik EJ. Annual summary of vital statistics: trends in the health of Americans during the 20th century. Pediatrics 2000;106:1307-1317.
2. Ergina PL, Gold SL, Meakins JL. Perioperative care of the elderly patient. World J Surg 1993;17:192-198.
3. Suttner SW, Surder C, Lang K, et al. Does age affect liver function and the hepatic acute phase response after major abdominal surgery? Intensive Care Med 2001;27:1762-1769.
4. Yancik R. Population aging and cancer: a cross-national concern. Cancer J 2005;11:437-441.
5. Pofahl WE. Geriatric general surgery. In Solomon DH, LoCicero J, 3rd, Rosenthal RA (eds): New Frontiers in Geriatrics Research: An Agenda for Surgical and Related Medical Specialties. New York: American Geriatrics Society, 2004, pp. 85-109 (online at http://www.frycomm.com/ags/rasp).
6. Tan KY, Chen CM, Ng C, et al. Which octogenarians do poorly after major open abdominal surgery in our Asian population? World J Surg 2006;30:547-552.
7. Bingener J, Richards ML, Schwesinger WH, et al. Laparoscopic cholecystectomy for elderly patients: gold standard for golden years? Arch Surg 2003;138:531-535; discussion 535-536.
8. Tambyraja AL, Kumar S, Nixon SJ. Outcome of laparoscopic cholecystectomy in patients 80 years and older. World J Surg 2004;28:745-748.
9. Waage A, Nilsson M. Iatrogenic bile duct injury: a population-based study of 152 776 cholecystectomies in the Swedish Inpatient Registry. Arch Surg 2006;141:1207-1213.
10. Kramer M, Franke C, Ohmann C, Yang Q. Acute appendicitis in late adulthood: incidence, presentation, and outcome. Results of a prospective multicenter acute abdominal pain study and a review of the literature. Langenbecks Arch Surg 2000;385:470-481.
11. Bickell NA, Aufses AH, Jr., Rojas M, Bodian C. How time affects the risk of rupture in appendicitis. J Am Coll Surg 2006;202:401-406.
12. Pavlidis TE, Marakis G, Ballas K, et al. Safety of bowel resection for colorectal surgical emergency in the elderly. Colorectal Dis 2006;8:657-662.
13. Muravchick S. The elderly outpatient: current anesthetic implications. Curr Opin Anaesthesiol 2002;15:621-625.
14. Feussner H. [Laparoscopy: potential and limitations in outpatient and short-term inpatient surgery]. Chirurg 2004;75:248-256.

15. Finley CR, McKernan JB. Laparoscopic antireflux surgery at an outpatient surgery center. Surg Endosc 2001;15:823-826.
16. Narain PK, Moss JM, DeMaria EJ. Feasibility of 23-hour hospitalization after laparoscopic fundoplication. J Laparoendosc Adv Surg Tech A 2000;10:5-11.
17. Ray S. Result of 310 consecutive patients undergoing laparoscopic Nissen fundoplication as hospital outpatients or at a free-standing surgery center. Surg Endosc 2003;17:378-380.
18. Stefanidis D, Sirinek KR, Bingener J. Gallbladder perforation: risk factors and outcome. J Surg Res 2006;131:204-208.
19. Cirillo DJ, Wallace RB, Rodabough RJ, et al. Effect of estrogen therapy on gallbladder disease. JAMA 2005;293:330-339.
20. Lin A, Stiven P, Bagshaw P, Connor S. Cholecystectomy following acute presentation to a major New Zealand metropolitan hospital: change to the timing of surgery is needed. N Z Med J 2006;119:U2104.
21. Cameron DR, Goodman AJ. Delayed cholecystectomy for gallstone pancreatitis: re-admissions and outcomes. Ann R Coll Surg Engl 2004;86:358-362.
22. Alvarez-Perez JA, Baldonedo-Cernuda RF, Garcia-Bear I, et al. [Risk factors in patients older than 70 years with complicated colorectal carcinoma]. Cir Esp 2006;79:36-41.
23. Brunt LM, Quasebarth MA, Dunnegan DL, Soper NJ. Outcomes analysis of laparoscopic cholecystectomy in the extremely elderly. Surg Endosc 2001;15:700-705.
24. Davidovic M, Svorcan P, Milanovic P, et al. Specifics of *Helicobacter pylori* infection/NSAID effects in the elderly. Rom J Gastroenterol 2005;14:253-258.
25. Paton C, Ferrier IN. SSRIs and gastrointestinal bleeding. BMJ 2005;331:529-530.
26. Yilmazlar T, Guner O, Yilmazlar A. Criteria to consider when assessing the mortality risk in geriatric surgery. Int Surg 2006;91:72-76.
27. Copeland GP, Jones D, Walters M. POSSUM: a scoring system for surgical audit. Br J Surg 1991;78:355-360.
28. Tambyraja AL, Kumar S, Nixon SJ. POSSUM scoring for laparoscopic cholecystectomy in the elderly. ANZ J Surg 2005;75:550-552.
29. Greutelaers B, Kullen K, Kollias J, et al. Pasieka Illness Questionnaire: its value in primary hyperparathyroidism. ANZ J Surg 2004;74:112-115.
30. Quiros RM, Alef MJ, Wilhelm SM, et al. Health-related quality of life in hyperparathyroidism measurably improves after parathyroidectomy. Surgery 2003;134:675-681; discussion 681-673.
31. Kebebew E, Duh QY, Clark OH. Parathyroidectomy for primary hyperparathyroidism in octogenarians and nonagenarians: a plea for early surgical referral. Arch Surg 2003;138:867-871.
32. Vestergaard P, Mosekilde L. Cohort study on effects of parathyroid surgery on multiple outcomes in primary hyperparathyroidism. BMJ 2003;327:530-534.
33. Emmelot-Vonk MH, Samson MM, Raymakers JA. [Cognitive deterioration in elderly due to primary hyperparathyroidism—resolved by parathyroidectomy]. Ned Tijdschr Geneeskd 2001;145:1961-1964.
34. Palazzo FF, Delbridge LW. Minimal-access/minimally invasive parathyroidectomy for primary hyperparathyroidism. Surg Clin North Am 2004;84:717-734.
35. Peto R, Boreham J, Clarke M, et al. UK and USA breast cancer deaths down 25% in year 2000 at ages 20-69 years. Lancet 2000;355:1822.
36. Yancik R, Wesley MN, Ries LA, et al. Effect of age and comorbidity in postmenopausal breast cancer patients aged 55 years and older. JAMA 2001;285:885-892.
37. McCarthy EP, Burns RB, Freund KM, et al. Mammography use, breast cancer stage at diagnosis, and survival among older women. J Am Geriatr Soc 2000;48:1226-1233.

38. McPherson CP, Swenson KK, Lee MW. The effects of mammographic detection and comorbidity on the survival of older women with breast cancer. J Am Geriatr Soc 2002;50:1061-1068.
39. American Geriatrics Society Clinical Practice Committee. Breast cancer screening in older women. J Am Geriatr Soc 2000;48:842-844.
40. Randolph WM, Goodwin JS, Mahnken JD, Freeman JL. Regular mammography use is associated with elimination of age-related disparities in size and stage of breast cancer at diagnosis. Ann Intern Med 2002;137:783-790.
41. Goldhirsch A, Glick JH, Gelber RD, et al. Meeting highlights: International Consensus Panel on the Treatment of Primary Breast Cancer. Seventh International Conference on Adjuvant Therapy of Primary Breast Cancer. J Clin Oncol 2001;19:3817-3827.
42. Silliman RA, Guadagnoli E, Rakowski W, et al. Adjuvant tamoxifen prescription in women 65 years and older with primary breast cancer. J Clin Oncol 2002;20:2680-2688.
43. Du XL, Jones DV, Zhang D. Effectiveness of adjuvant chemotherapy for node-positive operable breast cancer in older women. J Gerontol A Biol Sci Med Sci 2005;60:1137-1144.
44. Effects of chemotherapy and hormonal therapy for early breast cancer on recurrence and 15-year survival: an overview of the randomised trials. Lancet 2005;365:1687-1717.
45. Fentiman IS, Christiaens MR, Paridaens R, et al. Treatment of operable breast cancer in the elderly: a randomised clinical trial EORTC 10851 comparing tamoxifen alone with modified radical mastectomy. Eur J Cancer 2003;39:309-316.
46. Gazet JC, Markopoulos C, Ford HT, et al. Prospective randomised trial of tamoxifen versus surgery in elderly patients with breast cancer. Lancet 1988;1:679-681.
47. Grube BJ. Barriers to diagnosis and treatment of breast cancer in the older woman. J Am Coll Surg 2006;202:495-508.
48. Boccardo F, Rubagotti A, Puntoni M, et al. Switching to anastrozole versus continued tamoxifen treatment of early breast cancer: preliminary results of the Italian Tamoxifen Anastrozole Trial. J Clin Oncol 2005;23:5138-5147.
49. Belfiglio M, Valentini M, Pellegrini F, et al. Twelve-year mortality results of a randomized trial of 2 versus 5 years of adjuvant tamoxifen for postmenopausal early-stage breast carcinoma patients (SITAM 01). Cancer 2005;104:2334-2339.
50. Cole BF, Gelber RD, Gelber S, et al. Polychemotherapy for early breast cancer: an overview of the randomised clinical trials with quality-adjusted survival analysis. Lancet 2001;358:277-286.
51. Edge SB, Gold K, Berg CD, et al. Patient and provider characteristics that affect the use of axillary dissection in older women with stage I-II breast carcinoma. Cancer 2002;94:2534-2541.
52. McMahon LE, Gray RJ, Pockaj BA. Is breast cancer sentinel lymph node mapping valuable for patients in their seventies and beyond? Am J Surg 2005;190:366-370.
53. Jinno H, Ikeda T, Asaga S, et al. Increasing age does not affect efficacy of sentinel lymph node biopsy using smaller-sized technetium-99m tin colloids for breast cancer patients. Am J Surg 2005;190:51-54.
54. Greenwald DA. Aging, the gastrointestinal tract, and risk of acid-related disease. Am J Med 2004;117 Suppl 5A:8S-13S.
55. Fowler SF, Khoubian JF, Mathiasen RA, Margulies DR. Peptic ulcers in the elderly is a surgical disease. Am J Surg 2001;182:733-737.
56. Di Carlo I, Toro A, Sparatore F, et al. Emergency gastric ulcer complications in elderly: factors affecting the morbidity and mortality in relation to therapeutic approaches. Minerva Chir 2006;61:325-332.
57. Sharma SS, Mamtani MR, Sharma MS, Kulkarni H. A prospective cohort study of postoperative complications in the management of perforated peptic ulcer. BMC Surg 2006;6:8.

58. Baradarian R, Ramdhaney S, Chapalamadugu R, et al. Early intensive resuscitation of patients with upper gastrointestinal bleeding decreases mortality. Am J Gastroenterol 2004;99:619-622.
59. Di Martino N, Izzo G, Torelli F, et al. Gastric cancer in the elderly patient. Acta Biomed 2005;76 Suppl 1:29-30.
60. Kolodziejczyk P, Kulig J, Popiela T, et al. Outcome of gastric cancer surgery in elderly patients. Hepatogastroenterology 2005;52:1911-1915.
61. Bataille F, Rummele P, Dietmaier W, et al. Alterations in p53 predict response to preoperative high dose chemotherapy in patients with gastric cancer. Mol Pathol 2003;56:286-292.
62. Ramesh HS, Pope D, Gennari R, Audisio RA. Optimising surgical management of elderly cancer patients. World J Surg Oncol 2005;3:17.
63. Kunisaki C, Akiyama H, Nomura M, et al. Comparison of surgical outcomes of gastric cancer in elderly and middle-aged patients. Am J Surg 2006;191:216-224.
64. Mochiki E, Ohno T, Kamiyama Y, et al. Laparoscopy-assisted gastrectomy for early gastric cancer in young and elderly patients. World J Surg 2005;29:1585-1591.
65. Stupart DA, Panieri E, Dent DM. Gastrojejunostomy for gastric outlet obstruction in patients with gastric carcinoma. S Afr J Surg 2006;44:52-54.
66. Fiocca E, Ceci V, Donatelli G, et al. Palliative treatment of upper gastrointestinal obstruction using self-expansible metal stents. Eur Rev Med Pharmacol Sci 2006;10:179-182.
67. Yanai H, Kuroiwa Y, Shimizu N, et al. The pilot experience of immunotherapy-combined photodynamic therapy for advanced gastric cancer in elderly patients. Int J Gastrointest Cancer 2002;32:139-142.
68. Makela JT, Kiviniemi H, Laitinen S. Prognostic factors of perforated sigmoid diverticulitis in the elderly. Dig Surg 2005;22:100-106.
69. Aydin HN, Remzi FH, Tekkis PP, Fazio VW. Hartmann's reversal is associated with high postoperative adverse events. Dis Colon Rectum 2005;48:2117-2126.
70. Salem L, Anaya DA, Roberts KE, Flum DR. Hartmann's colectomy and reversal in diverticulitis: a population-level assessment. Dis Colon Rectum 2005;48:988-995.
71. Bell C, Asolati M, Hamilton E, et al. A comparison of complications associated with colostomy reversal versus ileostomy reversal. Am J Surg 2005;190:717-720.
72. Balducci L. The geriatric cancer patient: equal benefit from equal treatment. Cancer Control 2001;8:1-25; quiz 27-28.
73. Rios A, Montoya MJ, Rodriguez JM, et al. Acute lower gastrointestinal hemorrhages in geriatric patients. Dig Dis Sci 2005;50:898-904.
74. Burt RW. Colon cancer screening. Gastroenterology 2000;119:837-853.
75. Walter LC, de Garmo P, Covinsky KE. Association of older age and female sex with inadequate reach of screening flexible sigmoidoscopy. Am J Med 2004;116:174-178.
76. Frazier AL, Colditz GA, Fuchs CS, Kuntz KM. Cost-effectiveness of screening for colorectal cancer in the general population. JAMA 2000;284:1954-1961.
77. Duncan JE, Sweeney WB, Trudel JL, et al. Colonoscopy in the elderly: low risk, low yield in asymptomatic patients. Dis Colon Rectum 2006;49:646-651.
78. Clinical Outcomes of Surgical Therapy Study Group. A comparison of laparoscopically assisted and open colectomy for colon cancer. N Eng J Med 2004;350:2050-2059.
79. Fisichella PM, Di Stefano A, Di Carlo I, et al. Efficacy and safety of elective laparoscopic cholecystectomy in elderly: a case-controlled comparison with the open approach. Ann Ital Chir 2002;73:149-153; discussion 153-144.
80. Uecker J, Adams M, Skipper K, Dunn E. Cholecystitis in the octogenarian: is laparoscopic cholecystectomy the best approach? Am Surg 2001;67:637-640.
81. Annamaneni RK, Moraitis D, Cayten CG. Laparoscopic cholecystectomy in the elderly. JSLS 2005;9:408-410.

82. O'Connell JB, Maggard MA, Ko CY. Cancer-directed surgery for localized disease: decreased use in the elderly. Ann Surg Oncol 2004;11:962-969.
83. Jemal A, Clegg LX, Ward E, et al. Annual report to the nation on the status of cancer, 1975-2001, with a special feature regarding survival. Cancer 2004;101:3-27.
84. Petrowsky H, Clavien PA. Should we deny surgery for malignant hepato-pancreatico-biliary tumors to elderly patients? World J Surg 2005;29:1093-1100.
85. Ramesh HS, Jain S, Audisio RA. Implications of aging in surgical oncology. Cancer J 2005;11:488-494.
86. Neoptolemos JP, Dunn JA, Stocken DD, et al. Adjuvant chemoradiotherapy and chemotherapy in resectable pancreatic cancer: a randomised controlled trial. Lancet 2001;358:1576-1585.
87. Takada T, Amano H, Yasuda H, et al. Is postoperative adjuvant chemotherapy useful for gallbladder carcinoma? A phase III multicenter prospective randomized controlled trial in patients with resected pancreaticobiliary carcinoma. Cancer 2002;95:1685-1695.
88. Stocken DD, Buchler MW, Dervenis C, et al. Meta-analysis of randomised adjuvant therapy trials for pancreatic cancer. Br J Cancer 2005;92:1372-1381.
89. Brozzetti S, Mazzoni G, Miccini M, et al. Surgical treatment of pancreatic head carcinoma in elderly patients. Arch Surg 2006;141:137-142.
90. Suc B, Msika S, Fingerhut A, et al. Temporary fibrin glue occlusion of the main pancreatic duct in the prevention of intra-abdominal complications after pancreatic resection: prospective randomized trial. Ann Surg 2003;237:57-65.
91. Hruban RH, Goggins M, Parsons J, Kern SE. Progression model for pancreatic cancer. Clin Cancer Res 2000;6:2969-2972.
92. Goggins M. Molecular markers of early pancreatic cancer. J Clin Oncol 2005;23:4524-4531.
93. Lindsay JO, Andreyev HJ, Vlavianos P, Westaby D. Self-expanding metal stents for the palliation of malignant gastroduodenal obstruction in patients unsuitable for surgical bypass. Aliment Pharmacol Ther 2004;19:901-905.
94. Mittal A, Windsor J, Woodfield J, et al. Matched study of three methods for palliation of malignant pyloroduodenal obstruction. Br J Surg 2004;91:205-209.
95. Profili S, Feo CF, Meloni GB, et al. Combined biliary and duodenal stenting for palliation of pancreatic cancer. Scand J Gastroenterol 2003;38:1099-1102.
96. Andrawes WF, Bussy C, Belmin J. Prevention of cardiovascular events in elderly people. Drugs Aging 2005;22:859-876.
97. Ballotta E, Da Giau G, Militello C, et al. High-grade symptomatic and asymptomatic carotid stenosis in the very elderly. A challenge for proponents of carotid angioplasty and stenting. BMC Cardiovasc Disord 2006;6:12.
98. Villalobos HJ, Harrigan MR, Lau T, et al. Advancements in carotid stenting leading to reductions in perioperative morbidity among patients 80 years and older. Neurosurgery 2006;58:233-240; discussion 233-240.
99. Grego F, Lepidi S, Antonello M, et al. Is carotid endarterectomy in octogenarians more dangerous than in younger patients? J Cardiovasc Surg (Torino) 2005;46:477-483.
100. Amato B, Markabaoui AK, Piscitelli V, et al. Carotid endarterectomy under local anesthesia in elderly: is it worthwhile? Acta Biomed 2005;76 Suppl 1:64-68.
101. Chaer RA, Derubertis BG, Trocciola SM, et al. Safety and efficacy of carotid angioplasty and stenting in high-risk patients. Am Surg 2006;72:694-698; discussion 698-699.
102. Fitzpatrick CM, Chiou ÂC, DeCaprio JD, Kashyap VS. Carotid revascularization in the presence of contralateral carotid artery occlusion is safe and durable. Mil Med 2005;170:1069-1074.
103. Michael KM, Shaughnessy M. Stroke prevention and management in older adults. J Cardiovasc Nurs 2006;21:S21-S26.

104. Kurukulasuriya LR, Govindarajan G, Sowers J. Stroke prevention in diabetes and obesity. Expert Rev Cardiovasc Ther 2006;4:487-502.
105. Hankey GJ. Potential new risk factors for ischemic stroke: what is their potential? Stroke 2006;37:2181-2188.
106. Collins P, McKay I, Rajagoplan S, et al. Is carotid duplex scanning sufficient as the sole investigation prior to carotid endarterectomy? Br J Radiol 2005;78:1034-1037.
107. Amato B, Iuliano GP, Markabauoi AK, et al. Endovascular procedures in critical leg ischemia of elderly patients. Acta Biomed 2005;76 Suppl 1:11-15.
108. Galaria, II, Surowiec SM, Rhodes JM, et al. Implications of early failure of superficial femoral artery endoluminal interventions. Ann Vasc Surg 2005;19:787-792.
109. Keefer A, Davies MG, Illig KA. Can endovascular therapy of infrainguinal disease for claudication be justified? Expert Rev Cardiovasc Ther 2004;2:229-237.
110. Bashir EA. Aggressive revascularization in patients with critical lower limbs ischemia. J Ayub Med Coll Abbottabad 2005;17:36-39.
111. Chung J, Bartelson BB, Hiatt WR, et al. Wound healing and functional outcomes after infrainguinal bypass with reversed saphenous vein for critical limb ischemia. J Vasc Surg 2006;43:1183-1190.
112. Bosiers M, Deloose K, Verbist J, Peeters P. Percutaneous transluminal angioplasty for treatment of ''below-the-knee'' critical limb ischemia: early outcomes following the use of sirolimus-eluting stents. J Cardiovasc Surg (Torino) 2006;47:171-176.
113. Hynes N, Kok N, Manning B, et al. Abdominal aortic aneurysm repair in octogenarians versus younger patients in a tertiary referral center. Vascular 2005;13:275-285.
114. Upchurch GR, Jr., Schaub TA. Abdominal aortic aneurysm. Am Fam Physician 2006;73:1198-1204.
115. Fleming C. Screening and management of abdominal aortic aneurysm: the best evidence. Am Fam Physician 2006;73:1157-1158.
116. Lindholt JS, Juul S, Fasting H, Henneberg EW. Cost-effectiveness analysis of screening for abdominal aortic aneurysms based on five year results from a randomised hospital based mass screening trial. Eur J Vasc Endovasc Surg 2006;32:9-15.
117. Wanhainen A, Lundkvist J, Bergqvist D, Bjorck M. Cost-effectiveness of screening women for abdominal aortic aneurysm. J Vasc Surg 2006;43:908-914; discussion 914.
118. Conway KP, Byrne J, Townsend M, Lane IF. Prognosis of patients turned down for conventional abdominal aortic aneurysm repair in the endovascular and sonographic era: Szilagyi revisited? J Vasc Surg 2001;33:752-757.
119. Rutherford RB. Commentary. Endovascular aneurysm repair versus open repair in patients with abdominal aortic aneurysm (EVAR trial 1): randomized controlled trial. Perspect Vasc Surg Endovasc Ther 2006;18:74-76.
120. Greenhalgh RM, Brown LC, Kwong GP, et al. Comparison of endovascular aneurysm repair with open repair in patients with abdominal aortic aneurysm (EVAR trial 1), 30-day operative mortality results: randomised controlled trial. Lancet 2004;364:843-848.
121. Manis G, Feuerman M, Hines GL. Open aneurysm repair in elderly patients not candidates for endovascular repair (EVAR): comparison with patients undergoing EVAR or preferential open repair. Vasc Endovascular Surg 2006;40:95-101.
122. Rutherford RB. Commentary. Endovascular aneurysm repair and outcome in patients unfit for open repair of abdominal aortic aneurysm (EVAR trial 2): randomized controlled trial. Perspect Vasc Surg Endovasc Ther 2006;18:76-77.
123. Vemuri C, Wainess RM, Dimick JB, et al. Effect of increasing patient age on complication rates following intact abdominal aortic aneurysm repair in the United States. J Surg Res 2004;118:26-31.

124. Azizzadeh A, Sanchez LA, Miller CC, 3rd, et al. Glomerular filtration rate is a predictor of mortality after endovascular abdominal aortic aneurysm repair. J Vasc Surg 2006;43:14-18.
125. Okuwa M, Sanada H, Sugama J, et al. A prospective cohort study of lower-extremity pressure ulcer risk among bedfast older adults. Adv Skin Wound Care 2006;19:391-397.
126. Allen DB. Aesthetic and reconstructive surgery in the aging patient. Arch Surg 2003;138:1099-1105.
127. Lyder CH, Preston J, Grady JN, et al. Quality of care for hospitalized medicare patients at risk for pressure ulcers. Arch Intern Med 2001;161:1549-1554.
128. Bourdel-Marchasson I, Barateau M, Rondeau V, et al. A multi-center trial of the effects of oral nutritional supplementation in critically ill older inpatients. GAGE Group. Groupe Aquitain Geriatrique d'Evaluation. Nutrition 2000;16:1-5.
129. Hartgrink HH, Wille J, Konig P, et al. Pressure sores and tube feeding in patients with a fracture of the hip: a randomized clinical trial. Clin Nutr 1998;17:287-292.
130. Mathus-Vliegen EM. Old age, malnutrition, and pressure sores: an ill-fated alliance. J Gerontol A Biol Sci Med Sci 2004;59:355-360.
131. Lang BH, Lo CY. Total thyroidectomy for multinodular goiter in the elderly. Am J Surg 2005;190:418-423.
132. Pacini F, Burroni L, Ciuoli C, et al. Management of thyroid nodules: a clinicopathological, evidence-based approach. Eur J Nucl Med Mol Imaging 2004;31:1443-1449.
133. Sakorafas GH, Peros G. Thyroid nodule: a potentially malignant lesion; optimal management from a surgical perspective. Cancer Treat Rev 2006;32:191-202.
134. Cerutti JM, Delcelo R, Amadei MJ, et al. A preoperative diagnostic test that distinguishes benign from malignant thyroid carcinoma based on gene expression. J Clin Invest 2004;113:1234-1242.
135. Lee JC, Truong PT, Kader HA, et al. Postmastectomy radiotherapy reduces locoregional recurrence in elderly women with high-risk breast cancer. Clin Oncol (R Coll Radiol) 2005;17:623-629.
136. Plosker GL, Keam SJ. Trastuzumab: a review of its use in the management of HER2-positive metastatic and early-stage breast cancer. Drugs 2006;66:449-475.
137. Witherby SM, Muss HB. Special issues related to breast cancer adjuvant therapy in older women. Breast 2005;14:600-611.
138. Kemeny MM, Peterson BL, Kornblith AB, et al. Barriers to clinical trial participation by older women with breast cancer. J Clin Oncol 2003;21:2268-2275.
139. Velanovich V, Gabel M, Walker EM, et al. Causes for the undertreatment of elderly breast cancer patients: tailoring treatments to individual patients. J Am Coll Surg 2002;194:8-13.
140. Diab SG, Elledge RM, Clark GM. Tumor characteristics and clinical outcome of elderly women with breast cancer. J Natl Cancer Inst 2000;92:550-556.
141. Singh R, Hellman S, Heimann R. The natural history of breast carcinoma in the elderly: implications for screening and treatment. Cancer 2004;100:1807-1813.
142. Linder JD, Wilcox CM. Acid peptic disease in the elderly. Gastroenterol Clin North Am 2001;30:363-376.
143. Holt PR. Gastrointestinal diseases in the elderly. Curr Opin Clin Nutr Metab Care 2003;6:41-48.
144. Shimazu T, Matsui T, Furukawa K, et al. A prospective study of the prevalence of gastroesophageal reflux disease and confounding factors. J Gastroenterol 2005;40:866-872.
145. Bammer T, Hinder RA, Klaus A, et al. Safety and long-term outcome of laparoscopic antireflux surgery in patients in their eighties and older. Surg Endosc 2002;16:40-42.
146. Ward EM, Wolfsen HC, Achem SR, et al. Barrett's esophagus is common in older men and women undergoing screening colonoscopy regardless of reflux symptoms. Am J Gastroenterol 2006;101:12-17.

147. Manes G, Pieramico O, Uomo G, et al. Relationship of sliding hiatus hernia to gastroesophageal reflux disease: a possible role for *Helicobacter pylori* infection? Dig Dis Sci 2003;48:303-307.
148. Orr WC, Chen CL, Sloan S. The role of age and salivation in acid clearance in symptomatic patients with gastro-oesophageal reflux disease. Aliment Pharmacol Ther 2001;15:1385-1388.
149. Bardan E, Xie P, Brasseur J, et al. Effect of ageing on the upper and lower oesophageal sphincters. Eur J Gastroenterol Hepatol 2000;12:1221-1225.
150. Amano K, Adachi K, Katsube T, et al. Role of hiatus hernia and gastric mucosal atrophy in the development of reflux esophagitis in the elderly. J Gastroenterol Hepatol 2001;16:132-136.
151. Pilotto A, Franceschi M, Paris F. Recent advances in the treatment of GERD in the elderly: focus on proton pump inhibitors. Int J Clin Pract 2005;59:1204-1209.
152. Teramoto S, Ouchi Y. A possible pathologic link between chronic cough and sleep apnea syndrome through gastroesophageal reflux disease in older people. Chest 2000;117:1215-1216.
153. ten Brinke A, Sterk PJ, Masclee AA, et al. Risk factors of frequent exacerbations in difficult-to-treat asthma. Eur Respir J 2005;26:812-818.
154. Bacak BS, Patel M, Tweed E, Danis P. What is the best way to manage GERD symptoms in the elderly? J Fam Pract 2006;55:251-254, 258.
155. Pilotto A. Aging and upper gastrointestinal disorders. Best Pract Res Clin Gastroenterol 2004;18 Suppl:73-81.
156. Orr WC, Chen CL. Aging and neural control of the GI tract: IV. clinical and physiological aspects of gastrointestinal motility and aging. Am J Physiol Gastrointest Liver Physiol 2002;283:G1226-G1231.
157. Trus TL, Laycock WS, Wo JM, et al. Laparoscopic antireflux surgery in the elderly. Am J Gastroenterol 1998;93:351-353.
158. Tedesco P, Lobo E, Fisichella PM, et al. Laparoscopic fundoplication in elderly patients with gastroesophageal reflux disease. Arch Surg 2006;141:289-292; discussion 292.
159. Cowgill SM, Arnaoutakis D, Villadolid D, et al. Results after laparoscopic fundoplication: does age matter? Am Surg 2006;72:778-783; discussion 783-774.
160. Iqbal A, Salmas V, Filipi CJ. Endoscopic therapies of gastroesophageal reflux disease. World J Gastroenterol 2006;12:2641-2655.
161. Ferulano GP, Dilillo S, D'Ambra M, et al. Oesophageal achalasia in elderly people: results of the laparoscopic Heller-Dor myotomy. Acta Biomed 2005;76 Suppl 1:37-41.
162. Miki C, Inoue Y, Toiyama Y, et al. Deficiency in systemic interleukin-1 receptor antagonist production as an operative risk factor in malnourished elderly patients with colorectal carcinoma. Crit Care Med 2005;33:177-180.
163. Konishi T, Watanabe T, Kishimoto J, Nagawa H. Risk factors for anastomotic leakage after surgery for colorectal cancer: results of prospective surveillance. J Am Coll Surg 2006;202:439-444.
164. Pokorny H, Herkner H, Jakesz R, Herbst F. Mortality and complications after stoma closure. Arch Surg 2005;140:956-960, discussion 960.
165. Bufalari A, Giustozzi G, Burattini MF, et al. Rectal cancer surgery in the elderly: a multivariate analysis of outcome risk factors. J Surg Oncol 2006;93:173-180.
166. Mantello G, Berardi R, Cardinali M, et al. Feasibility of preoperative chemoradiation in rectal cancer patients aged 70 and older. J Exp Clin Cancer Res 2005;24:541-546.
167. Larsen SG, Wiig JN, Tretli S, Giercksky KE. Surgery and pre-operative irradiation for locally advanced or recurrent rectal cancer in patients over 75 years of age. Colorectal Dis 2006;8:177-185.
168. Brand MI, Saclarides TJ, Dobson HD, Millikan KW. Liver resection for colorectal cancer: liver metastases in the aged. Am Surg 2000;66:412-415; discussion 415-416.

169. Fong Y, Blumgart LH, Fortner JG, Brennan MF. Pancreatic or liver resection for malignancy is safe and effective for the elderly. Ann Surg 1995;222:426-434; discussion 434-427.
170. Nagano Y, Nojiri K, Matsuo K, et al. The impact of advanced age on hepatic resection of colorectal liver metastases. J Am Coll Surg 2005;201:511-516.
171. Tada K, Kokudo N, Seki M, et al. Hepatic resection for colorectal metastasis with macroscopic tumor thrombus in the portal vein. World J Surg 2003;27:299-303.
172. Yeh CN, Lee WC, Jeng LB, Chen MF. Hepatic resection for hepatocellular carcinoma in elderly patients. Hepatogastroenterology 2004;51:219-223.
173. Ferrero A, Vigano L, Polastri R, et al. Hepatectomy as treatment of choice for hepatocellular carcinoma in elderly cirrhotic patients. World J Surg 2005;29:1101-1105.
174. Hanazaki K, Kajikawa S, Shimozawa N, et al. Hepatic resection for large hepatocellular carcinoma. Am J Surg 2001;181:347-353.
175. Dimick JB, Cowan JA, Jr., Knol JA, Upchurch GR, Jr. Hepatic resection in the United States: indications, outcomes, and hospital procedural volumes from a nationally representative database. Arch Surg 2003;138:185-191.
176. Aldrighetti L, Arru M, Catena M, et al. Liver resections in over-75-year-old patients: surgical hazard or current practice? J Surg Oncol 2006;93:186-193.
177. Angus DC, Linde-Zwirble WT, Lidicker J, et al. Epidemiology of severe sepsis in the United States: analysis of incidence, outcome, and associated costs of care. Crit Care Med 2001;29:1303-1310.
178. Murphy K, Haudek SB, Thompson M, Giroir BP. Molecular biology of septic shock. New Horiz 1998;6:181-193.
179. Hotchkiss RS, Karl IE. The pathophysiology and treatment of sepsis. N Engl J Med 2003;348:138-150.
180. Fisher CJ, Jr., Agosti JM, Opal SM, et al. Treatment of septic shock with the tumor necrosis factor receptor:Fc fusion protein. The Soluble TNF Receptor Sepsis Study Group. N Engl J Med 1996;334:1697-1702.
181. Fisher CJ, Jr., Slotman GJ, Opal SM, et al. Initial evaluation of human recombinant interleukin-1 receptor antagonist in the treatment of sepsis syndrome: a randomized, open-label, placebo-controlled multicenter trial. Crit Care Med 1994;22:12-21.
182. Ziegler EJ, Fisher CJ, Jr., Sprung CL, et al. Treatment of gram-negative bacteremia and septic shock with HA-1A human monoclonal antibody against endotoxin: a randomized, double-blind, placebo-controlled trial. The HA-1A Sepsis Study Group. N Engl J Med 1991;324:429-436.
183. Oberholzer A, Oberholzer C, Moldawer LL. Sepsis syndromes: understanding the role of innate and acquired immunity. Shock 2001;16:83-96.
184. Marik PE. Management of the critically ill geriatric patient. Crit Care Med 2006;34:S176-S182.
185. Kaye KS, Sloane R, Sexton DJ, Schmader KA. Risk factors for surgical site infections in older people. J Am Geriatr Soc 2006;54:391-396.

5

GERIATRIC GENERAL THORACIC SURGERY

*Thomas A. D'Amico, MD; Joseph LoCicero, III, MD, FACS**

General thoracic surgery is a relatively complex surgical discipline in which outcomes have been closely associated with the experience of the hospital [1] and the surgeon. [2] Treatment guidelines and systems of care have been scrutinized and improved in order to optimize the outcome for all patients, particularly those with the highest surgical risk. [3] In addition to the development of and adherence to evidence-based guidelines, better understanding of the molecular biological aspects of thoracic malignancies will improve the outcomes for the many elderly patients who undergo general thoracic surgery.

The Key Questions in geriatric general thoracic surgery from *New Frontiers in Geriatrics Research* [4] are unchanged:

***ThoracicSurg KQ1*: How effective is preoperative preparation in improving the immediate surgical outcome for elderly patients?**

***ThoracicSurg KQ2*: What changes in perioperative care are needed to improve outcomes in the elderly thoracic surgical patient?**

***ThoracicSurg KQ3*: To what extent do thoracic surgical operations improve quality-of-life outcomes in the elderly patient population?**

In this update of the research agenda for general thoracic surgery in older adults, new research addressing agenda items proposed in *New Frontiers* is discussed in the section Progress in Geriatric General Thoracic Surgery. Suggestions for new agenda items in the field are presented in New Horizons in Geriatric General Thoracic Surgery at the end of the chapter.

METHODS

The search was conducted on the National Library of Medicine's PubMed database. In the previous review by LoCicero and Yee, [4] the time period covered was from January 1982 to October 2002. The current search was from October 2002 to December 2005. The search strategy combined various terms for general thoracic surgical procedures (general or specific commonly performed operations, including the esophagus, lung, and mediastinum), the terms *elective* and *emergency*, and various terms for perioperative care, complications, and outcomes. Additional requirements were either that the publication be a review, clinical trial, randomized controlled trial, or meta-analysis, and that terms for risk or age factors be present as title words or MeSH headings. Terms denoting advanced age were *age factors, age, aging, elderly, geriatric, gerontologic, older, or octogenarian, nonagenarian,* or *centenarian*. Finally, animal research was systematically excluded.

* D'Amico: Professor of Surgery, Program Director, Division of Thoracic Surgery, Department of Surgery, Duke University Medical Center, Durham, NC; LoCicero: Director of Surgical Oncology and Chief of General Thoracic Surgery, Maimonides Medical Center, Brooklyn, NY.

PROGRESS IN GERIATRIC GENERAL THORACIC SURGERY

LUNG CANCER

See *New Frontiers,* pp. 112–121.

ThoracicSurg 1 (Level A): **Randomized controlled trials are needed of the effect on mortality and morbidity of the use of computed tomography screening for elderly patients with high-risk factors for the development of cancer.**

New Research Addressing This Question: The high mortality rate of lung cancer, existence of a recognizable preclinical stage of disease, and efficacy of surgical therapy for early-stage disease of lung cancer has suggested the potential for decreasing lung cancer mortality by the employment of screening strategies. To date, the role of screening for lung cancer has been considered investigational, and several current trials involving spiral computed tomography (CT) scanning have been designed to evaluate the clinical efficacy and cost-effectiveness of this strategy. The Early Lung Cancer Action Project performed yearly low-dose spiral CT scans and chest x-ray in a single-arm study of 1000 smokers. One to six noncalcified lung nodules were found at baseline (ie, prevalence) in 233 participants, 27 (12% or 2.7% of the total screened population) of which had a malignancy. Among these 27 nodules with malignancy, 20 (74%) were not found on standard chest x-ray, while no malignant nodules were detected by chest x-ray that were not also seen on CT scan. The majority (23 of 27, 85%) of malignancies were stage I, and all but one (97%) were resectable. [5]

Subsequently, the group published follow-up on the patients who had a new stage I lung cancer discovered as a result of the study. Screening resulted in a diagnosis of lung cancer in 484 participants. Of these participants, 412 (85%) had clinical stage I lung cancer, and the estimated 10-year survival rate was 88% in this subgroup (95% confidence interval [CI], 84 to 91). Among the 302 participants with clinical stage I cancer who underwent surgical resection within 1 month after diagnosis, the survival rate was 92% (95% CI, 88 to 95). The 8 participants with clinical stage I cancer who did not receive treatment died within 5 years after diagnosis. [6]

Randomized studies of low-dose spiral CT scan screening are under way at other centers in North America and Europe.

Modification of This Question in Light of New Research: This question should remain unmodified on the research agenda.

ThoracicSurg 2 (Level B): **An instrument to assess age-specific outcomes, functional status, and quality of life for elderly lung cancer patients that is applicable to both preoperative and postoperative situations needs to be developed and validated.**

New Research Addressing This Question: No new research addressing this question reported during the current search period from October 2002 to December 2005 has come to light.

Modification of This Question in Light of New Research: This question should remain unmodified on the research agenda.

> *ThoracicSurg 3 (Level A)*: **Ongoing large therapeutic lung cancer trials need to incorporate the age-specific instrument described in ThoracicSurg 2.**

New Research Addressing This Question: No new research addressing this question reported during the current search period from October 2002 to December 2005 has come to light.

Modification of This Question in Light of New Research: This question should remain unmodified on the research agenda.

> *ThoracicSurg 4 (Level B)*: **A preoperative tool to assess the general function of the elderly patient having a major pulmonary procedure needs to be developed and validated.**

New Research Addressing This Question: No new research addressing this question reported during the current search period from October 2002 to December 2005 has come to light.

Modification of This Question in Light of New Research: This question should remain unmodified on the research agenda.

> *ThoracicSurg 5 (Level B)*: **A multivariate analysis using the Society of Thoracic Surgeons Database or other collections of cases and aimed at defining the most important risk factors for adverse surgical outcomes should be performed. The instrument should include measures of the patient's functional capacity as well as pulmonary functions.**

New Research Addressing This Question: No new research addressing this question reported during the current search period from October 2002 to December 2005 has come to light.

Modification of This Question in Light of New Research: This question should remain unmodified on the research agenda.

> *ThoracicSurg 6 (Level B)*: **A method of preoperative optimization that addresses the most important risk factors for morbidity and mortality from pneumonectomy should be developed and tested.**

New Research Addressing This Question: No new research addressing this question reported during the current search period from October 2002 to December 2005 has come to light.

Modification of This Question in Light of New Research: This question should remain unmodified on the research agenda.

> *ThoracicSurg 7 (Level A)*: **Randomized controlled trials are needed to compare the efficacy of preoperative optimization methods with current best medical practices.**

New Research Addressing This Question: For patients with T2 or T3 tumors or with mediastinal adenopathy on chest CT or positron-emission tomography (PET), cervical mediastinoscopy is recommended prior to exploration for pulmonary resection. [3,7] Reliance on the CT or PET scan alone for this group of patients is unacceptably inaccurate. [8,9] In a recent multi-institutional study (American College of Surgeons Oncology Group Z0050 trial), the utility of PET in staging potentially operable non–small cell lung cancer patients was assessed in 287 patients (22 institutions). In the assessment of mediastinal lymph nodes, the sensitivity was only 61%, specificity 84%, positive predictive value 56%, and negative predictive value 87%. [9] Thus, PET may be used to direct biopsies, but mediastinoscopy is required to confirm or exclude mediastinal lymph node involvement in patients with potentially operable lung cancer.

The power of large databases used to derive the staging system in predicting prognosis is self-evident. Nevertheless, there is an inherent inaccuracy of this staging process that is attributable to the presence of undetectable metastatic disease at presentation. Molecular biological staging refers to the assessment tumor markers associated with various oncogenic mechanisms in order to improve the risk stratification provided by conventional tumor, nodes, and metastasis (TNM) staging. Biological staging may target oncogenes, oncogenic protein products, growth factors, or receptors. The biological techniques that are utilized include analysis of DNA, RNA, or protein products. Molecular biological staging may potentially be applied to the primary tumor, lymph nodes, bone marrow, or serum in order to establish the diagnosis of malignancy at earlier stage, to assess prognosis, to detect occult metastases, to select therapy, and to predict chemotherapy sensitivity or resistance. [10]

Characterization of the primary tumor may be made using various molecular markers. Trials of biological parameters that may be used to select patients who would most benefit from surgical therapy and to predict whether patients respond to chemotherapy are currently being conducted. [11]

The treatment of non–small cell lung cancer is based on the stage of disease, as determined by the TNM staging system. [3] In general, surgical resection is the standard treatment of patients with stage I disease, and surgery with postoperative chemotherapy is used for stage II disease. Determination of operability must include assessment of the medical risk of thoracotomy as well as the risk of removal of the requisite pulmonary parenchyma. The degree of cardiopulmonary disease, usually a consequence of tobacco use, represents the most significant medical factor in determining operability and the major cause of postoperative morbidity and mortality. Contraindications to surgical resection include pulmonary insufficiency and untreated cardiovascular or cerebrovascular disease. Age is not considered a contraindication, and surgery is considered a viable option in patients with good performance status and reasonable chance for cure into the 9th and 10th decades of life. Sullivan et al assessed 140 patients who underwent lobectomy for non–small cell lung cancer at a Veterans Affairs Medical Center to compare the effect of lobectomy in elderly patients (aged 70 and older) and younger patients (younger than 70 years) on pulmonary function, as measured by forced expiratory volume at 1 second (FEV_1), and functional status, as measured by Karnofsky Status (KS), 1 year following surgery. FEV_1 decreased by 19% in elderly patients and by 13% in younger patients. Functional status declined for two older patients (8%), whose KS dropped from 80%–100% (normal activity without limitation) to 40%–70% (unable to work, but able to take care of self at home). Nine of the younger patients (24%) had a KS drop from 80%–100% to 40%–70%. Thus, elderly patients undergoing lobectomy for non–small cell lung cancer had similar pulmonary function test results and functional status as younger patients 1 year after undergoing surgery, and curative resection should not be denied on the basis of age alone.[12] In another study, the outcomes of 40 consecutive patients (aged 80 to 88 years) with non–small cell lung cancer who underwent complete resection were analyzed. There was no perioperative mortality, and patients had nonlethal complications (20%). The actuarial survival rates of the 40 patients, including deaths from all causes, were 92.4%, 71.6%, and 56.9% at 1, 3, and 5 years, respectively. In patients with stage I disease, the respective survival rates were 94.3%, 74.3%, and 57.3%.[13] A retrospective study of 1114 patients with lung cancer classified patients as younger (< 75 years) and elderly (75 years and older). Regarding treatment, 51.0% of those in the younger group and 36.1% of those in the elderly group underwent surgery. The perioperative mortality rates for the younger and elderly groups were 0.9% and 4.1%, respectively, with no significant difference, and the overall survival was similar in the two groups.[14] Despite these data, it is clear that age may inappropriately influence treatment selection. In a study from the Netherlands, de Rijke et al asked whether age, comorbidity, performance status, or pulmonary function influenced treatment in patients with newly diagnosed non–small cell lung cancer (N = 803). In this series, 82% with stage I or II disease and 48% with stage IIIA disease received treatment according to the guidelines. For all stages, this proportion decreased with increasing age. Multivariate analyses showed associations between comorbidity and treatment choice, but none with performance status. Age of 75 years or older appeared to be the most important factor for not receiving treatment according to guidelines.[15]

Although chemotherapy has clearly been demonstrated to improve survival for patients with stage III and stage IV non–small cell lung cancer, its efficacy and use in patients with early-stage disease has been controversial. A meta-analysis suggests that cisplatin-based regimens could improve 5-year survival by approximately 5%, but that there is no survival advantage for regimens without platinum.[16] The International Adjuvant Lung Cancer Trial Collaborative Group enrolled 1867 patients with completely resected stage I, II, or III non–small cell lung cancer. In this study, the use of adjuvant chemotherapy was associated with significantly improved overall and disease-free survival: the 5-year overall survival was 44.5% in the adjuvant chemotherapy group and 40.4% in the control group—an absolute benefit of 4.1% ($P < .03$).[17] In a study conducted by the Cancer and Leukemia Group B, 344 patients with completely resected stage IB (T2N0) non–small cell lung cancer were randomized to treatment with paclitaxel and carboplatin or observation. After 4 years of follow-up, overall survival was 71% in the adjuvant treatment group and 59% in the observation group ($P = .028$), a 12% absolute improvement and 49% relative improvement. Failure-free survival and lung cancer mortality were also significantly improved in the adjuvant chemotherapy group. The therapy was well tolerated, with no toxicity-related deaths and grade 3–4 neutropenia in only 36% of patients.[18] Finally, in a study conducted by the National Cancer Institute of Canada, 482 patients with completely resected stage IB (T2N0) or II (T1-2N0) non–small cell lung cancer were randomized to adjuvant treatment with vinorelbine and cisplatin or follow-up alone. Overall survival was found to be significantly prolonged in the adjuvant treatment group (94 months versus 73 months; $P = .011$). These results translated to a 5-year survival rate of 69% with adjuvant treatment compared with 54% for the control group.[19]

The selection of patients to proceed to surgery after preoperative therapy is also important. For patients with stage III disease, it has been demonstrated that nodal downstaging is strongly associated with survival. Betticher et al, for example, examined the effects of preoperative docetaxel and cisplatin in patients with stage IIIA non–small cell lung cancer. In this small study, 90 patients were treated with docetaxel and cisplatin before surgical resection; 33 patients also received adjuvant radiotherapy. Mediastinal downstaging (N0, N1 versus N2) was the most powerful predictive factor for survival.[20]

Modification of This Question in Light of New Research: This question should remain unmodified on the research agenda. However, over the previous two decades, a large amount of clinical experience has been gained regarding the use of induction therapy for non–small cell lung cancer. There are several controversial issues that should be addressed in clinical trials:

- The selection of patients for resection after induction therapy
- The use of induction chemotherapy versus chemoradiotherapy
- The use of induction chemotherapy for early-stage disease
- The use of induction therapy as opposed to adjuvant therapy

***ThoracicSurg 8 (Level A)*: Randomized controlled trials are needed to evaluate video-assisted thoracic surgery techniques for lobectomy; the trials should compare outcomes, including long-term survival in elderly patients, with those of standard open procedures.**

New Research Addressing This Question: Thoracoscopic lobectomy has emerged as a viable strategy for resection in patients with non–small cell lung cancer. Advantages of a thoracoscopic approach to anatomic lung resection include decreased blood loss, less postoperative pain, shorter length of stay, more rapid return to preoperative activity, preserved postoperative pulmonary function, fewer overall complications, and decreased inflammatory response (which may confer superior immunologic function). These benefits are achieved with equivalent oncologic effectiveness.[21,22]

Thoracoscopic lobectomy has also been found to be safe and effective in selected patients after induction chemotherapy, with or without radiation therapy.[23] Current areas of interest include the investigation of the potential immunoprotective effects of minimally invasive lobectomy and the advantages regarding the delivery of postoperative chemotherapy in patients after thoracoscopic lobectomy. A registry trial is planned to compare the overall effectiveness, including survival and quality of life, between thoracoscopic lobectomy and conventional lobectomy (thoracotomy).

Modification of This Question in Light of New Research: This question should remain unmodified on the research agenda.

Benign Diseases of the Lungs

See *New Frontiers*, pp. 122–123.

***ThoracicSurg 9*: (*Levels B, A*): The effects of lung volume reduction procedures and their complications on elderly patients with chronic obstructive pulmonary disease need to be investigated in cohort**

studies that compare younger and older patients. Subsequently, a randomized controlled trial might be needed to compare outcomes in elderly patients who undergo a standard volume-reduction procedure with similar patients who do not.

New Research Addressing This Question: Currently, lung volume reduction surgery is most commonly performed bilaterally, via thoracoscopy or median sternotomy using linear staple reduction techniques, with or without buttressing materials. Given the evidence that this procedure can be beneficial in well-selected patients, investigators have been vigorously pursuing research into innovative alternative methods for achieving lung volume reduction. Many of these new methods are reaching the stage of clinical trials. Currently, three new general conceptual approaches to lung volume reduction surgery are under evaluation: surgical resection with banding devices, endobronchial volume-reducing methods, and endobronchial bronchial bypass approaches. [24] There are theoretical approaches and technical issues that must be investigated for each approach, and studies are under way to evaluate the relative risk and benefit of these procedures, as compared with lung volume reduction surgery, in patients with emphysema.

Modification of This Question in Light of New Research: This question should remain unmodified on the research agenda.

ThoracicSurg 10 (Level A): **Randomized trials are needed to evaluate the efficacy of minimally invasive techniques and compare them with standard thoracotomy for the management of empyema in elderly patients.**

New Research Addressing This Question: No new research addressing this question reported during the current search period from October 2002 to December 2005 has come to light.

Modification of This Question in Light of New Research: This question should remain unmodified on the research agenda.

Esophageal Cancer

See *New Frontiers,* pp. 123–132.

ThoracicSurg 11 (Level B): **Screening endoscopic trials should be performed for elderly patients with longstanding reflux or a history of Barrett's esophagus to determine if early detection and treatment of high-grade dysplasia is cost-effective.**

New Research Addressing This Question: Medical management of Barrett's esophagus with no dysplasia or with metaplasia is based on the symptomatic control of gastroesophageal reflux using histamine-receptor antagonists or proton-pump inhibitors. Medical management may also include lifestyle modifications, such as weight loss, sleeping with the head of the bed elevated, avoidance of late-night meals, and dietary exclusion of fat and alcohol. The aim of medical therapy is based on symptomatic control of gastroesophageal reflux. Endoscopic surveillance must also be performed to evaluate progression to high-grade dysplasia or adenocarcinoma. Endoscopy is performed on patients with severe symptoms of gastroesophageal reflux, especially those with a family history of

Barrett's esophagus or esophageal cancer. Once the diagnosis of metaplasia is established, routine endoscopic screening with biopsy every 1 to 2 years is indicated. The interval is decreased to 6 months if low-grade dysplasia is present. [25]

Surgical management for uncomplicated Barrett's esophagus (metaplasia or low-grade dysplasia, without stricture) consists of fundoplication for gastroesophageal reflux in the appropriate patient. Patients with high-grade dysplasia may be candidates for mucosal ablative therapy, with photodynamic therapy [26] or with radio frequency ablation. [27] Esophagectomy with cervical esophagogastrostomy may be performed in patients with Barrett's esophagus who present with bleeding, perforation, or fistulization.

Modification of This Question in Light of New Research: This question should remain unmodified on the research agenda.

> *ThoracicSurg 12 (Levels B, A)*: **Nonrandomized chemoprevention trials targeted specifically toward at-risk elderly patients should be continued, to be followed by a randomized controlled trial of chemoprevention using the most promising agent and comparing it with usual care.**

New Research Addressing This Question: No new research addressing this question reported during the current search period from October 2002 to December 2005 has come to light.

Modification of This Question in Light of New Research: This question should remain unmodified on the research agenda.

> *ThoracicSurg 13 (Level B)*: **The Society of Thoracic Surgeons database and other similar databases should be used to gather data on the impact of age-related comorbidities and other factors related to operative management on the outcomes of esophagectomy for elderly patients.**

New Research Addressing This Question: No new research addressing this question reported during the current search period from October 2002 to December 2005 has come to light.

Modification of This Question in Light of New Research: This question should remain unmodified on the research agenda.

> *ThoracicSurg 14 (Level B)*: **A national database for collecting morbidity and long-term survival rates of minimally invasive techniques for esophageal cancer should be established.**

New Research Addressing This Question: No new research addressing this question reported during the current search period from October 2002 to December 2005 has come to light.

Modification of This Question in Light of New Research: This question should remain unmodified on the research agenda.

> *ThoracicSurg 15 (Level B)*: **Esophagectomy needs to be evaluated for effectiveness as a procedure for improving quality of life and preventing complications of aspiration in elderly patients.**

New Research Addressing This Question: It is recommended that operable patients with T1-T2 esophageal carcinoma proceed with surgery.[28] The choice of surgical procedure depends on the preferences of the surgeon, and choices include transhiatal, Ivor Lewis, and McKeown esophagogastrectomy. Advocates of the transhiatal approach (in which a cervical and celiac lymph node dissection may still be performed) have demonstrated that overall survival is equivalent and that overall morbidity is less.[28]

Rice et al reported their results with preoperative chemotherapy and radiation therapy for esophageal cancer in elderly patients. In this study, 312 consecutive patients underwent esophagectomy for esophageal cancer. Outcomes of patients aged 70 years and older who underwent preoperative therapy were compared with those of patients younger than 70 years who received preoperative therapy. There were no differences between the two groups in the rates of postoperative cardiac, pulmonary, neurologic, gastrointestinal, or anastomotic complications.[29]

Despite surgical and anesthetic advances over the years, morbidity and mortality rates of esophageal resection have been consistently higher than those associated with other commonly performed general and thoracic surgical procedures. Birkmeyer et al analyzed the effect of hospital volume on outcome from complex surgical procedures using information from the national Medicare claims database. Mortality was found to decrease as volume increased for all types of procedures analyzed, but the relative importance of volume varied markedly according to the type of procedure. For esophageal resection, adjusted mortality rates at very-low-volume hospitals were 11.9% higher than at very-high-volume hospitals.[1] In a subsequent study, the effect of surgeon volume was investigated. In this study, surgeon volume was found to be inversely related to operative mortality for all procedures studied. The adjusted odds ratio for operative death (for patients with a low-volume surgeon versus those with a high-volume surgeon) varied widely according to the procedure, and surgeon volume accounted for a large proportion of the apparent effect of the hospital volume, accounting for 46% of mortality for esophagectomy. For most procedures, including esophageal resection and lung resection, the mortality rate was found to be higher among patients of low-volume surgeons than among those of high-volume surgeons, regardless of the surgical volume of the hospital in which they practiced.[2]

Improvements in perioperative care, surgical techniques, and anesthetic techniques have consistently led to decreased complication rates, but esophagectomy remains a formidable operation. Many analyses have been performed to identify the most important risk factors for esophagectomy.[30–36] Perhaps the most important contributor to morbidity and mortality after esophagectomy is the development of pulmonary complications.[37–43] Other factors have been demonstrated in individual studies to be associated with increased mortality after esophagectomy: age, atrial fibrillation, operative approach, extent of resection, genetic and immune factors, nutrition, the use of induction therapy, and pain management.[37] However, the importance of these factors varies across studies, with the exception of age.[44]

Several factors have been associated with pulmonary complications after esophagectomy, including issues related to the preoperative status (age, nutritional status, induction therapy, baseline pulmonary function, ethanol use, smoking history, poor performance status), intraoperative details (stage and location of tumor, surgical approach, estimated blood loss, length of surgical procedure, entry into two separate body cavities, disruption of bronchial innervation and lymphatic circulation), and postoperative details (pulmonary toilet, vocal cord paralysis or recurrent laryngeal nerve palsy, postoperative respiratory muscle dysfunction). In one series, pulmonary morbidity was the primary cause of death in 54.5% of patients, and respiratory failure associated with pneumonia was an important component of the clinical course in over 80% of deaths.[37] Similarly, Dumont et al also noted that 2/3 of all fatal complications were respiratory in nature.[39] In the Avendano et al study of 61 patients after esophagectomy, all patients who died postoperatively experienced pneumonia.[38] Kinugasa et al found the development of pneumonia after esophagectomy to be associated with worse prognosis for overall survival ($P < .01$), along with pathologic tumor stage, and they showed that those with pneumonia had 5-year survival of 26.7%, while those without pneumonia had 53.4% survival at 5 years.[41]

One of the most consistently proven preoperative factors associated with postoperative pulmonary morbidity is advanced age. Sauvanet et al showed pulmonary morbidity to be associated with age above 60 years.[35] Kozlow et al also show a strong association between aspiration pneumonia and age.[45] In addition, advanced age has also been shown to be an independent predictor of mortality after esophagectomy.[30,37,42]

Modification of This Question in Light of New Research: This question should remain unmodified on the research agenda.

***ThoracicSurg 16 (Level B)*: Instruments to measure age-specific outcomes of surgery for esophageal cancer need to be developed and validated. Functional status and quality of life should be among the outcomes assessed.**

New Research Addressing This Question: No new research addressing this question reported during the current search period from October 2002 to December 2005 has come to light.

Modification of This Question in Light of New Research: This question should remain unmodified on the research agenda.

***ThoracicSurg 17 (Level A)*: Large clinical esophageal cancer trials should incorporate the age-specific instruments described in ThoracicSurg 16.**

New Research Addressing This Question: No new research addressing this question reported during the current search period from October 2002 to December 2005 has come to light.

Modification of This Question in Light of New Research: This question should remain unmodified on the research agenda.

***ThoracicSurg 18 (Level B)*: Esophagectomy could be used as a model for highly complex surgical procedures in the elderly patient to answer the following questions:**

- **What makes the high-volume center able to provide better care for elderly esophagectomy patients?**
- **Do high-volume centers achieve better surgical outcomes with the oldest-old patients?**

- **In what ways can care be improved for the elderly patient after esophagectomy?**
- **Once a formula for success is characterized, is it applicable to the care of elderly patients receiving other types of major operations?**

New Research Addressing This Question: No new research addressing this question reported during the current search period from October 2002 to December 2005 has come to light.

Modification of This Question in Light of New Research: This question should remain unmodified on the research agenda.

BENIGN ESOPHAGEAL DISEASE

See *New Frontiers,* pp. 133–134.

ThoracicSurg 19 (Level B): **A structured literature review should be performed and a consensus conference between gastroenterologists and surgeons should be organized to establish criteria, based on symptoms and quality of life, for intervention in the management of gastroesophageal reflux disease, particularly in elderly patients.**

New Research Addressing This Question: No new research addressing this question reported during the current search period from October 2002 to December 2005 has come to light.

Modification of This Question in Light of New Research: This question should remain unmodified on the research agenda.

ThoracicSurg 20 (Level A): **A prospective trial of laparoscopic antireflux surgery comparing elderly patients with younger matched control patients operated on during the same period should be performed to determine the suitability of this operation for the elderly patient.**

New Research Addressing This Question: The advisability of such aggressive antireflux therapy for all patients with gastroesophageal reflux disease remains controversial, although advocates of this aggressive approach argue that acid reflux is the main factor contributing to carcinogenesis and that its elimination should prevent cancer.[25]

Modification of This Question in Light of New Research: This question should remain unmodified on the research agenda.

RESEARCH IN SUPPORT OF IMPROVED CARE

See *New Frontiers,* pp. 134–135. This discussion contained no research agenda items.

NEW HORIZONS IN GERIATRIC GENERAL THORACIC SURGERY

New technologies just emerging may make major changes in the way that we diagnose and stage lung and esophageal cancer. These techniques include magnetic navigation bronchoscopy,[46] endoscopic bronchoscopic ultrasound biopsy,[47] and endoscopic confocal microscopy.[48] It is conceivable that a simple bronchoscopy or CT-guided biopsy may obtain enough tissue to confirm cancer and develop a genetic footprint of the tumor. On the basis of current studies, some patients may go straight to chemotherapy or combined modality therapy. The endoscopic bronchoscopic ultrasound biopsy may replace mediastinoscopy for staging locally advanced cancers. The endoscopic confocal microscopy may allow in-situ diagnosis of cancer both in the esophagus and in the airway. We may be able to detect such early cancers as to allow curative therapies that are concentrated at the surface of the mucosa. Clinical studies are necessary to confirm the reproducibility of the results before therapeutic trials may begin. These diagnostic techniques are especially suitable to the elderly population.

ThoracicSurg 21 (Level A): **Genetic profiles should be collected on lung and esophageal cancer and paired with data on long-term survival to assess traditional staging and revise the staging system as needed.**

ThoracicSurg 22 (Level B): **Observational studies are needed to compare new technologies for diagnosis and staging of lung and esophageal cancer with traditional methods.**

REFERENCES

1. Birkmeyer JD, Siewers AE, Finlayson EV, et al. Hospital volume and surgical mortality in the United States. N Engl J Med 2002;346:1128-1137.
2. Birkmeyer JD, Stukel TA, Siewers AE, et al. Surgeon volume and operative mortality in the United States. N Engl J Med 2003;349:2117-2127.
3. Ettinger DS, Bepler G, Bueno R, et al. Non-small cell lung cancer clinical practice guidelines in oncology. J Natl Compr Canc Netw 2006;4:548-582.
4. LoCicero J, 3rd, Yee J. Geriatric general thoracic surgery. In Solomon DH, LoCicero J, 3rd, Rosenthal RA (eds): New Frontiers in Geriatrics Research: An Agenda for Surgical and Related Medical Specialties. New York: American Geriatrics Society, 2004, pp. 111-145 (online at http://www.frycomm.com/ags/rasp).
5. Henschke CI, McCauley DI, Yankelevitz DF, et al. Early Lung Cancer Action Project: overall design and findings from baseline screening. Lancet 1999;354:99-105.
6. Henschke CI, Yankelevitz DF, Libby DM, et al. Survival of patients with stage I lung cancer detected on CT screening. N Engl J Med 2006;355:1763-1771.
7. Lemaire A, Nikolic I, Petersen T, et al. Nine-year single center experience with cervical mediastinoscopy: complications and false negative rate. Ann Thorac Surg 2006;82:1185-1189; discussion 1189-1190.
8. Gonzalez-Stawinski GV, Lemaire A, Merchant F, et al. A comparative analysis of positron emission tomography and mediastinoscopy in staging non-small cell lung cancer. J Thorac Cardiovasc Surg 2003;126:1900-1905.
9. Reed CE, Harpole DH, Posther KE, et al. Results of the American College of Surgeons Oncology Group Z0050 trial: the utility of positron emission tomography in staging potentially operable non-small cell lung cancer. J Thorac Cardiovasc Surg 2003;126:1943-1951.
10. D'Amico TA. Molecular staging and the selection of therapy for non-small cell lung cancer. Semin Thorac Cardiovasc Surg 2005;17:180-185.

11. Brooks KR, To K, Joshi MB, et al. Measurement of chemoresistance markers in patients with stage III non-small cell lung cancer: a novel approach for patient selection. Ann Thorac Surg 2003;76:187-193; discussion 193.
12. Sullivan V, Tran T, Holmstrom A, et al. Advanced age does not exclude lobectomy for non-small cell lung carcinoma. Chest 2005;128:2671-2676.
13. Matsuoka H, Okada M, Sakamoto T, Tsubota N. Complications and outcomes after pulmonary resection for cancer in patients 80 to 89 years of age. Eur J Cardiothorac Surg 2005;28:380-383.
14. Sawada S, Komori E, Nogami N, et al. Advanced age is not correlated with either short-term or long-term postoperative results in lung cancer patients in good clinical condition. Chest 2005;128:1557-1563.
15. de Rijke JM, Schouten LJ, ten Velde GP, et al. Influence of age, comorbidity and performance status on the choice of treatment for patients with non-small cell lung cancer; results of a population-based study. Lung Cancer 2004;46:233-245.
16. Non-small Cell Lung Cancer Collaborative Group. Chemotherapy for non-small cell lung cancer. Cochrane Database Syst Rev 2000:CD002139.
17. Arriagada R, Bergman B, Dunant A, et al. Cisplatin-based adjuvant chemotherapy in patients with completely resected non-small-cell lung cancer. N Engl J Med 2004;350:351-360.
18. Strauss GM, Jerndon J, Maddaus MA, et al. Randomized clinical trial of adjuvant chemotherapy with paclitaxel and carboplatin following resection in Stage 1B non-small cell lung cancer (NSCLC): Report of Cancer and Leukemia Group B (CALGB) Protocol 9633. ASCO Annual Meeting Proceedings (Post-Meeting Edition). J Clin Oncol 2004;22:7019.
19. Winton T, Livingston R, Johnson D, et al. Vinorelbine plus cisplatin vs. observation in resected non-small-cell lung cancer. N Engl J Med 2005;352:2589-2597.
20. Betticher DC, Hsu Schmitz SF, Totsch M, et al. Mediastinal lymph node clearance after docetaxel-cisplatin neoadjuvant chemotherapy is prognostic of survival in patients with stage IIIA pN2 non-small-cell lung cancer: a multicenter phase II trial. J Clin Oncol 2003;21:1752-1759.
21. Daniels LJ, Balderson SS, Onaitis MW, D'Amico TA. Thoracoscopic lobectomy: a safe and effective strategy for patients with stage I lung cancer. Ann Thorac Surg 2002;74:860-864.
22. Onaitis MW, Petersen RP, Balderson SS, et al. Thoracoscopic lobectomy is a safe and versatile procedure: experience with 500 consecutive patients. Ann Surg 2006;244:420-425.
23. Petersen RP, Pham D, Toloza EM, et al. Thoracoscopic lobectomy: a safe and effective strategy for patients receiving induction therapy for non-small cell lung cancer. Ann Thorac Surg 2006;82:214-218; discussion 219.
24. Brenner M, Hanna NM, Mina-Araghi R, et al. Innovative approaches to lung volume reduction for emphysema. Chest 2004;126:238-248.
25. Spechler SJ. Clinical practice. Barrett's esophagus. N Engl J Med 2002;346:836-842.
26. Overholt BF, Panjehpour M, Halberg DL. Photodynamic therapy for Barrett's esophagus with dysplasia and/or early stage carcinoma: long-term results. Gastrointest Endosc 2003;58:183-188.
27. Bergman JJ, Sondermeijer C, Peters FP, et al. Circumferential balloon-based radiofrequency ablation of Barrett's esophagus in patients with low-grade dysplasia or high-grade dysplasia with and without a prior endoscopic resection using the HALO360 ablation system. Gastrointest Endosc 2006;63:Abstract 137.
28. Ajani J, Bekaii-Saab T, D'Amico TA, et al. Esophageal Cancer Clinical Practice Guidelines. J Natl Compr Canc Netw 2006;4:328-347 (available online: http://www.nccn.org/professionals/physician_gls/PDF/esophageal.pdf).

29. Rice DC, Correa AM, Vaporciyan AA, et al. Preoperative chemoradiotherapy prior to esophagectomy in elderly patients is not associated with increased morbidity. Ann Thorac Surg 2005;79:391-397; discussion 391-397.
30. Bailey SH, Bull DA, Harpole DH, et al. Outcomes after esophagectomy: a ten-year prospective cohort. Ann Thorac Surg 2003;75:217-222; discussion 222.
31. Bartels H, Stein HJ, Siewert JR. Risk analysis in esophageal surgery. Recent Results Cancer Res 2000;155:89-96.
32. Ferguson MK, Martin TR, Reeder LB, Olak J. Mortality after esophagectomy: risk factor analysis. World J Surg 1997;21:599-603; discussion 603-594.
33. Jamieson GG, Mathew G, Ludemann R, et al. Postoperative mortality following oesophagectomy and problems in reporting its rate. Br J Surg 2004;91:943-947.
34. Rizk NP, Bach PB, Schrag D, et al. The impact of complications on outcomes after resection for esophageal and gastroesophageal junction carcinoma. J Am Coll Surg 2004;198:42-50.
35. Sauvanet A, Mariette C, Thomas P, et al. Mortality and morbidity after resection for adenocarcinoma of the gastroesophageal junction: predictive factors. J Am Coll Surg 2005;201:253-262.
36. Whooley BP, Law S, Murthy SC, et al. Analysis of reduced death and complication rates after esophageal resection. Ann Surg 2001;233:338-344.
37. Atkins BZ, Shah AS, Hutcheson KA, et al. Reducing hospital morbidity and mortality following esophagectomy. Ann Thorac Surg 2004;78:1170-1176.
38. Avendano CE, Flume PA, Silvestri GA, et al. Pulmonary complications after esophagectomy. Ann Thorac Surg 2002;73:922-926.
39. Dumont P, Wihlm JM, Hentz JG, et al. Respiratory complications after surgical treatment of esophageal cancer: a study of 309 patients according to the type of resection. Eur J Cardiothorac Surg 1995;9:539-543.
40. Ferguson MK, Durkin AE. Preoperative prediction of the risk of pulmonary complications after esophagectomy for cancer. J Thorac Cardiovasc Surg 2002;123:661-669.
41. Kinugasa S, Tachibana M, Yoshimura H, et al. Postoperative pulmonary complications are associated with worse short- and long-term outcomes after extended esophagectomy. J Surg Oncol 2004;88:71-77.
42. Law S, Wong KH, Kwok KF, et al. Predictive factors for postoperative pulmonary complications and mortality after esophagectomy for cancer. Ann Surg 2004;240:791-800.
43. Leo F, Venissac N, Palihovici R, et al. Aristotle, esophagectomy, and pulmonary complications. Ann Thorac Surg 2004;77:1503.
44. Poon RT, Law SY, Chu KM, et al. Esophagectomy for carcinoma of the esophagus in the elderly: results of current surgical management. Ann Surg 1998;227:357-364.
45. Kozlow JH, Berenholtz SM, Garrett E, et al. Epidemiology and impact of aspiration pneumonia in patients undergoing surgery in Maryland, 1999-2000. Crit Care Med 2003;31:1930-1937.
46. Gildea TR, Mazzone PJ, Karnak D, et al. Electromagnetic navigation diagnostic bronchoscopy: a prospective study. Am J Respir Crit Care Med 2006;174:982-989.
47. Yasufuku K, Nakajima T, Motoori K, et al. Comparison of endobronchial ultrasound, positron emission tomography, and CT for lymph node staging of lung cancer. Chest 2006;130:710-718.
48. Hoffman A, Goetz M, Vieth M, et al. Confocal laser endomicroscopy: technical status and current indications. Endoscopy 2006;38:1275-1283.

6

GERIATRIC CARDIAC SURGERY

*Joseph C. Cleveland, Jr., MD; Nicola A. Francalancia, MD, FACS**

Cardiovascular disease remains the leading cause of death among adults aged 65 and over in the United States and other Western populations. As the older age group continues to increase rapidly, the treatment of cardiovascular disease will become an increasingly important factor in the health of older persons. In fact, of the over 6 million cardiovascular procedures performed during 2002 in the United States, more than half were carried out in patients aged 65 or over. [1,2] Cardiovascular surgical interventions are offered to older patients to improve both length and quality of life. The challenges of thoracic aortic procedures and of providing surgical therapy for coronary artery disease (CAD) and valvular disease in older patients are increasing. The field of cardiac surgery faces a demand for continual improvement in the processes and structures of care to address the unique problems encountered in older patients undergoing cardiac surgery.

This chapter updates the research agenda for cardiac surgery for the older adult that was presented in *New Frontiers in Geriatrics Research.* [3] Discussion of the more recent research for each cluster of agenda items from *New Frontiers* is found in the section Progress in Geriatric Cardiac Surgery. The Key Questions for research in geriatric cardiac surgery remain as stated in that publication, with one addition. For the new Key Question and discussion, see the section New Horizons in Geriatric Cardiac Surgery at the end of the chapter.

Elderly patients still require greater resources and are more likely to suffer stroke and a prolonged length of stay following cardiac surgery. Improvement in anesthesia, postoperative care, better myocardial protection, and perhaps preoperative prehabilitation require continual refinement to yield better outcomes. The care of elderly patients will best be delivered by continual close collaboration between cardiac surgeons and geriatricians to synergistically offer different perspectives and skill sets, with the goal of optimizing outcomes for elders who undergo cardiac surgery.

CardiacSurg KQ1: **To what extent do cardiac surgical operations improve functional outcomes in an elderly patient population?**

CardiacSurg KQ2: **How can stroke and neurocognitive deterioration following cardiac surgical procedures be reduced among elderly patients?**

CardiacSurg KQ3: **What changes in peri-operative care are needed to improve outcomes in the elderly cardiac surgical patient?**

METHODS

To update the review of issues that affect decisions about the role and potential benefits of surgery for heart disease in older adults, we searched the National Library of Medicine's

* Cleveland: Associate Professor of Surgery and Surgical Director, Cardiac Transplantation and MCS, Department of Surgery, Division of Cardiothoracic Surgery, University of Colorado at Denver Health Sciences Center, Denver, CO; Francalancia: Cardiac Surgery Associates, St. Francis Heart Center, Indianapolis, IN.

PubMed database for the period from April 2000 to December 2005. This time frame covers the period from the end of the searches for *New Frontiers* to the writing of this update. The search strategy combined terms for specified cardiac surgery procedures with terms for complications, and it was further qualified by adding the various terms for risk factors, age factors, outcomes, quality of life, and rehabilitation. The search resulted in 10,742 references. From among the relevant papers, we chose those that emphasize the management of such issues as peri-operative care, postoperative complications, and quality of life for the elderly cardiac surgical patient. Age as a risk factor for specific cardiac surgical procedures was also examined.

PROGRESS IN GERIATRIC CARDIAC SURGERY

THE CHANGING PATTERN OF PATIENTS UNDERGOING HEART SURGERY

See *New Frontiers,* pp. 147–149.

CardiacSurg 1 (Level B): **Risk profiles must be revised to accurately reflect current medical and surgical practices with regard to advanced age and heart surgery. Existing databases must be expanded to include functional outcomes in elderly patients and to monitor cardiac care patterns for elderly patients. This will yield important outcome data to guide clinical decision making for the aging population.**

CardiacSurg 2 (Level A): **Intervention studies (clinical trials) of specific geriatric clinical pathways in cardiac surgery are needed to identify possible beneficial effects on outcomes.**

CardiacSurg 3 (Level D): **Methods for estimating future total costs of cardiac surgery in elderly patients, including the peri-operative and rehabilitative periods, need to be developed.**

CardiacSurg 4 (Level A): **Multicenter randomized controlled trials comparing catheter-based interventions and coronary artery bypass grafting for the treatment of coronary artery disease in geriatric cardiac patients is needed.**

CardiacSurg 5 (Level D): **Studies are needed to review resources that accommodate potential longer length of hospital stays by elderly heart surgery patients who present with greater acuity and complications following surgery.**

CardiacSurg 6 (Level B): **Predictive models are needed to estimate the numbers of patients with risk factors for heart disease who may ultimately require surgical care (eg, the current diabetic population that will require surgery in their 60s through their 80s).**

CardiacSurg 7 (Level B): **Prospective cohort studies are needed that investigate the potential role of cardiac assist devices in the treatment**

of congestive heart failure in elderly patients deemed unlikely to undergo heart transplantation.

CardiacSurg 8 (Level B): **Further investigation of the senescent myocardium and age-specific physiologic response to stress is needed to identify reasons for pump failure or for low-output syndrome.**

New Research Addressing These Questions: The characteristics of patients undergoing cardiac surgery have continued to change over the past five decades. Succinctly stated, the profiles of patients who are referred for cardiac surgery indicate that they are older and have more comorbid conditions. Ferguson et al reviewed the Society of Thoracic Surgeons National Adult Cardiac Surgical Database during the period 1990 through 1999 for patients undergoing coronary artery bypass grafting (CABG) procedure. Several important findings emerged from this observational analysis of over 1.1 million patient records. The mean age of patients undergoing CABG increased from 63.7 years in 1990 to 65.1 years in 1999. Other comorbidities, such as diabetes mellitus and prior stroke, also increased during this study period. Interestingly, although the predicted operative risk increased from 2.6% in 1990 to 3.4% in 1999, the observed operative mortality decreased from 3.4% in 1990 to 3.0% in 1999. There was, however, no analysis of the cohort of patients aged 65 or older to determine whether the improvement in operative mortality was also enjoyed by the geriatric patients. Similarly, if one examines the Coronary Artery Surgery Study registry of patients undergoing CABG from 1975 to 1979, only 12.2% were 65 years of age and older. Two decades later, over half (56%) of the patients undergoing CABG were aged 65 years and older.[2]

Analysis of valvular heart surgery trends reveal similar patterns to those observed for CABG. Nowicki et al examined data from the Northern New England Cardiovascular Disease Study Group data registry from the period of 1990 to 1999. In patients undergoing mitral valve surgery, the mean age increased from 64.7 years of age in 1990 to 67.0 in 1999. More striking was the proportion of patients aged 80 years or older undergoing mitral valve surgery. The data show that mitral valve operations were infrequently performed in octogenarians prior to 1990, but by 1999 that age group represented 12.4% of all patients undergoing this surgery. Over the course of this study, the majority of patients underwent surgery for mitral regurgitation rather than stenosis. This report demonstrates the shifting patient population who receive cardiac surgery and highlights that older patients with poorer left ventricular function are increasingly offered mitral valve surgery.[4]

Though one can question whether this phenomenon is observed only in New England, other reports substantiate this trend toward increasingly offering older patients valve surgery. Collart et al from France describe a similar pattern of referring patients aged 80 and older for valvular surgery.[5]

Modification of These Questions in Light of New Research: No changes or additions to the research agenda are recommended.

Coronary Artery Disease

See *New Frontiers,* pp. 150–154.

CardiacSurg 9 (Level B): **Prospective studies of young and elderly patients are needed to investigate lung function as a risk for coronary**

artery bypass grafting by determining the degree of pulmonary compromise that would shift risk from surgical to medical management of coronary artery disease.

CardiacSurg 10 (Level B): **Cohort studies on various cardiopulmonary bypass techniques are needed, with morbidity in elderly patients as the chief outcome measure.**

CardiacSurg 11 (Level A): **Randomized controlled trials are needed that select the most promising cardiopulmonary bypass techniques and compare them, again with morbidity in elderly patients as the chief outcome measure.**

CardiacSurg 12 (Level B): **Cohort studies are needed to identify risk factors and benefit predictors of myocardial protective techniques for both on- and off-pump coronary artery bypass in elderly patients. This includes myocardial protective strategies aimed specifically at the aged myocardium and mechanical or chemical protective techniques when off-pump procedures are used.**

CardiacSurg 13 (Level A): **Randomized controlled trials are needed that select the most promising myocardial protective techniques and compare them with each other and with traditional bypass techniques; morbidity, need for reintervention, and relief of symptoms in elderly patients should be the main outcome measures. The best on-pump method could also be compared with the best off-pump method.**

CardiacSurg 14 (Level B): **Cohort studies are needed of innovative and emerging therapies for coronary artery disease (eg, gene therapy, transmyocardial laser revascularization), as well as of other complementary treatments in the elderly patient population.**

CardiacSurg 15 (Level B): **Cohort studies are needed to investigate the profiles and clinical course of elderly patients who undergo angioplasty and to establish future risks of reintervention or need for coronary artery bypass grafting.**

CardiacSurg 16 (Level B): **Outcome studies are needed of conduit use (mammary artery, radial artery, saphenous vein graft) in elderly patients, specifically to analyze a possible selection bias by surgeon in the choice of conduit.**

CardiacSurg 17 (Level B): **Studies are needed that apply and test minimally invasive techniques that may reduce cost, decrease length of stay, and yield good long-term outcome in elderly coronary artery bypass grafting patients.**

New Research Addressing These Questions: Advances in the treatment of CAD, including early intervention, prevention, risk modification, and general public awareness, have resulted in improved clinical outcomes in myocardial ischemia. Patients presenting with acute coronary syndromes (ACS) deserve prompt reperfusion for myocardium at risk. The entire scope of defining practice patterns for elderly patients presenting with ACS is outside the scope of this chapter; however, a brief consideration of this topic seems warranted. The overarching theme in the management of elderly patients with ACS is presented in an analysis of the Global Registry of Acute Coronary Events (GRACE) data. Avezum et al examined over 200,000 patients reported to this observational registry and found that seemingly standard therapies such as aspirin, β-blockers, thrombolytic therapy, statins, and glycoprotein IIb/IIIa inhibitors were prescribed less in patients aged 65 or older, whereas calcium channel antagonists were not. Coronary angiography and percutaneous coronary intervention rates also significantly decreased with age. [6] In summary, elderly ACS patients do not receive evidence-based therapies, and the inconsistent utilization of standard invasive therapies argues strongly for the need for clinical trials that examine the use of these therapies in elderly patients. (See the new Key Question, CardiacSurg KQ4, in the section New Horizons in Geriatric Cardiac Surgery at the end of the chapter.)

The treatment paradigm for CAD has changed dramatically during the past decade. In essence, a shift toward increasing utilization of percutaneous coronary intervention (PCI) has occurred, particularly for multivessel CAD. Concurrently, the number of CABG procedures has decreased, particularly in the past 3 years. Mack et al reviewed the HCA Casemix Database for the years 1999 to 2002. This database is utilized by the 76 HCA hospitals performing cardiac surgery. During this period, PCI accounted for 65% of all coronary revascularization, with an annual growth rate of nearly 7%, whereas CABG volume declined at 2% annually. [7] If one examines these trends over a longer period, even greater differences emerge. Ulrich et al queried the rate of PCI versus CABG in Washington State from 1987 to 2001. While CABG rates remained stable until 1997 and then declined by 20%, PCI rates demonstrated an explosion—with an increase of PCI rates by 128%. [8] In summary, multiple reports substantiate the relatively rapid growth and acceptance of PCI for multivessel coronary revascularization, with a concomitant decline in the utilization of CABG in the treatment of CAD.

Three randomized controlled trials have been conducted and are widely cited to support PCI as an equivalent therapy to CABG for the treatment of multivessel CAD. When reading these trials, one must realize that the term *multivessel* does not necessarily mean three-vessel CAD, as a great proportion of these patients in these trials have single- or double-vessel disease with preserved left ventricular function. The Arterial Revascularization Therapies Studies (ARTS) group randomized 1205 patients to either CABG or PCI; the primary clinical endpoint of this study examined freedom from major adverse cardiac or cerebrovascular events at 1 year. Assessment at 1 year showed no difference in rates of death, myocardial infarction, or stroke between the two groups. However, the PCI group was more likely to have undergone another intervention (16.8 % PCI versus 3.5% CABG). Although not cited as an endpoint, relief of angina was substantially greater in the CABG group (89.5%) than in the PCI group (78.9%) at 1 year. It is noteworthy, however, that the mean age of patients in this study was 61 years for both groups, and the mean ejection fraction was 61% in both groups—suggesting that patients were carefully selected for enrollment in the study. The 5-year follow-up of the ARTS study revealed that there was no difference in mortality between stenting and surgery. However, the disparity in revascularization rates widened further, with a 30.3% re-intervention rate in the stent group versus 8.8% in the CABG group. [9] The SoS (Stent or Surgery) trial similarly randomized 988 patients with symptomatic multivessel CAD to PCI or to CABG. Again, like other randomized trials, the population studied was relatively young (mean age 61 years) and predominantly male (79%). In this study, a mortality difference favoring CABG was observed, with a 2% death rate in CABG patients compared with 5% in the PCI group. Also, the rate of repeat revascularization for PCI, although lower than other studies, remained at 21%, compared with 6% in the CABG group. All patients were followed for a minimum of 1 year, and the median follow-up was 2 years. [10] Lastly, the ERACI II study examined both 30-day and 1-year outcomes in 450 patients randomized to receive either stenting (PCI) or CABG. Although the mean age of both groups was approximately 62 years, 38% of the patients were older than 65 years. At 30 days' follow-up the composite major adverse rate (death, myocardial infarction, repeat revascularization, and stroke) favored PCI with a 3.6% rate versus 12.3% for the CABG patients. At 1 year, the mortality advantage enjoyed by the PCI group remained, with a 96.9% survival in PCI group versus 92.5% in the CABG group. In concert with the other two studies, the rate of repeat revascularization was 16.8% for PCI but 4.8% for CABG. [11]

Though multicenter randomized trials are considered the gold standard for comparing therapies, these trials must be considered in the perspective of other investigations and for the populations of patients in these trials. When one considers the population used in these randomized trials, concerns arise regarding the applicability of their findings to "real world" practice patterns for PCI and CABG. This statement is supported by the reporting of the ERACI II trial—in which nearly 2800 patients were screened to obtain 500 for study (roughly 20% eligibility). Two other retrospective studies add further controversy to the role of PCI versus CABG for the treatment of multivessel CAD. Brener et al at the Cleveland Clinic examined 6603 patients undergoing revascularization at their center in the 1990s; 872 underwent PCI and 5161 underwent CABG. Nearly half the patients had significant left ventricular dysfunction or diabetes mellitus. This group of investigators utilized propensity analysis to attempt to control for selection bias and match the groups as evenly as possible. At 5 years, the unadjusted mortality rate for CABG was 14% versus 16% for PCI. However, when PCI was adjusted for mortality with the propensity model, PCI was found to be associated with an increased risk of death (hazard ratio 2.3, 95% confidence interval [CI] 1.9 to 2.9, $P < .0001$). Thus, in this group of patients with multivessel CAD and many high-risk characteristics, CABG was associated with better survival than PCI. [12] Again, one must also consider the clinical setting of this study to appropriately frame these results. The Cleveland Clinic is a large-volume center with a very low operative mortality rate for CABG.

Perhaps the most intriguing and controversial study to fuel this controversy was conducted by Hannan et al. This retrospective study examined the two mandatory reporting registries for cardiac intervention in New York State. The Cardiac Surgery Reporting System and the Percutaneous Coronary Intervention Reporting System were examined for the endpoint of death or the composite endpoint of death or revascularization over a 3-year period from January 1997 to December 2000. It is remarkable that the median age of PCI patients was 65 versus 67 for CABG patients, and that 38.1% of the PCI patients were aged 70 or older and 42.4% of CABG patients were aged 70 or older. Again, the older age of patients examined reflected the "real world" practice in New York State, unlike the younger patients selected for the randomized studies. The analysis of the survival in both cohorts yielded an advantage for CABG over PCI. For three-vessel disease involving the proximal left anterior descending artery, the adjusted hazard ratio favoring CABG was

0.64. Also, 3-year rates of revascularization were considerably higher for PCI patients than for CABG patients. In the stenting group, 7.8% underwent CABG and 27.3% underwent a subsequent PCI, compared with 0.3% of the CABG group undergoing another CABG and 4.6 % of the CABG group undergoing PCI. [13] These studies will not settle the controversy that continues in the management of the patient with multivessel CAD. The advent of drug-eluting stents has not been fully evaluated yet, but preliminary analyses suggest a much lower rate of need of subsequent revascularization.

The surgical management of CAD has undergone a significant paradigm shift with the advent and development of "beating-heart" or "off-pump" coronary artery bypass (CAB) surgery. On the basis principally of descriptions by Benetti et al [14] and Buffolo et al, [15] surgeons began exploring techniques for conducting multivessel revascularization without the use of cardiopulmonary bypass—so called off-pump CAB. Even though advocates of this technology firmly believe that off-pump CAB is associated with superior outcomes, available data suggest that the avoidance of cardiopulmonary bypass does not necessarily improve outcomes. [16] The use of off-pump CAB has not been extensively studied in elderly patients, although advocates of off-pump surgery often state that this group of patients may benefit from off-pump CAB.

Athanasiou et al published a meta-analysis of nine studies which examined off-pump CAB in patients aged 70 years or older. All nine studies were observational and were published between 1999 and 2002. Noteworthy was the fact that the total number of subjects included was 4475, of which 1253 (28%) underwent off-pump CAB and 3222 (72%) underwent CAB with cardiopulmonary bypass. The overall analysis focused upon neurologic outcomes; stroke was chosen as the primary endpoint. This analysis documented a lower incidence of stroke in elderly patients who had off-pump CAB (1%) versus CAB performed with cardiopulmonary bypass (3%). Several limitations of this study bear comment. Unfortunately, because of the observational nature of this study, it was impossible to match the groups for baseline neurologic function. Second, bias in selection of patients for off-pump CAB is also a potential confounding variable. Last, rigorous definition of stroke varied between studies. [17]

Other studies have shown some specific increased risk profiles in elderly patients undergoing surgical revascularization. CAB following acute myocardial infarction carries added risk for mortality. Kaul et al observed that age 70 years is an independent predictor of early mortality for patients who undergo CAB within 30 days of an acute myocardial infarction. [18] In a study of over 4500 patients undergoing CAB at the Toronto Hospital, patients who had low-output syndrome were found to be aged 70 years or older, resulting in an odds ratio increase of 1.5. [19] This suggests that efforts to reduce myocardial ischemia, a known precipitating factor for low-output syndrome, should be investigated, with particular emphasis on the aging myocardium. In multivariate analysis of 2264 patients undergoing CAB, Del Rizzo et al noted that age above 70, re-do surgery, poor left ventricular function, renal impairment, and the presence of preoperative intra-aortic balloon pump are predictors of mortality. [20]

For elderly patients undergoing CAB, time to recovery may determine needs for postoperative resources and rehospitalization. Paone et al studied 146 patients aged 70 and over with the expectation that these patients would progress through the postoperative clinical pathway in much the same way as a younger comparison group. Although age was found to be one significant factor in contributing to increased length of stay, the study suggests that extraordinary modifications of the clinical pathways are not necessary for success with elderly patients. Advanced age was not found to be significantly associated with 30-day hospital readmission following CAB. [21] With regard to the health status of elderly patients following CAB, Conaway et al examined the symptoms, function, and quality of life in elderly patients and younger patients following CAB. This group administered the Seattle Angina Questionnaire to 690 patients (156 were aged 75 years or older, 534 were younger than 75 years) at baseline and at 1 year post-CAB. The first 224 patients were given the questionnaire monthly for 1 year; the remainder had the questionnaire only at baseline and at 1 year. Of interest, although initial peri-operative mortality was similar (2.6% versus 2.2%) at 1 year, the elderly cohort had a mortality of 11.5% versus 5.4% for the younger group. Recovery of physical function was slower in the elderly group, and a significant age-time interaction existed in the elderly patients, showing a slower time to recovery. At 1 year post-CAB, however, angina relief and quality of life did not differ by age. [22] Hedeshian et al examined whether increasing age has impacts on 6-month functional outcome after CAB. They utilized the Duke Activity Status Index (DASI) and analyzed age-specific cohorts for functional outcomes following CAB. Although the mean baseline DASI score was lower in patients undergoing CAB who were 70 years or older, the 6-month change in DASI scores did not differ between the patients aged 70 or older and those who were younger. Further, when three separate terciles of age were analyzed (age 31–60, age 61–70, and age 71–90), the 6-month changes in DASI did not differ. The authors concluded that patients older than 70 present for CAB with a lower functional level, and they remain at a lower functional level at 6 months post-CAB. The change in functional improvement following CAB, however, does not appear to be affected by age. [23]

Cognitive decline after CAB constitutes a great source of concern for both physicians and patients who undergo the procedure. Indeed, a recent report by van Dijk et al [24] estimated the incidence to be 22.5% of patients following CAB; however, others have estimated the incidence to approach nearly 50%. Ho et al identified several predictors of cognitive decline following CAB. They utilized 994 patients in the VA Processes Structures and Outcomes of Care in Cardiac Surgery study. These patients completed a short battery of cognitive tests at baseline and 6 months following CAB surgery. In this multivariate analysis, patient characteristics associated with cognitive decline included cerebrovascular disease, peripheral vascular disease, history of chronic disabling neurologic illness, and living alone. Years of education and cardiopulmonary bypass time were found to be inversely associated with the risk of cognitive decline. Age did not emerge in the risk model to predict cognitive decline. [25] In contrast, Tuman et al have noted age to be an important risk factor for cognitive decline after CAB. [26]

Another entity that consumes great resources and prolongs hospital length of stay is postoperative atrial fibrillation. Mathew et al examined risk factors for the development of atrial fibrillation after CAB surgery. This study was a prospective observational study involving 4657 patients at multiple centers. The endpoint studied was new-onset atrial fibrillation after CAB. Overall, 1503 patients (32.3%) developed atrial fibrillation after CAB. Risk factors for the development of atrial fibrillation after CAB in this study included a history of atrial fibrillation, chronic obstructive pulmonary disease, postoperative withdrawal of either a β-blocker or angiotensin-converting enzyme inhibitor, and advanced age. Advanced age was quantified by a 10-year increase, with an odds ratio of 1.75

for each 10-year increase.[27] On the basis of this study, anyone older than 70 years of age would be considered to be at high risk of developing atrial fibrillation. When all other preoperative risk factors are considered, advanced age is the most consistent predictor for the development of atrial fibrillation after CAB.[28–30] Multiple hypotheses are offered to explain this increased risk, including structural changes in the atria that occur with age, as well as nonuniform anisotropic conduction in the atria of elderly patients.[31] It bears comment, however, that advanced age alone is a risk factor for the development of atrial fibrillation independently of cardiac surgery, as observed in the Framingham population.

Modification of These Questions in Light of New Research: Research in coronary artery surgery should continue to focus on technical aspects of the operations that allow safer peri-operative management of the elderly CAB patient. In addition, future research should focus specifically on the processes of peri-operative management of sedation, analgesia, arrhythmias, physical and occupational therapies, and cardiac rehabilitation strategies that optimize the physiologic recovery of aged patients undergoing CAB.

Valve Surgery

See *New Frontiers,* pp. 155–157.

CardiacSurg 18 (Level A): **Prospective randomized trials are needed to compare regimens of anticoagulant therapy for elderly patients with a mechanical prosthesis to minimize valvular complications and thromboembolic complications. Such studies may require cost-benefit analysis of decreasing anticoagulation as a function of age in patients with valvular prostheses.**

CardiacSurg 19 (Level A): **Prospective randomized trials comparing minimally invasive aortic valve replacement with conventional methods in elderly patients are needed to assess the benefits of improved morbidity and decreased hospitalization.**

CardiacSurg 20 (Level A): **Prospective randomized trials comparing minimally invasive with conventional mitral valve operations in elderly patients are needed. These studies should include the efficacy and duration of repair and outcomes with respect to operative and peri-operative morbidity when thoracoscopic and robotic techniques are employed.**

New Research Addressing These Questions: Aortic stenosis is the most common adult heart valve condition in the Western world. Although the pathophysiology of the development of aortic stenosis is incompletely understood, the pathologic findings include the deposition of calcium about the aortic valve leaflets, in the aortic annulus, and with extension into the aortic sinuses. It is very likely that aortic sclerosis precedes stenosis, with stenosis marking the end stage of this process. Epidemiologic data suggest that aortic sclerosis is present in 20% to 30% of persons aged 65 years or older and 48% of those aged 85 and older. Aortic stenosis is present in 2% and 4%, respectively.[32] Clinical risk factors for aortic stenosis include age, male sex, smoking, diabetes mellitus, hypertension, CAD, and chronic renal failure. Once a patient is diagnosed with aortic stenosis, progression in gradients and velocities are 7 to 8 mm Hg per year and 0.3 meters per second.

These gradients correspond to a decrease in aortic valve area by approximately 0.2 cm^2 per year.[33] The natural history for patients with asymptomatic aortic stenosis closely parallels age- and sex-matched controls. However, with the onset of symptoms of angina, dyspnea, or heart failure, the prognosis changes dramatically without surgery; survival without surgery is only 50% at 2 years. Data regarding elderly patients who progress to symptoms with aortic stenosis are scarce; however, it is suggested that patients aged 70 or over have a worse prognosis without surgery of 2-year survival of only 37%.[34]

The decision process regarding referral of elderly patients for aortic valve replacement (AVR) remains clouded with controversy. Bouma et al surveyed 530 cardiologists in the Netherlands with a six-point scale questionnaire to determine patterns of referral for AVR in elderly patients. This survey with 32 case vignettes contained a scale from 1 to 6 regarding recommendation for AVR (1 = certainly no and 6 = certainly yes) in symptomatic aortic stenosis patients 70 years of age. Of 530 cardiologists, 275 (52%) responded to the survey. A wide variability was observed in the advice scores given. However, by the use of latent class regression analysis, six groups of cardiologists could be identified who within each group arrived at similar recommendations regarding valve replacement. Of these groups, 41% of the cardiologists were principally influenced by age of the patient rather than other clinical variables (valve area, left ventricular function, and comorbidities). Interestingly, comorbid conditions had very little effect on the decision to refer elderly patients for surgery across all cardiologists who participated in this study. The authors concluded that prospective observational studies are needed to appropriately characterize elderly patients who should undergo AVR for aortic stenosis.[35]

Several observational studies regarding outcomes for AVR in elderly patients have been reported. Collart et al sought to assess the pre- and postoperative mortality and morbidity factors in octogenarian patients undergoing AVR in Marseilles, France, during the period 1993 to 2003. They prospectively created a database that yielded 215 patients for study; the average age of patients operated on was 83 years. They further calculated the EuroSCORE for the patients and divided them into three groups—low risk, medium risk, and high risk—on the basis of the scores. Overall, operative mortality for this group was 8.8%; cardiogenic shock with low cardiac output compromising was the principal cause of death. The only preoperative factor that emerged as significant in a multivariate analysis was moderate depression in left ventricular function. Postoperative complications were experienced by 63% of patients; the onset of atrial fibrillation in 31% of patients was the most common complication. From the standpoint of quality-of-life indicators, 65% of patients had an Outcomes Management System (OMS) scale of 0 or 1 (0 = normal life without restriction, 4 = bedridden). Importantly, 77% of patients returned home, and 38% were able to live independently. The 5-year survival curve for this group was similar to the age-matched population without aortic valve surgery.[36]

Chiappini et al retrospectively analyzed outcomes after AVR in octogenarians in Italy. This series consisted of 115 patients treated between 1983 and April 2003 with AVR or AVR with concomitant CAB. The operative mortality was 8.5%, similar to Collart's findings, and the majority of peri-operative deaths occurred secondarily to low cardiac output with peri-operative myocardial infarction. Of interest, mechanical bioprostheses were implanted in 28% of these 115 patients. The 5-year actuarial survival in this group was strongly affected by the choice of prosthesis—it was a relatively robust 82% at 5 years in the bioprosthesis group versus 57% in the mechanical valve group. Among patients undergoing mechanical valve implantation, 22% experienced valve-related complications such as thromboembolic or bleeding events. In their analysis of their outcomes, the researchers identified preoperative ejection fraction, preoperative heart failure, and type of implanted prosthesis (bioprosthetic versus mechanical) as predictors of late death. This group did not undertake a systematic, rigorous analysis of quality-of-life indicators but reported that in telephone follow-up 98% of patients who underwent AVR were satisfied with this decision. [37]

Proponents of minimally invasive cardiac surgical procedures advocate the avoidance of sternotomy in performing AVR to potentially reduce morbidity. Sharony et al reported their experience with minimally invasive AVR in elderly patients. They performed a case-control study analyzing 515 patients aged 65 years or older. Their study cohort included patients who underwent isolated AVR from 1995 to 2002 at their institution. They matched 189 patients who had minimally invasive AVR with 189 patients undergoing AVR with conventional sternotomy. The minimally invasive group had either a small third intercostal space thoracotomy or a mini-sternotomy. Overall in-hospital mortality was identical in both groups—6.9%. Similar to other investigations, this analysis, by the use of multivariate analysis, showed that preoperative congestive heart failure, urgent or emergent status of operation, ejection fraction, and increasing age are risk factors for mortality. Complication rates also were similar in the two groups; however, the hospital length of stay was lower in the minimally invasive group—11 days versus 14 days in the conventional sternotomy group. A greater percentage of patients with minimally invasive AVR were discharged home—53% versus 38% in the group receiving conventional treatment. Acknowledging the limitations in retrospective case-control studies, these researchers concluded that minimally invasive techniques can be safely applied to AVR patients aged 65 and older. [38]

Mitral valve surgery in the elderly patient is much less well characterized than AVR. The natural history of mitral valve disease does not seem to have the same proclivity for aging-related changes with sclerosis and stenosis as is seen in the aortic valve. Kolh et al describe peri-operative outcomes and long-term results in patients undergoing cardiac surgery operations. Of the 182 patients reviewed who had cardiac operations from 1992 to 1998, only 12 patients had mitral valve surgery. Of this subgroup of 12 patients, mitral valve replacement was performed in 9 (75%) of these patients. This group could not offer any statistical insights into mitral valve surgery in the elderly age group with this small number of patients. However, peri-operative mortality was substantial: 25% of patients died. Despite the low number of patients, the authors conclude that mitral valve surgery should be offered only to patients without any other therapeutic option who remain without any other significant comorbid conditions. [39]

Mitral valve repair has become the preferred method of cardiac surgeons for addressing mitral valve regurgitation. Lee et al examined the feasibility and outcomes for mitral repair in elderly patients by reviewing their experience with 140 patients operated upon for mitral regurgitation, 44 of whom who were aged 70 years or older. Multivariate analysis indicated that preoperative cardiogenic shock but not age was a risk factor for death. The older patients in this group suffered more atrial fibrillation, prolonged ventilation, and hospital stay. The overall mortality approached 9.1% in those aged 70 or over versus 5.2% in the younger group. The researchers concluded that mitral valve surgery should not be denied to appropriate candidates on the basis of age alone. [40] (See also the new Key

Question in the section New Horizons in Geriatric Cardiac Surgery at the end of the chapter.)

Modification of These Questions in Light of New Research: Valvular heart surgery can be safely conducted in the elderly patient. No change in the research agenda is recommended.

REOPERATIVE CARDIAC SURGERY

See *New Frontiers,* pp. 158–159.

CardiacSurg 21 (Level B): **Cohort studies are needed that focus on patency and outcomes related to conduit choice in elderly patients who have had prior coronary artery bypass grafting and who require reoperation.**

CardiacSurg 22 (Level A): **Randomized trials of myocardial protective strategies in reoperative heart surgery in the elderly patient are needed to identify the optimal approach in recurrent coronary disease.**

CardiacSurg 23 (Level B): **Feasibility and outcomes analyses of off-pump techniques in elderly patients are needed to define morbidity and mortality in repeat revascularization procedures.**

CardiacSurg 24 (Level B): **Cohort studies are needed of outcomes in elderly patients who have undergone reoperative coronary artery bypass grafting with arterial grafts after venous conduits developed stenosis or other flow-limiting changes occurred.**

CardiacSurg 25 (Level B): **Longitudinal studies are needed to determine outcomes in valvular repair or replacement operations in elderly patients who have had prior coronary revascularization procedures.**

New Research Addressing These Questions: Reoperative surgery in elderly patients carries a profound risk for morbidity and mortality. In a comparison of younger and older (aged 70 and above) patients undergoing reoperative CABG, Christenson et al noted that the older patients had poorer New York Heart Association functional classification and more generalized atherosclerosis. These older patients had a higher occurrence of low cardiac output syndrome, a higher incidence of gastrointestinal and renal complications, and longer cardiopulmonary bypass times. Hospital mortality rates for the older patients were 17.9% and 7.1% for younger patients; however, the 5-year survival rates and cardiac event–free survival rates for the older and younger patients were 76.2% and 69.9%, respectively.[41] In an analysis comparing reoperative CABG and primary CABG, Christenson et al also noted that age above 80 years, urgent operation, poor ventricular function, and generalized atherosclerosis are among the independent risk factors for postoperative death in both the primary and reoperative CABG patients.[42] Weintraub et al reviewed the course of 2030 patients who underwent CABG and noted that in-hospital mortality increases from 5.7% for patients younger than 50 years to 10% for patients aged 70 and older. Neurologic events were found to occur at a significantly higher rate in older patients undergoing reoperative surgery, with an incidence of 4.1% for those patients aged 70 and older.[43] Pellegrini et al noted higher mortality, occurrence of low-output syndrome, renal failure, and sepsis in reoperative CABG patients aged 70 to 79 than in those 60 to 69 years of age.[44] With regard to long-term survival, Noyez and van Eck studied 541 patients with reoperative CABG. They found age lower than 65 years to be associated with greater cardiac survival, but impaired left ventricular function to be the only independent variable predicting late cardiac-related mortality.[45]

Modification of These Questions in Light of New Research: Reoperation carries increased risk for the elderly patient, and research in this area remains very important. No change in the research agenda is recommended.

AORTIC DISSECTION

See *New Frontiers*, p. 159.

CardiacSurg 26 (Level B): **Longitudinal studies of elderly patients treated nonoperatively for aortic dissection are needed to determine the profile of patients at greatest risk of early death that is related to initial dissection.**

CardiacSurg 27 (Level B): **Outcome analyses of operative treatment for ascending and descending aortic dissection in elderly patients are needed to further clarify risk profiles. Emphasis should be on comparison of acute and chronic presentation.**

CardiacSurg 28 (Levels B, A): **Cohort studies and ultimately randomized clinical trials of cerebral protection techniques in elderly patients are needed to identify surgical techniques that lead to fewer neurologic complications, transfusion requirements, and other peri-operative complications.**

New Research Addressing These Questions: Type A aortic dissection constitutes a true surgical emergency with an extremely poor prognosis for patients who do not undergo operative management with replacement of the ascending aorta. Many studies have evaluated both CAB and AVR in the elderly patient, but aortic dissection has not been examined in great detail. Indeed, Mehta et al were the first to examine the International Registry of Acute Aortic Dissection (IRAD) to compare the outcomes in patients younger than 70 with patients aged 70 years or older. This retrospective study covered the period of January 1996 to December 1999. A total of 550 patients were reviewed, 174 (32%) of whom constituted the older cohort. With regard to the presentation, the older patients with type A dissection are much less likely than their younger counterparts to present with abrupt onset of chest or back pain and lower systolic blood pressure. Relatively fewer elderly patients were managed surgically (64% versus 87%), and comorbid conditions were listed as the principal reason that surgical therapy was deferred. Peri-operative complications (coma, myocardial infarction, acute renal failure, and cardiac tamponade) were similar in the two groups. Mortality for the younger patients undergoing surgical repair was 38% versus 27% for the older patients. Logistic regression analysis identified age above 70 as an independent risk factor for death with type A aortic dissection. The limitations of this analysis are consistent with those of most retrospective studies; however, this investigation provides multicenter data regarding higher mortality in patients aged 70 and older with type A aortic dissection.[46]

Contrasting findings were reported by Chiappini et al in their retrospective analysis of single-center experience with type A aortic dissection. This group analyzed 315 patients who underwent surgery for type A dissection between 1976 and 2001; of this sample, 245 patients were younger than 70, and 70 were aged 70 years or older. The data show that in-hospital mortality did not differ between the two groups—20.5% in those younger than 70 and 17.6% in those 70 and older. Longer term actuarial survival did not differ between groups—77.1% in the younger patients and 80% in the older patients. These researchers concluded that surgery for type A aortic dissection can be performed with acceptable results in patients aged 70 and older. Furthermore, they concluded that surgery should not be withheld in this group of patients solely because of age. [47]

Type B aortic dissections traditionally include older patients with comorbid conditions. The management of type B aortic dissections usually involves medical therapy unless specific complications develop to mandate operative intervention. Mehta et al investigated the outcomes of elderly patients with type B aortic dissection in the IRAD registry. They examined 383 patients with type B aortic dissection and compared a group of 161 patients (42%) who were aged 70 or older with 222 patients (58%) who were younger than 70. This analysis was retrospective, as well. The comorbid conditions of hypertension, diabetes mellitus, prior aneurysms, and arteriosclerosis were more common in elderly patients. Overall, in-hospital mortality was higher in the elderly cohort—16% versus 10% in the younger group. Multivariate logistic regression analysis identified three risk factors that greatly increase mortality in the elderly cohort. The presence of shock with hypotension, the involvement of a branch vessel in the dissection, or the presence of a periaortic hematoma places the patient aged 70 or older in a high-risk category, in which mortality is 35%. Without one of these three adverse predictors, the mortality was found to be less than 2%. It is also noteworthy that the older group with an operation fared least well, which is in agreement with other investigations regarding the surgical results with type B aortic dissection. [48]

Another increasingly common clinical scenario for type A aortic dissection involves patients with prior cardiac surgical procedures presenting with acute type A dissection. Collins et al retrospectively examined a group of 100 patients in the IRAD registry with acute type A dissection and prior cardiac surgery. This group was more likely to be male and elderly. Multivariate analysis revealed that age above 70 years, previous AVR, shock, and acute renal failure were all independent predictors of in-hospital mortality. [49]

Modifications of These Questions in Light of New Research: The treatment of aortic dissection in the elderly patient remains an important issue, and more studies of the types described here are needed. No change in the research agenda is recommended.

COMPLICATIONS OF CARDIAC SURGERY

See *New Frontiers*, pp. 160–161.

CardiacSurg 29 (Levels B, A): **Exploratory cohort studies are needed to seek evidence of success with treatments designed to reduce peri-operative arrhythmias associated with a large percentage of cardiac operations. It would be important to establish whether postoperative atrial arrhythmias in elderly patients lead to lessened mobility and subsequent added risk for pneumonia, deep-vein**

thrombosis, and other complications. Subsequently, randomized controlled trials might be carried out to compare success rates and possible benefits from the treatments that show promise.

CardiacSurg 30 (Level B): **Outcome studies of specific technical aspects of operations are needed to identify potential means of reducing wound complications in elderly patients. The use of minimally invasive techniques for both cardiac exposure and vein harvest to reduce surgical trauma in elderly patients should be evaluated.**

CardiacSurg 31 (Level B): **Cohort studies are needed to establish the incidence of and risk factors for complications in the geriatric cardiac patient, including delirium, bowel dysfunction, and swallowing difficulties.**

CardiacSurg 32 (Level B): **Studies of the susceptibility to hospital-acquired infections of elderly cardiac patients are needed. This should include efforts to determine if wound complications in the older patient are a result of prolonged hospital stay, lessened mobility, or age-related depression of the immune system.**

New Research Addressing These Questions: Atrial fibrillation after cardiac surgery is arguably the most common complication following cardiac surgery. The exact incidence of postoperative atrial fibrillation varies, as different studies document a rate from as low as 20% to over 60%. The reasons for this wide variation principally include differing methods of diagnosis in studies, lack of a consistent definition for postoperative atrial fibrillation, differing rates with type of cardiac surgery, and patient demographics. The onset of atrial fibrillation is generally between the second and fourth postoperative days; however, this complication can occur at any time during the peri-operative period. In fact, this complication is also the leading cause of readmission following cardiac surgery. [50]

Mechanisms of atrial fibrillation are not universally agreed upon and are incompletely understood. A unifying hypothesis suggests that re-entry is the central mechanism whereby the atria become chaotic, and there is a lack of uniformity to dispersion of the atrial impulse. Multiple factors may promote atrial fibrillation, including operative trauma during manipulation of the heart, pericardial inflammation, endogenous and exogenous heightened levels of circulating catecholamines (epinephrine), anemia, pain, local atrial stretch with volume changes, and alteration of sympathetic or vagal tone.

Risk factors for atrial fibrillation have been extensively investigated. Overall, the literature is somewhat inconsistent because of a lack of uniformity in patient monitoring for atrial fibrillation, differing definitions of what constitutes atrial fibrillation, and heterogeneous patient populations. However, accepting these limitations, the variable that most consistently appears as an independent risk for atrial fibrillation following cardiac surgery is increasing patient age. A common hypothesis for relating patient age to the development of postoperative atrial fibrillation is age-associated changes in the atria of elderly patients. As patients age, the deposition of lipofuscin increases greatly in the atria, and this phenomenon may be related to alterations in atrial electrophysiology. Another potent risk factor that is modifiable is the withdrawal of β-blockers. Ali et al noted that withholding β-blockers after cardiac surgery doubles the incidence of atrial fibrillation from 17% to 38%. [51]Though atrial enlargement is noted in population-based studies to be a risk factor for the development of atrial fibrillation, its role as a causative factor for atrial fibrillation following cardiac surgery is less clear. Shore-Lesserson et al measured left atrial dimensions with transesophageal echocardiography during cardiac surgery and found that size of left atrial chamber was not predictive of postoperative atrial fibrillation.[52] Last, speculation abounds that postoperative atrial fibrillation occurs in patients who are prone to develop atrial arrhythmias. Steinberg et al analyzed signal-averaged electrocardiograms in patients undergoing cardiac surgery. They established that a p-wave duration > 140 ms identified risk for atrial fibrillation.[53] Others have also reported that a history of atrial fibrillation predisposes a patient to postoperative atrial fibrillation.

A paradigm shift in cardiac surgery has recently included the realization that atrial fibrillation is not a "benign" condition. Mathew et al[27] analyzed outcomes in patients developing atrial fibrillation after cardiac surgery and found a nearly threefold increase in peri-operative stroke. Lahtinen et al also documented that 36% of postoperative strokes result from the development of atrial fibrillation. Their data suggested, on average, 2.5 episodes of atrial fibrillation that preceded the stroke.[54] In addition to contributing to poor outcomes, the postoperative atrial fibrillation entails the use of considerable extra resources. Aranki et al provided a very thorough analysis of 570 patients undergoing CAB and investigated postoperative length of stay and hospital charges associated with the development of atrial fibrillation. They noted that the development of postoperative atrial fibrillation increases the length of stay by 4.9 days. In addition, the excess charges incurred by a patient who develops atrial fibrillation were approximately $11,000.[55] When one considers the large number of patients who develop postoperative atrial fibrillation, the enormous societal costs of this arrhythmia become apparent.

Pharmacologic prophylaxis against atrial fibrillation has proven difficult. In total, 91 randomized controlled trials have examined a variety of agents, including β-blockers (propranolol, atenolol), antiarrhythmic drugs with β-adrenergic receptor blocking effects (sotalol, amiodarone), digitalis, magnesium, and various other agents. On the basis of a review of these trials, the American College of Chest Physicians released guidelines for pharmacologic prophylaxis. Essentially, the use of Vaughn-Williams β-blockers is recommended, with consideration being given to sotalol and amiodarone if therapy with Vaughn-Williams Class II β-blockers is contraindicated. Digitalis, magnesium, and calcium channel antagonists (diltiazem and verapamil) were not recommended as prophylactic agents to prevent postoperative atrial fibrillation.[56]

Wound complications following any surgical procedure may significantly increase the length of hospital stay, overall costs, and even mortality rates. In a retrospective study of 12,267 consecutive patients over a 5-year period, Borger et al noted that advanced age is an independent risk factor for the development of serious sternal wound infection.[57]

Delirium in elderly patients following heart surgery is often attributable to multiple causes. The chapter on cross-cutting issues addresses this common geriatric surgical complication. (See *New Frontiers,* pp. 401–402.)

Modification of These Questions in Light of New Research: Complications associated with cardiac surgical procedures unfortunately are far too prevalent, and they have a profoundly negative impact upon outcomes in the elderly population. Further research in this area is needed and no modification of the research agenda is recommended.

Stroke, Neurologic Deficits, and Cardiac Surgery

See *New Frontiers,* pp. 162–163.

CardiacSurg 33 (Level A): **Randomized clinical trials are needed to compare the neurologic results of coronary artery bypass grafting alone with the results of this procedure preceded by carotid endarterectomy when carotid stenosis > 50% is present.**

CardiacSurg 34 (Level A): **More randomized clinical trials should be conducted to investigate the occurrence of stroke and neurocognitive behavioral symptoms in elderly patients on whom coronary artery bypass grafting is performed with or without the use of cardiopulmonary bypass. This would include the development of widely acceptable neurobehavioral assessment tools (eg, cognitive tests) to be used as benchmarks in the evaluation of elderly patients before and after cardiac surgery.**

CardiacSurg 35 (Level B): **To identify possible modifiable risk factors for stroke in elderly patients undergoing cardiac surgery, investigation is needed of available and novel techniques (eg, epi-aortic ultrasound, cerebral oximetry, and transesophageal echocardiography) in elderly patients. Studies of the role of pharmacologic agents as risk factors are also needed.**

New Research Addressing These Questions: Stroke is a leading cause in the United States of serious long-term disability. The vast majority of strokes occur in people aged 65 and older. With the increasing age of patients undergoing cardiac surgical operations, the aged population is certainly at higher risk for age-related adverse cerebrovascular events.

Determining the incidence of stroke after cardiac surgical procedures remains imprecise because of the different methods used to calculate neurologic events after cardiac surgery. McKhann et al reviewed this subject and illustrate the variance in reported rates of stroke. They note that, depending on whether stroke incidence is obtained prospectively or retrospectively, the incidence following CAB can vary considerably. Prospective risk of stroke is estimated at 1.5% to 5.2%, whereas the retrospective incidence is estimated at 0.8% to 3.2%. Further, the timing of postoperative stroke is quite difficult to estimate when retrospective methods are applied. These researchers have found, however, that the 65% to 85% of strokes following CAB or CAB with valve or valve surgery appear within the first 2 days of surgery. [58]

Identifying patient groups at higher risk for cerebrovascular accident following cardiac surgery has inherent advantages. Patients can be adequately informed of their risk in discussions regarding surgery, and other intraoperative and postoperative maneuvers can be undertaken to mitigate this risk. Nearly all studies uniformly confirm that a history of prior stroke remains as one of the most robust risk factors for stroke after cardiac surgery. Baker et al reviewed a large experience with 4380 patients undergoing CABG in their center. They identified seven predictors of postoperative stroke: previous stroke, diabetes mellitus, age, hypertension, the presence of cerebrovascular disease, elevated creatinine, and preoperative atrial fibrillation. Of these risk factors, the odds ratio for prior stroke was 6.3, and it far outweighed the other factors with regard to predictive ability. Increasing age had a modest odds ratio of 1.1. Noteworthy in this report was the excess in resources that patients who developed stroke consumed. A postoperative stroke increased the intensive care unit (ICU) length of stay by 4 times, doubled the overall length of hospital stay, and increased the mortality at 30 days by a factor of 10.[59]

If a patient does incur a stroke following cardiac surgery, the short- and long-term outcomes are poor. Salazar et al analyzed the Johns Hopkins Cardiac Surgery Stroke Database and determined what the early and late outcomes were for patients with stroke. Their overall incidence of stroke following CAB was 3.2%, with combined CAB–carotid endarterectomy having the highest incidence of 17.3% of peri-operative stroke. The impact of stroke upon early outcomes was impressive. Stroke doubled the ICU length of stay from 3.6 to 7.3 days, nearly tripled the overall hospital length of stay from 10 to 25 days, doubled the hospital charges from $30,000 to $60,000, and more than quadrupled the mortality from 4% to 19%. These researchers were able to follow up via telephone interview with 99% of the stroke patients, at a mean of 1.89 years following cardiac surgery. Overall survival after stroke was 67% at 1 year and 47% at 5 years; this survival was not compared with an age-matched population cohort, but it would appear that the occurrence of stroke significantly compromised long-term survival. Functional status was assessed at the time of telephone interview by Rankin Scale. Of the 81% of patients who survived to discharge following stroke, only 39% lead a life with minimal disability. Stated differently, nearly two thirds of patients who sustain a stroke after cardiac surgery will die early or be significantly disabled.[60]

The cause of stroke following cardiac surgery is usually multifactorial and not likely to be pinpointed on one specific factor. The leading culprits include embolic debris, hypoperfusion during cardiopulmonary bypass, and perhaps the early postoperative development of atrial fibrillation. Although large embolic events during cardiac surgery are much less common, the persistence of microembolic debris remains problematic. Embolic debris can include gaseous or particulate matter. Particulate matter includes microscopic thrombi (despite anticoagulation with heparin), lipid material, and atherosclerotic material from the ascending or transverse aorta. Indeed, Djaiani et al performed TEE, transcranial Doppler (TCD), and epiaortic scanning during the conduct of CAB in their institution. Patients then underwent postoperative brain magnetic resonance imaging (MRI) on days 3 to 7 after their CAB. These researchers divided the patients into those at low risk (intimal thickness on TEE and epiaortic scan $\leq$ 2 mm) and at high risk ($>$ 2 mm) for cerebral events. A strong correlation was observed between the high-risk group and number of embolic episodes by TCD, and only the high-risk group had changes seen on MRI consistent with ischemic injury. The researchers concluded that at least mild to moderate atheromatous burden in the thoracic aorta correlates with brain injury following CAB. With regard to when embolic events occur, they are most likely to occur during manipulation of the aorta for cannulation for cardiopulmonary bypass or cross-clamping or unclamping the aorta.[61]

Cerebral hypoperfusion during cardiopulmonary bypass (CPB) invariably occurs; however, firm evidence is still lacking to determine the level of hypoperfusion necessary to produce reversible injury. It is widely theorized that risk factors such as diabetes mellitus and hypertension contribute to a microvascular dysautoregulation in the brain during CPB that can produce ischemic brain injury. However, investigative efforts to either affirm or disprove this hypothesis remain inconclusive. In fact, the optimal mean arterial pressure that should be maintained during CPB is still unknown. Gold et al actually randomized

124 patients to a low mean arterial pressure (50 to 60 mm Hg) and compared them with a group with high mean arterial pressure (80 to 100 mm Hg) during CPB. These researchers observed a lower incidence of combined cardiac and neurologic complications—4.8% versus 13% in the higher mean arterial pressure group.[62] Further investigation of this area, however, is needed to more clearly refine the relationship between risk factors for cerebral hypoperfusion and ischemic brain injury after cardiac surgery.

Encephalopathy or diffuse brain injury following cardiac surgery remains an equally vexing and troublesome complication. This complication is variably known as confusion, delirium, coma, seizures, prolonged alteration in mental status, combativeness, and agitation. The incidence of encephalopathy varies widely; reports range from 8% to over 30% following cardiac surgery. McKhann et al prospectively examined the impact and risk factors for encephalopathy in patients undergoing CAB. They identified five risk factors for the development of encephalopathy: prior stroke, the presence of a carotid bruit, diabetes mellitus, hypertension, and incremental age > 65 and age > 75. The development of encephalopathy after CAB, in a similar manner to stroke, doubled hospital stay from 6 days (no encephalopathy) to 15 days, and increased mortality from 1.7% (no encephalopathy) to 7.5%.[58] The mechanisms underlying the development of encephalopathy remain largely unknown. These five risk factors likely point toward a vascular mechanism whereby either an ischemic or inflammatory insult is inflicted upon the brain, which then exhibits a spectrum of functional impairments.

Modification of These Questions in Light of New Research: Review of the available data indicates that either stroke or encephalopathy following cardiac surgery profoundly and negatively impacts both short- and long-term outcomes for older patients. No modification of the research agenda for this important area is recommended.

THE OCTOGENARIAN AS CARDIAC SURGICAL PATIENT

See *New Frontiers,* pp. 163–165.

CardiacSurg 36 (Level A): **Randomized clinical trials comparing percutaneous coronary intervention techniques (angioplasty plus stenting) and coronary artery bypass grafting in patients aged 80 and over are needed, with emphasis on the presentation of acute myocardial infarction or congestive heart failure, or both, to clarify selection criteria for this patient group.**

CardiacSurg 37 (Level A): **Randomized clinical trials are needed that compare outcomes with conventional and beating-heart coronary artery bypass grafting in patients aged 80 and over.**

CardiacSurg 38 (Level B): **Longitudinal outcome studies are needed of octogenarians who are treated by surgery, percutaneous interventions, or medically only to suggest the functional and neurologic long-term results and the need for reintervention.**

CardiacSurg 39 (Level B): **Follow-up studies should be performed to determine the need for readmission, repeat intervention, and functional outcomes in patients aged 80 and over who have undergone cardiac surgery.**

CardiacSurg 40 (Level B): **The development of cardiac treatment protocols specifically aimed at patients aged 80 and over is a critical need. This might include prospective trials to allow earlier surgical intervention when risk profile is favorable for good outcomes, particularly for coronary artery bypass grafting.**

New Research Addressing These Questions: Although the majority of contemporary health care providers do not exclude patients from being considered for a cardiac operation on the basis of age alone, Rady et al questioned whether elderly patients are capable of making an informed decision regarding cardiac surgery. They conducted a cohort study of 96 octogenarians undergoing cardiac surgery and compared their outcomes with those of a younger group of 687 patients undergoing cardiac surgery. They also examined the use of hospital and Medicare expenses for both groups of patients. The cohorts examined differed in that the octogenarians were more likely female, and the comorbid conditions of pulmonary hypertension, previous malignancy, cerebral vascular disease, valvular heart disease, and congestive heart failure were more common in octogenarians. The rate of postoperative complications—cardiovascular, neurologic, and renal complications and nosocomial infections—was substantially greater in the elderly cohort than in the younger group. Most striking was the rate of death or discharge to a nursing facility: 53% in the over-80 group compared with 14% in the younger group. Hospital charges were greater in the elderly group. In multivariate analysis, these researchers found female sex, age 80 or older, congestive heart failure, and surgical re-exploration to be independent factors for death or discharge to a nursing facility. Given these outcomes, these investigators appropriately questioned the cost-effectiveness of referring elders aged 80 or older for cardiac surgery.[63]

Great strides have been undertaken to optimize outcomes following cardiac surgery in elderly patients. Though much attention has been focused on postoperative processes of care, growing interest in optimizing physical functional reserve before surgery now exists. This concept of enhancing physical function prior to elective surgery is now termed *prehabilitation*. Carli and Zavorsky reviewed the available literature and noted striking improvements in 275 elderly patients undergoing cardiac or abdominal surgery. In various programs of aerobic training and strength conditioning, improvement was noted in fewer complications, shortened time in the hospital postoperatively, and improvement in health-related quality of life.[64] It remains cogent to remember that prehabilitation can be offered only to patients undergoing elective cardiac surgical operations. Though limited, this therapy is intuitively attractive and is likely to offer an important adjunct to all other therapies directed at improving surgical outcomes for elderly patients.

Modification of These Questions in Light of New Research: No change in the research agenda in this important topic is recommended.

QUALITY OF LIFE AFTER CARDIAC SURGERY

See *New Frontiers,* pp. 166–167.

CardiacSurg 41 (Level B): **Survey tools to assess quality of life after cardiac surgery in elderly patients need to be refined, to determine the contribution of surgical intervention to long-term disability. This**

should include cohort studies to clarify the impact of surgical treatment on caregivers.

CardiacSurg 42 (Level B): **Long-term study of elderly cardiac surgical patients who had prolonged peri-operative course is needed to determine the degree to which functional and symptomatic improvement occurs when operative therapy is complicated by stroke, infection, or other medical condition commonly associated with surgery in elderly patients.**

CardiacSurg 43 (Level B): **Comparison studies of outcomes of acute and elective cardiac surgery in elderly patients are needed to identify high-risk groups of elderly patients and to develop potential exclusion criteria for operative therapy.**

New Research Addressing These Questions: A primary indication for undergoing cardiac surgery is to relieve symptoms of angina (CAB) or valvular-related pathology (aortic and mitral valve surgery). Until recently, data addressing quality of life after cardiac surgery was limited. As our population of aging patients is increasingly being considered for these invasive operations, it is desirable to offer improvement in health-related quality of life as well as improvement in survival.

Data derived from the Department of Veterans Affairs Processes, Structures, and Outcomes in Cardiac Surgery study yielded important insights into quality of life after CABG. Rumsfeld et al administered the Medical Outcomes Study Short Form 36-item health survey (SF-36) to elective CAB patients at baseline (preoperatively) and at 6 months or more after CAB; 1744 patients responded. The SF-36 variables were divided into a physical component summary (PCS) and a mental component summary (MCS). Both the PCS and the MCS were scored from 0 to 100, with a higher value reflecting better health status. On average, both physical and mental health status improved following CAB. The major determinant of change in quality of life following CAB was the preoperative health status. Patients with lower PCS or MCS scores were likely to enjoy the greatest positive change in quality of life after surgery, whereas patients with a higher preoperative score were less likely to have an improvement in quality in life. [65] In counseling patients about surgery, one should therefore perhaps offer patients with good preoperative health status CAB primarily for improved survival.

While many resources and much attention are devoted to the early outcomes and optimization of in-hospital outcomes following cardiac surgery for the elderly patient, outcomes in the longer term are important as well. Herlitz et al administered three separate quality-of-life questionnaires to the patients undergoing CABG. Patients answered three self-administered questionnaires—the Physical Activity Score, the Nottingham Health Profile, and the Psychological General Well-Being Index—at the time of their coronary angiography and postoperatively at 3 months and 1, 2, 5, and 10 years. Of the 2235 patients undergoing CAB, 637 responded before their surgery and at 10 years following CAB. Two factors independently predicted an inferior quality of life after 10 years with all three instruments: history of diabetes mellitus and chronic obstructive pulmonary disease. Not surprisingly, when these investigators introduced the variable of an inferior quality of life preoperatively, it was found to independently and strongly predict inferior quality of life at 10 years follow-up. Age did not consistently emerge as a strong predictor of impaired quality of life.[66]

Investigations specifically addressing long-term quality of life in elderly patients after cardiac surgery remain limited. Sjogren and Thulin undertook an analysis regarding the quality of life in octogenarians after cardiac surgery. SF-36 questionnaires were completed by 41 octogenarian patients at a mean follow-up of 8 years after their cardiac surgery, either CAB, AVR, or AVR with CAB. The results from this cohort were compared with an age-matched population. Two of the SF-36 headings differed significantly between the cardiac surgical patients and their age-matched cohorts: bodily pain and physical functioning. Although the cardiac surgery group had lower physical function scores, they had less pain in comparison with the overall population. On the basis of these results, these authors concluded that a selected population of elderly patients may undergo heart surgery with good long-term quality of life.[67]

NEW HORIZONS IN GERIATRIC CARDIAC SURGERY

With the explosion in the aging population and the prevalence of cardiac disease in the aged population, more cardiac surgical procedures will be performed in elderly patients. Even though the paradigm for the treatment of CAD continues to shift toward percutaneous approaches, a need for coronary artery surgery will remain in our older population. The impacts of newer technologies, such as off-pump surgery, are yet to be determined, and whether elderly patients will benefit from these techniques is still unknown. Cardiac surgical operations can be offered to elderly patients safely and with reasonable results—assuming that patients are appropriately selected.

Accurate data are needed to determine the population at risk for heart disease and to target groups who will benefit from surgical intervention. Primary care for elderly patients should include surveys and population-based data to ensure that referral bias is not excluding aged patients for surgery because of their age alone. Close collaboration between cardiologists, geriatricians, and cardiac surgeons must also occur to ensure optimal delivery of appropriate care for the management of heart disease in these patients.

***CardiacSurg KQ4*: Does ageism adversely affect appropriate consideration of patients for cardiac surgical procedures?**

REFERENCES

1. Heart disease and stroke statistics—2006 Update. Dallas, TX: American Heart Association, 2006 (online at http://www.americanheart.org/downloadable/heart/1136308648540Statupdate 1136308642006.pdf).
2. Ferguson TB, Jr., Hammill BG, Peterson ED, et al. A decade of change—risk profiles and outcomes for isolated coronary artery bypass grafting procedures, 1990-1999: a report from the STS National Database Committee and the Duke Clinical Research Institute. Society of Thoracic Surgeons. Ann Thorac Surg 2002;73:480-489; discussion 489-490.
3. Francalancia N, LoCicero J, 3rd. Geriatric cardiac surgery. In Solomon DH, LoCicero J, 3rd, Rosenthal RA (eds): New Frontiers in Geriatrics Research: An Agenda for Surgical and Re-

lated Medical Specialties. New York: American Geriatrics Society, 2004, pp.147-176 (online at http://www.frycomm.com/ags/rasp).

4. Nowicki ER, Weintraub RW, Birkmeyer NJ, et al. Mitral valve repair and replacement in northern New England. Am Heart J 2003;145:1058-1062.
5. Collart F, Feier H, Kerbaul F, et al. Primary valvular surgery in octogenarians: perioperative outcome. J Heart Valve Dis 2005;14:238-242; discussion 242.
6. Avezum A, Makdisse M, Spencer F, et al. Impact of age on management and outcome of acute coronary syndrome: observations from the Global Registry of Acute Coronary Events (GRACE). Am Heart J 2005;149:67-73.
7. Mack MJ, Brown PP, Kugelmass AD, et al. Current status and outcomes of coronary revascularization 1999 to 2002: 148,396 surgical and percutaneous procedures. Ann Thorac Surg 2004;77:761-766; discussion 766-768.
8. Ulrich MR, Brock DM, Ziskind AA. Analysis of trends in coronary artery bypass grafting and percutaneous coronary intervention rates in Washington state from 1987 to 2001. Am J Cardiol 2003;92:836-839.
9. Serruys PW, Ong AT, van Herwerden LA, et al. Five-year outcomes after coronary stenting versus bypass surgery for the treatment of multivessel disease: the final analysis of the Arterial Revascularization Therapies Study (ARTS) randomized trial. J Am Coll Cardiol 2005;46:575-581.
10. Coronary artery bypass surgery versus percutaneous coronary intervention with stent implantation in patients with multivessel coronary artery disease (the Stent or Surgery trial): a randomised controlled trial. Lancet 2002;360:965-970.
11. Rodriguez A, Bernardi V, Navia J, et al. Argentine Randomized Study: Coronary Angioplasty with Stenting versus Coronary Bypass Surgery in patients with Multiple-Vessel Disease (ERACI II): 30-day and one-year follow-up results. ERACI II Investigators. J Am Coll Cardiol 2001;37:51-58.
12. Brener SJ, Lytle BW, Casserly IP, et al. Propensity analysis of long-term survival after surgical or percutaneous revascularization in patients with multivessel coronary artery disease and high-risk features. Circulation 2004;109:2290-2295.
13. Hannan EL, Racz MJ, Walford G, et al. Long-term outcomes of coronary-artery bypass grafting versus stent implantation. N Engl J Med 2005;352:2174-2183.
14. Benetti FJ, Naselli G, Wood M, Geffner L. Direct myocardial revascularization without extracorporeal circulation: experience in 700 patients. Chest 1991;100:312-316.
15. Buffolo E, Andrade JC, Branco JN, et al. Myocardial revascularization without extracorporeal circulation: seven-year experience in 593 cases. Eur J Cardiothorac Surg 1990;4:504-507; discussion 507-508.
16. Sellke FW, DiMaio JM, Caplan LR, et al. Comparing on-pump and off-pump coronary artery bypass grafting: numerous studies but few conclusions: a scientific statement from the American Heart Association council on cardiovascular surgery and anesthesia in collaboration with the interdisciplinary working group on quality of care and outcomes research. Circulation 2005;111:2858-2864.
17. Athanasiou T, Al-Ruzzeh S, Kumar P, et al. Off-pump myocardial revascularization is associated with less incidence of stroke in elderly patients. Ann Thorac Surg 2004;77:745-753.
18. Kaul TK, Fields BL, Riggins SL, et al. Coronary artery bypass grafting within 30 days of an acute myocardial infarction. Ann Thorac Surg 1995;59:1169-1176.
19. Rao V, Ivanov J, Weisel RD, et al. Predictors of low cardiac output syndrome after coronary artery bypass. J Thorac Cardiovasc Surg 1996;112:38-51.
20. Del Rizzo DF, Fremes SE, Christakis GT, et al. The current status of myocardial revascularization: changing trends and risk factor analysis. J Card Surg 1996;11:18-29.

21. Paone G, Higgins RS, Havstad SL, Silverman NA. Does age limit the effectiveness of clinical pathways after coronary artery bypass graft surgery? Circulation 1998;98:II41-II45.
22. Conaway DG, House J, Bandt K, et al. The elderly: health status benefits and recovery of function one year after coronary artery bypass surgery. J Am Coll Cardiol 2003;42:1421-1426.
23. Hedeshian MH, Namour N, Dziadik E, et al. Does increasing age have a negative impact on six-month functional outcome after coronary artery bypass? Surgery 2002;132:239-244.
24. van Dijk D, Keizer AM, Diephuis JC, et al. Neurocognitive dysfunction after coronary artery bypass surgery: a systematic review. J Thorac Cardiovasc Surg 2000;120:632-639.
25. Ho PM, Arciniegas DB, Grigsby J, et al. Predictors of cognitive decline following coronary artery bypass graft surgery. Ann Thorac Surg 2004;77:597-603; discussion 603.
26. Tuman KJ, McCarthy RJ, Najafi H, Ivankovich AD. Differential effects of advanced age on neurologic and cardiac risks of coronary artery operations. J Thorac Cardiovasc Surg 1992;104:1510-1517.
27. Mathew JP, Fontes ML, Tudor IC, et al. A multicenter risk index for atrial fibrillation after cardiac surgery. JAMA 2004;291:1720-1729.
28. Hravnak M, Hoffman LA, Saul MI, et al. Predictors and impact of atrial fibrillation after isolated coronary artery bypass grafting. Crit Care Med 2002;30:330-337.
29. Almassi GH, Schowalter T, Nicolosi AC, et al. Atrial fibrillation after cardiac surgery: a major morbid event? Ann Surg 1997;226:501-511; discussion 511-503.
30. Mathew JP, Parks R, Savino JS, et al. Atrial fibrillation following coronary artery bypass graft surgery: predictors, outcomes, and resource utilization. MultiCenter Study of Perioperative Ischemia Research Group. JAMA 1996;276:300-306.
31. Spach MS, Dolber PC. Relating extracellular potentials and their derivatives to anisotropic propagation at a microscopic level in human cardiac muscle. Evidence for electrical uncoupling of side-to-side fiber connections with increasing age. Circ Res 1986;58:356-371.
32. Lindroos M, Kupari M, Heikkila J, Tilvis R. Prevalence of aortic valve abnormalities in the elderly: an echocardiographic study of a random population sample. J Am Coll Cardiol 1993;21:1220-1225.
33. Otto CM, Burwash IG, Legget ME, et al. Prospective study of asymptomatic valvular aortic stenosis: clinical, echocardiographic, and exercise predictors of outcome. Circulation 1997;95:2262-2270.
34. Cowell SJ, Newby DE, Boon NA, Elder AT. Calcific aortic stenosis: same old story? Age Ageing 2004;33:538-544.
35. Bouma BJ, van der Meulen JH, van den Brink RB, et al. Variability in treatment advice for elderly patients with aortic stenosis: a nationwide survey in The Netherlands. Heart 2001;85:196-201.
36. Collart F, Feier H, Kerbaul F, et al. Valvular surgery in octogenarians: operative risks factors, evaluation of Euroscore and long term results. Eur J Cardiothorac Surg 2005;27:276-280.
37. Chiappini B, Camurri N, Loforte A, et al. Outcome after aortic valve replacement in octogenarians. Ann Thorac Surg 2004;78:85-89.
38. Sharony R, Grossi EA, Saunders PC, et al. Minimally invasive aortic valve surgery in the elderly: a case-control study. Circulation 2003;108 Suppl 1:II43-II47.
39. Kolh P, Kerzmann A, Lahaye L, et al. Cardiac surgery in octogenarians: peri-operative outcome and long-term results. Eur Heart J 2001;22:1235-1243.
40. Lee R, Sundt TM, 3rd, Moon MR, et al. Mitral valve repair in the elderly: operative risk for patients over 70 years of age is acceptable. J Cardiovasc Surg (Torino) 2003;44:157-161.
41. Christenson JT, Simonet F, Schmuziger M. The influence of age on the results of reoperative coronary artery bypass grafting. Coron Artery Dis 1997;8:91-96.
42. Christenson JT, Schmuziger M, Simonet F. Reoperative coronary artery bypass procedures: risk factors for early mortality and late survival. Eur J Cardiothorac Surg 1997;11:129-133.

43. Weintraub WS, Jones EL, Craver JM, et al. In-hospital and long-term outcome after reoperative coronary artery bypass graft surgery. Circulation 1995;92:II50-II57.
44. Pellegrini RV, Di Marco RF, Werner AM, Marrangoni AG. Recurrent ischemic heart disease: the effect of advancing age. J Cardiovasc Surg (Torino) 1994;35:371-376.
45. Noyez L, van Eck FM. Long-term cardiac survival after reoperative coronary artery bypass grafting. Eur J Cardiothorac Surg 2004;25:59-64.
46. Mehta RH, O'Gara PT, Bossone E, et al. Acute type A aortic dissection in the elderly: clinical characteristics, management, and outcomes in the current era. J Am Coll Cardiol 2002;40:685-692.
47. Chiappini B, Tan ME, Morshuis W, et al. Surgery for acute type A aortic dissection: is advanced age a contraindication? Ann Thorac Surg 2004;78:585-590.
48. Mehta RH, Bossone E, Evangelista A, et al. Acute type B aortic dissection in elderly patients: clinical features, outcomes, and simple risk stratification rule. Ann Thorac Surg 2004;77:1622-1628; discussion 1629.
49. Collins JS, Evangelista A, Nienaber CA, et al. Differences in clinical presentation, management, and outcomes of acute type A aortic dissection in patients with and without previous cardiac surgery. Circulation 2004;110:II237-II242.
50. Hogue CW, Jr., Creswell LL, Gutterman DD, Fleisher LA. Epidemiology, mechanisms, and risks: American College of Chest Physicians guidelines for the prevention and management of postoperative atrial fibrillation after cardiac surgery. Chest 2005;128:9S-16S.
51. Ali IM, Sanalla AA, Clark V. Beta-blocker effects on postoperative atrial fibrillation. Eur J Cardiothorac Surg 1997;11:1154-1157.
52. Shore-Lesserson L, Moskowitz D, Hametz C, et al. Use of intraoperative transesophageal echocardiography to predict atrial fibrillation after coronary artery bypass grafting. Anesthesiology 2001;95:652-658.
53. Steinberg JS, Zelenkofske S, Wong SC, et al. Value of the P-wave signal-averaged ECG for predicting atrial fibrillation after cardiac surgery. Circulation 1993;88:2618-2622.
54. Lahtinen J, Biancari F, Salmela E, et al. Postoperative atrial fibrillation is a major cause of stroke after on-pump coronary artery bypass surgery. Ann Thorac Surg 2004;77:1241-1244.
55. Aranki SF, Shaw DP, Adams DH, et al. Predictors of atrial fibrillation after coronary artery surgery: current trends and impact on hospital resources. Circulation 1996;94:390-397.
56. Bradley D, Creswell LL, Hogue CW, Jr., et al. Pharmacologic prophylaxis: American College of Chest Physicians guidelines for the prevention and management of postoperative atrial fibrillation after cardiac surgery. Chest 2005;128:39S-47S.
57. Borger MA, Rao V, Weisel RD, et al. Deep sternal wound infection: risk factors and outcomes. Ann Thorac Surg 1998;65:1050-1056.
58. McKhann GM, Grega MA, Borowicz LM, Jr., et al. Encephalopathy and stroke after coronary artery bypass grafting: incidence, consequences, and prediction. Arch Neurol 2002;59:1422-1428.
59. Baker RA, Hallsworth LJ, Knight JL. Stroke after coronary artery bypass grafting. Ann Thorac Surg 2005;80:1746-1750.
60. Salazar JD, Wityk RJ, Grega MA, et al. Stroke after cardiac surgery: short- and long-term outcomes. Ann Thorac Surg 2001;72:1195-1201; discussion 1201-1192.
61. Djaiani G, Fedorko L, Borger M, et al. Mild to moderate atheromatous disease of the thoracic aorta and new ischemic brain lesions after conventional coronary artery bypass graft surgery. Stroke 2004;35:e356-e358.
62. Gold JP, Charlson ME, Williams-Russo P, et al. Improvement of outcomes after coronary artery bypass: a randomized trial comparing intraoperative high versus low mean arterial pressure. J Thorac Cardiovasc Surg 1995;110:1302-1311; discussion 1311-1304.

63. Rady MY, Johnson DJ. Cardiac surgery for octogenarians: is it an informed decision? Am Heart J 2004;147:347-353.
64. Carli F, Zavorsky GS. Optimizing functional exercise capacity in the elderly surgical population. Curr Opin Clin Nutr Metab Care 2005;8:23-32.
65. Rumsfeld JS, Magid DJ, O'Brien M, et al. Changes in health-related quality of life following coronary artery bypass graft surgery. Ann Thorac Surg 2001;72:2026-2032.
66. Herlitz J, Brandrup-Wognsen G, Caidahl K, et al. Determinants for an impaired quality of life 10 years after coronary artery bypass surgery. Int J Cardiol 2005;98:447-452.
67. Sjogren J, Thulin LI. Quality of life in the very elderly after cardiac surgery: a comparison of SF-36 between long-term survivors and an age-matched population. Gerontology 2004;50:407-410.

7

GERIATRIC OPHTHALMOLOGY

*David S. Friedman, MD, MPH, PhD; Andrew G. Lee, MD**

As the United States shifts toward an older population, the specialty of ophthalmology will be impacted disproportionately, since many common eye disorders occur with increasing frequency and severity with older age. This chapter updates the chapter on geriatric ophthalmology in *New Frontiers in Geriatrics Research* by evaluating the more recent literature on the eye care of older persons. [1] Research addressing agenda items that were proposed in *New Frontiers* is described in the section Progress in Geriatric Ophthalmology; research suggesting the need for additions to the research agenda is described in the section New Horizons in Geriatric Ophthalmology at the end of the chapter. The Key Questions for geriatric ophthalmology highlighted in *New Frontiers* are unchanged:

> ***Ophth KQ1*: Does visual improvement or stabilization, including low-vision rehabilitation, reduce the severity, incidence, and prevalence of depression, dementia, delirium, falls, driving accidents, loss of function or quality of life, and hospital complications in the elderly population?**
>
> ***Ophth KQ2*: What is the best timing for and what are the best methods for intervention in visual loss in the elderly person, and what are the best outcome measures for documenting success?**
>
> ***Ophth KQ3*: What are the risk factors for functional vision impairment in the elderly person, and what screening intervals and methods and what instruments for measuring visual function would be best for identifying an older person's risks for such impairment?**

METHODS

Articles on geriatric ophthalmology from 2000 to 2005 were reviewed systematically. Two searches of the National Library of Medicine's PubMed database were conducted in June and July 2005. Three topics (search 1) were searched as major medical subject headings (MeSH): *ophthalmology, ophthalmologic surgical procedures,* and *vision, low*. These headings were combined with the following MeSH terms denoting advanced age: *age, geriatric assessment, aged, 80 and over, frail, elderly, longevity*, and *geriatrics*. The limits placed on all searches were as follows: aged 65+ years, English language, humans, and the years 2000–2005. A second search of the National Library of Medicine database was performed in June 2005 using the topic *ophthalmology* combined with the following terms denoting advanced age: *65 or older*, *aged*, and *geriatric*. Limits placed on this search were English language, core clinical journals, and the years 2000–2005.

The first search strategy yielded 71 articles in ophthalmology, 3054 articles in ophthalmologic surgical procedures, and 125 articles in low vision. The second search yielded 83 articles. The senior writer (AGL) reviewed the titles and abstracts in the search

* Friedman: Associate Professor, Department of Ophthalmology, The Wilmer Eye Institute, The Johns Hopkins University, Baltimore, MD; Lee: Professor of Ophthalmology, Neurology, and Neurosurgery, University of Iowa Hospitals and Clinics, Iowa City, IA.

results for relevance, type of study, and application to the research agenda. Case reports, editorials, and letters to the editor were included only if they added significant new information. The lists of eligible articles were also reviewed by the senior writer for articles that might have been missed by the searches. Finally, additional articles were obtained by using the PubMed search term *visual loss* combined with *dementia*, *depression*, *hearing loss*, *functional impairment*, and *falls*, limiting results to English language only, abstracted items, and years 2000–2005.

PROGRESS IN GERIATRIC OPHTHALMOLOGY

ASSESSING VISUAL LOSS IN AGE

Scope of the Problem

See *New Frontiers*, p. 178.

Although the emphasis of *New Frontiers* was on the increasing prevalence of vision loss in the United States (see p. 178), the problem is in fact occurring globally as a consequence of the large increase in the numbers of elderly persons throughout the world.[2–8] Some of the vision loss associated with aging is irreversible (eg, late age-related macular degeneration [ARMD]), but much of it is treatable, and the impact of some conditions on vision (eg, glaucoma) can be reduced through preventive efforts. In a striking finding, one cross-sectional population-based study of nearly 5000 elderly persons in Australia found uncorrected refractive error to be the most common cause of bilateral visual impairment.[6] Supporting this finding that uncorrected refractive error is a significant problem in older populations is a report from England in which vision was found to improve with pinhole (indicating likely improvement with eyeglasses) in 21% of those studied (persons aged 65 years or older and without mental impairment). These researchers also reported that visual impairment is very common in the oldest persons, with over 35% of the population aged 85 or older being visually impaired.[9] Another study from England found that among persons aged 75 years or older attending general health clinics, 13% were visually impaired (visual acuity less than 20/60). Over 25% of this impairment improved with pinhole.[3] In a separate report on older community-dwelling residents in the United States, Munoz et al found that over half of those with bilateral visual impairment had treatable or preventable disorders.[4]

Since most major eye diseases occur with much greater frequency among older adults, the rates of visual impairment will increase as the population ages and people live longer. A recent meta-analysis using data from most of the major US population-based eye disease prevalence studies conducted in the past 20 years reported that 937,000 (0.78%) Americans older than age 40 years are blind and 2.4 million (1.98%) have low vision (using the US definitions). Among white Americans the leading cause of blindness was ARMD, but for black Americans the leading causes were cataract and glaucoma. Although persons aged 80 years and older make up 7.7% of the US population 40 years and older, they account for 69% of the blindness. Again, because of the aging of the population and not an increase in the incidence or age-specific prevalence of eye disease, it is estimated that the number of blind persons in the United States will increase 70%, to 1.6 million by

2020 (using the criterion of visual acuity of 6/60 or worse). The number of older adults with visual impairment will increase from 7 million at present to 11.2 million in 2020, and possibly as high as 15 million in 2030. [10]

Much has been published about eye diseases among whites and blacks in Western countries, but data have only recently been published on the prevalence of eye disease among Hispanics, and data continues to be refined for Asian populations. Rodriguez et al reported that Hispanics in Arizona have higher rates of vision impairment than non-Hispanic whites, and that primary open-angle glaucoma (POAG) is the leading cause of blindness in this population. [5] A strong association of visual impairment with age was confirmed in a Japanese population, where 1.8% of those aged 40 to 79 years were found to be visually impaired. This study also reported that myopia is an independent risk factor for visual impairment, as is lower education level. [11] Myopia associated with retinal detachment, myopic retinal degeneration, glaucoma, and cataract was not as recognized previously to be such an important factor. [12,13] The association of myopia with visual impairment raises the possibility that the prevalence of low vision may increase in the coming decades in countries where myopia rates appear to be increasing (such as China and other parts of Asia).

Among Chinese persons in Hong Kong, 35% of persons aged 60 years or older had visual impairment in at least one eye, with a substantial proportion improving with pinhole. Bilateral blindness was present in 1.1%, but this decreased to 0.5% with pinhole. [14] Chinese in Taiwan were found to have similar rates of blindness (0.6%); the investigators examined only slightly over half of those eligible, so the true prevalence rate for the population may be higher or lower. The leading causes of visual impairment were found to be cataract (41.7%), myopic degeneration (12.5%), and ARMD (10.4%). [15] Such a high proportion of visual impairment caused by myopic degeneration has not been reported previously in European-derived populations, was not seen in the Hong Kong study, and awaits confirmation in other Asian populations.

A large population-based study in south India reported higher rates of visual impairment than those seen in more developed countries, with 52% of persons aged 60 to 69 years and 71% of persons aged 70 years or older visually impaired, using as the standard vision worse than 6/18 in the eye with better vision. Once again, refractive error accounted for a high proportion of this vision loss (nearly 10%), and cataract was responsible for about 25%. Cataract was a common cause of visual impairment even in persons in their 50s. [2]

Measures and Levels of Visual Loss

See *New Frontiers,* pp. 178–179.

Measuring Impact of Loss on Visual Function

See *New Frontiers,* p. 179.

Measuring Impact of Loss on Functional Ability

See *New Frontiers,* pp. 179–180.

***Ophth 1 (Level B)*: Future research in the treatment of ocular disease in the older person or rehabilitation for older persons with low vision**

should, wherever possible, make use of tools for assessing functional outcomes.

New Research Addressing This Question: One challenge in ophthalmic research is determining how diseases and interventions to prevent or cure them affect quality of life (QOL). QOL instruments are becoming an increasingly accepted outcome measure in ophthalmologic research; at least 29 different visual function rating scale questionnaires were documented in a review conducted in 2001. [16] Probably the most widely used and validated visual function assessment tool is the National Eye Institute Visual Function Questionnaire (NEI-VFQ), which asks 51 questions in 11 domains of visual function. [17] More recently, the NEI-VFQ 25, a reduced version, was demonstrated to work well in evaluating the impact of a wide variety of eye diseases. [18] The Age-Related Eye Disease Study (AREDS), a large clinical trial assessing the benefit of supplementation with beta-carotene and vitamins A and E along with zinc for the prevention of late ARMD and cataract, administered the NEI-VFQ 25 to 4077 participants and reported moderate to high internal consistency of NEI VFQ subscales. [19] Low NEI-VFQ 25 scores were associated with the presence of cataract or macular degeneration or reduced visual acuity. The NEI-VFQ 25 was also found in the AREDS study to be responsive to the progression of ARMD—that is, changes in scores indicated losses of function. Mean changes over the median of more than 3 years of follow-up ranged from 11 to 25 points for the subscales for general vision, near and distance activities, social functioning, mental health, role difficulties, dependency, and driving. The NEI-VFQ 25 was not found to be responsive to lens opacity progression. However, when lens opacity progressed in the eye with the best vision, the researchers found moderate responsiveness in the color vision (effect size = 0.62) and driving (effect size = 0.66) subscales. The progression of some participants to advanced ARMD with visual acuity loss contributed significantly to the variation in the mean difference in NEI-VFQ 25 scores over the course of the study. The authors concluded that changes in the NEI-VFQ 25 overall and subscale scores of 10 points or more indicate clinically significant changes in visual function resulting from ARMD. Given these findings, interventional studies of ARMD and loss of visual acuity might well include the NEI-VFQ 25 as an outcome measure. [20]

Others have also used the NEI-VFQ in studies of ARMD, diabetic retinopathy, optic neuritis, glaucoma, uveitis, and low vision. [19,21–23] The authors of one study [23] cautioned that adjustment of the NEI-VFQ scores for general health may be advisable and that using the adjustments from the physical and mental components of the Medical Outcomes Study Short Form 36-item health survey (SF-36) summary scores might be useful.

Work has continued on QOL measures among older persons. Some researchers have attempted to better define utility measures for visual impairment. Sharma et al cross-sectionally studied 239 patients with a variety of ocular disorders. [24] In contrast to previous reports that found patients to be unwilling to trade time for better vision, [25] the average patient in Sharma's study was willing to trade 2.8 years of every 10 remaining years of life to obtain perfect vision in both eyes. The authors concluded that utility values for vision loss from these patients were strongly associated with visual acuity and could be estimated mathematically. [24] Brown et al demonstrated good test-retest reliability for utility analysis in 115 patients with ophthalmic disease. [26]

Although studies have found only weak associations between measures of general health and visual status, [27] Tsai et al found visual impairment among older Chinese residents of Taiwan to be associated with significantly lower SF-36 physical and social functioning scores. In addition, the authors reported lower QOL for those with visual impairment and found that the use of eye care services is associated with a higher QOL.[28]

In a study of longitudinal household survey data, Sloan et al found that a self-reported decline from excellent or good vision to fair or poor near and distance vision has statistically significant effects on several limitations of instrumental activities of daily living (IADLs) and some activities of daily living (ADLs). The largest effects were for driving (odds ratio [OR] for no limitation: 0.55, $P = .003$), managing money (OR: 0.61, $P < .001$), and preparing hot meals (OR: 0.61, $P < .001$). Onset of fair to poor near vision increases the likelihood of onset of at least one IADL limitation (OR for no limitation: 0.71, $P < .01$) and ADL limitation (OR: 0.74, $P = .003$). Incident legal blindness results in a 78% increase in IADL limitation (OR for no limitation: 0.22, $P < .001$). The effects of vision declines on cognition and depressive symptoms were found to be statistically significant but small. Furthermore, self-reported declines in vision increase the probability of nursing home residence. The authors argued that visual impairment leads to important declines in function among older persons, concluding that preventing vision loss might improve their functioning.[29]

In a study of QOL measures in patients with low vision, Stelmack reported that the Veterans Affairs Low-Vision Visual Functioning Questionnaire has good psychometric properties, concluding that the instrument is valid and reliable for measuring the visual abilities of low-vision patients across many diverse clinical settings.[30]

Modification of This Question in Light of New Research: We are encouraged by the development of and increasing use of functional outcomes assessments in the evaluation and treatment of ocular disease in older persons, and we recommend continued use of these tools in the assessment of rehabilitation for older persons with low vision.

VISUAL LOSS AND SPECIFIC GERIATRIC CONDITIONS

See the section New Horizons in Geriatric Ophthalmology at the end of the chapter for added agenda items under new topics regarding the impacts of visual loss.

Visual Loss and Falls

See *New Frontiers*, pp. 180–181. For a new agenda item, see the subsection on visual loss and falls in New Horizons in Geriatric Ophthalamology at the end of the chapter.

***Ophth 2 (Level A)*: Elderly patients with visual impairment treated with low-vision rehabilitation or whose vision has improved following a specific intervention (eg, cataract surgery, refraction) should be compared with an untreated group or a treated group without visual improvement. The change in incidence of falls over time in the two groups should be prospectively studied.**

***Ophth 3 (Level B)*: Cross-sectional or prospective cohort studies should be performed to determine if certain ocular disorders are more or less likely to be associated with falls by elderly persons and whether multiple ocular disorders are synergistic or additive risk factors.**

***Ophth 4 (Level B)*: Time-series studies of correlations between level of visual function and likelihood of falls should be carried out in cohort studies.**

***Ophth 5 (Levels B, A)*: Prospective interventional studies are needed to establish whether interventions to reduce environmental hazards are cost-effective and practical. Prospective interventional randomized or nonrandomized studies should be performed to determine if the incidence of falls in older patients with visual impairment decreases among those for whom home safety improvements are performed.**

New Research Addressing These Questions: Vision plays an important part in stabilization of posture, and visual impairment may increase the risk for falls independently of environmental hazards. Lord and Menz assessed the impact on sway of contrast sensitivity, depth perception, stereopsis, and lower visual field in 156 older persons aged 63 to 90 years. They concluded that vision and in particular contrast sensitivity and stereopsis are important for posture control under challenging conditions (no effect was seen on a stable surface).[31] Lord and Dayhew found that wearers of multifocal glasses have impaired edge-contrast sensitivity and depth perception, and that the use of multifocal eyeglasses substantially increases the risk of a fall. Furthermore, the population-attributable risk of falls in this cohort was found to be 35% for those wearing multifocal eyeglasses.[32] The same authors also performed a prospective cohort study (N = 156 community-dwelling elderly persons) and reported that impaired vision is an important and independent risk factor for falls, with depth perception and distant-edge-contrast sensitivity being particularly important for maintaining balance as well as detecting and avoiding environmental hazards.[33] This study demonstrates that parameters of visual function other than visual acuity and visual field may be important in the study and prevention of falls and fractures in visually impaired older adults.

De Boer et al examined contrast sensitivity in 1509 older men and women and prospectively (3 years) evaluated the cohort for falls and fractures, finding that visual impairment is an independent risk factor for falls and fractures.[34] In the Blue Mountains Eye Study, a prospective population-based study of eye disease conducted in Australia, the 2-year risk of fractures in patients with visual acuity loss, the visual field deficits, and the presence of posterior subcapsular cataracts were found to be significantly higher than in persons without these findings at baseline.[35]

In order to assess more accurately how the visual system affects balance, Buckley et al studied the impact of visual impairment on the mechanics of landing during stepping down by elderly patients (N = 12) and concluded that correcting common visual problems might be an important intervention strategy for elderly persons negotiating stairs.[36] A separate study reported that stair negotiation appears to be an important hazard for older persons.[37]

In a randomized controlled trial from New Zealand, Campbell et al assessed the efficacy and cost-effectiveness of a home safety program and a home exercise program to reduce falls and injuries in community-dwelling older people with low vision (391 women and men aged 75 years or older with visual acuity of 6/24 or worse). Participants received a home safety assessment and modification program delivered by an occupational therapist (n = 100), an exercise program prescribed at home by a physiotherapist plus vitamin D supplementation (n = 97), both interventions (n = 98), or social visits (n = 96). The main outcome measure was the number of falls and injuries resulting from falls. These authors found fewer falls occurring in the group randomized to the home safety program but not in the exercise program—incidence rate ratios 0.59 (95% confidence interval [CI]: 0.42 to 0.83) and 1.15 (0.82 to 1.61), respectively. [38]

In another prospective cohort study assessing the impact of vision on likelihood of falling, women with declines in visual acuity over 4 to 6 years were found to have significantly greater odds of experiencing frequent falling during the subsequent year. Odds ratios after adjustment for baseline acuity and other confounders were 2.08 (95% CI: 1.39 to 3.12) for loss of 1 to 5 letters, 1.85 (95% CI: 1.16 to 2.95) for loss of 6 to 10 letters, 2.51 (95% CI: 1.39 to 4.52) for loss of 11 to 15 letters, and 2.08 (95% CI: 1.01 to 4.30) for loss of > 15 letters. This study lends further support to the conclusion that loss of vision among elderly women increases the risk of frequent falls and that prevention or correction of visual loss may help reduce the number of future falls. [39] Yet another study of falls risk assessed 1285 persons over 65 years of age and found previous falls, visual impairment, urinary incontinence, and the use of benzodiazepines to be the strongest predictors of fall risk. [40] In support of these findings from multiple studies reported here, one systematic review reported that visual intervention strategies to improve visual function and prevent falls in older people are warranted. [41]

Modification of These Questions in Light of New Research: No change in these agenda items is recommended, but the addition of one new item is proposed. See the section New Horizons in Geriatric Ophthalmology at the end of the chapter.

Visual Loss and Hearing Loss

See *New Frontiers*, p. 182.

Ophth 6 (Level B): **Research is needed to quantify the effect of multisensory loss in elderly patients (eg, hearing and vision) on functional outcomes. Observational cohort studies should be performed to determine which ocular disorders (eg, age-related macular degeneration, cataract, glaucoma) are more likely to be associated with hearing loss and whether or not these ocular disorders have an additive or synergistic effect on functional outcome.**

Ophth 7 (Level A): **Prospective, focused cohort studies with appropriate comparison groups or nonrandomized controlled trials of interventions for multisensory loss, including visual or hearing rehabilitation, should be performed to test for improved functional outcomes.**

New Research Addressing These Questions: In a large cohort study of risk factors for cognitive and functional decline, visual impairment alone was found to be associated with declines in both, but combined hearing and visual loss was found to be associated with the greatest likelihood of cognitive and functional decline. [42] These and other authors emphasized again the need for studies regarding whether treatment of both vision and hearing impairment can decrease these declines. [43,44] Wallhagen et al also found that vision and hearing loss self-reported by patients have strong independent effects on disability, physical functioning, mental health, and social function 1 year after initial evaluation. [45]

Modification of These Questions in Light of New Research: The more recent research adds to our knowledge of the synergistic negative effects of the comorbidities, but further research is still needed to determine the efficacy and impact of any low-vision or other rehabilitation interventions that might improve functional outcomes in the older patient with vision and hearing loss.

Visual Loss and Depression

See *New Frontiers*, p. 182.

Ophth 8 (Level B): **Research is needed to establish what types and what level of visual impairment might be associated with clinical depression in elderly patients. Observational cohort studies should be performed to determine the interaction of visual impairment and depression on the health-related quality of life or other studies of function in older persons.**

Ophth 9 (Level B): **Interventional studies of the evaluation and treatment of depression in older patients with visual impairment should be performed to determine the best timing for intervention.**

Ophth 10 (Level A): **Interventional studies of the effect in elderly patients of specific treatments of visual loss on depression should be performed to determine if improvement in the vision-related depression might lead to improved health-related quality of life and overall functioning.**

New Research Addressing These Questions: Galaria et al reported on the development of a shorter version of the Geriatric Depression Scale (GDS) for visually impaired older patients (N = 70).[46] Horowitz et al conducted a descriptive study of the effects of specific vision rehabilitation services (eg, low-vision clinical services, skills training, counseling, optical device use, and adaptive device use) on depression among 95 older adults with age-related vision impairments. Hierarchical regression analyses indicated that low-vision clinical services, counseling, and the use of optical devices, in separate models, each significantly contributed to a decline in depression (after controlling for age, health status, vision status, functional disability, and baseline depression). The authors concluded that vision rehabilitation interventions impact both physical and psychological functioning, and they underscored the need for future controlled research on rehabilitation service models that address mental health issues.[47]

Brody et al assessed the effectiveness of a self-management program (ie, health education and enhancement of problem-solving skills) on mood and function in 231 community-dwelling cognitively intact patients with vision loss from ARMD. Patients were randomly assigned to a 12-hour self-management program, a series of 12 hours of tape-recorded health lectures, or to a waiting list. The primary outcome measured was emotional distress. The secondary outcomes measured were self-reported function, social support, outlook on life, and self-confidence to handle ARMD-specific challenges in daily life. Clinical depression was determined with the Structured Clinical Interview of *The Diagnostic and Statistical Manual of Mental Disorders*, Axis I (4th edition, research version). The self-management group showed significant improvement in measures of mood and function in comparison with the control patients, and the changes were found to be significantly greater for those who were depressed than for those who were not. Decreases in emotional distress were found to be associated with increases in self-efficacy, and improvements in function were found to be associated with increases in self-efficacy and the perception of social support. The authors concluded that the ARMD self-management program effectively enhances well-being in older persons with poor eyesight and ARMD, particularly those with initial depression.[48]

Modification of These Questions in Light of New Research: The recent research on visual loss and depression continues to add to our knowledge of the impact of the comorbidities of vision loss and depression. Further work is still needed to determine if interventional strategies aimed at both comorbidities might improve functional outcomes for elderly persons.

Visual Loss and Dementia

See *New Frontiers,* p. 183.

Ophth 11 (Level B): **Observational cohort studies should be performed to determine if there is any association between type or severity of visual loss and the major causes of dementia (eg, Alzheimer's disease, multi-infarct dementia).**

Ophth 12 (Level B): **Large population studies should be performed to determine if dementia and visual loss are associated in elderly persons and if the association is independent of other important variables (eg, age could explain the entire association).**

Ophth 13 (Level A): **If an association between dementia and visual loss is found (Ophth 12), especially a severity-related one, then interventional studies should be performed to determine if improvement or stabilization of vision might reduce the incidence or severity of dementia in older persons.**

Ophth 14 (Level A): **In elderly patients with visual loss and dementia, the type and timing of specific interventions should be compared to determine the most effective for improving visual function that leads to improved health-related quality of life or overall functioning.**

New Research Addressing These Questions: Reyes-Ortiz et al found that over 2 years the scores of the blind version of the Mini–Mental State Examination (MMSE-blind) declined more among older Hispanics with near-vision impairment than among those with normal near vision. Distance vision and hearing impairment were not found to be associated with cognitive decline. On average, the MMSE-blind scores of the Hispanic subjects decreased 0.62 points over 2 years and decreased 0.13 points more per year than the scores of normal near-vision subjects.[49] In a population-based study of 2087 very old adults, Anstey et al reported an association between memory loss over 2 years with vision impairment but did not see an association with hearing.[50] Sloan et al also reported on a large cohort followed over nearly a decade and reported small but significant associations of self-reported vision decline with declines in cognition and increases in depressive symptoms.[29]

Modification of These Questions in Light of New Research: The recent studies of visual impairment and cognitive impairment confirm the association and negative impact of these comorbidities, but further research is necessary to determine the efficacy of interventions that might improve functional outcome in older persons.

Visual Loss and Overall Function

See *New Frontiers*, p. 184.

Ophth 15 (Level B): **Single-time observational or time-series observational studies should be performed in elderly patients to determine the relationship between loss of independence or decreases in measures of overall function and the type (eg, cataract, glaucoma), timing of onset (eg, early or late), and severity of loss of vision.**

New Research Addressing This Question: No new research addressing this question has come to light since the publication of *New Frontiers.*

Modification of This Question in Light of New Research: This item should remain unchanged on the research agenda, as findings from research addressing this question will contribute to improved ophthalmologic care of older adults.

Ophth 16 (Level A): **Interventional studies should be performed to determine whether stabilization or improvement in vision or visual function (eg, with low-vision rehabilitation) in elderly patients leads to increased independence and improved overall functioning.**

New Research Addressing This Question: No new research addressing this question has come to light since the publication of *New Frontiers.*

Modification of This Question in Light of New Research: This item should remain unchanged on the research agenda, as findings from research addressing this question will contribute to improved ophthalmologic care of older adults.

Visual Loss and Driving Impairment

See *New Frontiers*, pp. 184–185.

Ophth 17 (Level B): **Single-time or time-series observational studies are needed to determine if mandatory vision screening of elderly drivers appears beneficial in decreasing or preventing traffic accidents.**

New Research Addressing This Question: No new research addressing this question has come to light since the publication of *New Frontiers.*

Modification of This Question in Light of New Research: This item should remain unchanged on the research agenda, as findings from research addressing this question will contribute to improved ophthalmologic care of older adults.

Ophth 18 (Level A): **Interventional cohort studies should be performed to determine whether improvement in vision decreases the frequency and severity of traffic accidents by elderly drivers.**

New Research Addressing This Question: No new research addressing this question has come to light since the publication of *New Frontiers.*

Modification of This Question in Light of New Research: This item should remain unchanged on the research agenda, as findings from research addressing this question will contribute to improved ophthalmologic care of older adults.

Ophth 19 (Level B): **Single-time or cross-sectional observational studies of a suitable cohort are needed to determine whether there is a relationship between the older person's driving performance and the type, severity, and onset of loss of vision.**

New Research Addressing This Question: No new research addressing this question has come to light since the publication of *New Frontiers.*

Modification of This Question in Light of New Research: This item should remain unchanged on the research agenda, as findings from research addressing this question will contribute to improved ophthalmologic care of older adults.

Ophth 20 (Level B): **Observational cohort studies should be performed to determine the interaction between visual loss and other comorbidities or risk factors for unsafe driving such as physical impairments, decreased hearing, and decreased cognition.**

New Research Addressing This Question: No new research addressing this question has come to light since the publication of *New Frontiers.*

Modification of This Question in Light of New Research: This item should remain unchanged on the research agenda, as findings from research addressing this question will contribute to improved ophthalmologic care of older adults.

Ophth 21 (Level A): **Interventional studies of treatments to improve vision or stabilize vision loss in older patients with visual impairment should be performed to determine whether improvement in vision decreases the frequency and severity of traffic accidents among elderly drivers.**

New Research Addressing This Question: No new research addressing this question has come to light since the publication of *New Frontiers.*

Modification of This Question in Light of New Research: This item should remain unchanged on the research agenda, as findings from research addressing this question will contribute to improved ophthalmologic care of older adults.

Visual Loss and Hospitalization

See *New Frontiers*, p. 186.

Ophth 22 (Level B): **Single-time or time-series observational studies are needed to establish the relationship in elderly patients of the type and severity of visual loss to the length of hospital stay and to the incidence and severity of in-hospital comorbidities (eg, delirium and depression).**

New Research Addressing This Question: No new research addressing this question has come to light since the publication of *New Frontiers.*

Modification of This Question in Light of New Research: This item should remain unchanged on the research agenda, as findings from research addressing this question will contribute to improved ophthalmologic care of older adults.

Ophth 23 (Level A): **Interventional studies of treatments to improve or stabilize vision prior to or during hospitalization should be performed to determine if such treatments decrease the length of hospital stay or reduce the incidence or severity of delirium in hospitalized elderly patients.**

New Research Addressing This Question: A retrospective study of the charts of 93 inpatients (half of whom had suffered strokes) who were referred to a low-vision rehabilitation clinic found that on average the visual acuity was moderately impaired and that this interfered with activities of daily living. A high proportion of those referred were believed to benefit from new eyeglasses correction or vision aids. [51]

Modification of Question in Light of New Research: This study does not provide insight into assessment of vision among the hospitalized older patients. Research as described in Ophth 23 is still needed.

Comprehensive Eye Evaluation and Screening

See *New Frontiers*, pp. 186–187.

Ophth 24 (Level B): **Prospective observational studies are needed to validate the current recommendations for visual screening and to establish the most cost-effective and reliable means for detecting treatable pathology in elderly persons. Prospective cost-effectiveness studies of vision screening of elderly populations at risk are needed to establish the efficacy of such programs. Prospective observational studies should define the leading approaches to screening (eg, Snellen testing, J-scale, visual function scales, comprehensive examinations), and comparative studies should be performed to determine cost-effectiveness, validity, reliability, and feasibility.**

New Research Addressing This Question: No new research addressing this question has come to light since the publication of *New Frontiers.*

Modification of This Question in Light of New Research: This item should remain unchanged on the research agenda, as findings from research addressing this question will contribute to improved ophthalmologic care of older adults.

Ophth 25 (Level A): **Interventional studies should be performed in elderly persons to compare no screening with different screening methods, measuring efficacy on the basis of visual and functional outcome.**

New Research Addressing This Question: No new research addressing this question has come to light since the publication of *New Frontiers.*

Modification of This Question in Light of New Research: This item should remain unchanged on the research agenda, as findings from research addressing this question will contribute to improved ophthalmologic care of older adults.

IMPORTANT EYE DISORDERS IN GERIATRIC POPULATIONS

Cataract

See *New Frontiers*, pp. 187–189.

***Ophth 26 (Level A)*: Interventional studies with elderly patients are needed to determine if there are differences in the amount of functional improvement that are based on the timing of cataract surgery, the initial and final visual outcome, whether one or both eyes are operated on, and the age of the patient at the time of the surgery.**

***Ophth 27 (Level A)*: Meta-analyses of existing data from previously performed interventional studies and clinical trials of cataract extraction should be performed to provide age-specific and age-stratified data for the elderly age group and to identify any age-specific differences in functional outcome.**

New Research Addressing These Questions: Friedman et al found low vision to be highly prevalent among nursing home residents (37% worse than 20/40 in the better eye) and black Americans to be more likely to have one or two cataracts (a potentially treatable cause of vision loss).[52] In a Scandinavian population, Buch et al concluded that adequate implementation of cataract surgery can reduce visual impairment by 33.3%.[53] The benefits of cataract extraction on function were confirmed in one small study that reported improvement in cognitive function after cataract surgery in elderly Japanese patients (n = 20) who were compared with controls (n = 20).[54] Though not directly addressing the impact of cataract surgery on function, an observational prospective study in Sweden of cataract surgery in 757 patients aged 85 years or older reported overall good visual outcomes.[55]

Modification of These Questions in Light of New Research: Although these studies are important and helpful, we encourage further data mining of existing databases for age-stratified information.

Age-Related Macular Degeneration

See *New Frontiers*, pp. 189–190.

***Ophth 28 (Level A)*: Interventional studies are needed to define the efficacy, cost-effectiveness, and functional outcomes of specific treatments for age-related macular degeneration.**

***Ophth 29 (Level A)*: Interventional studies are needed to determine the differences made, if any, by the timing of the treatment of age-related macular degeneration, with results stratified by age of the patient or timing of onset.**

***Ophth 30 (Level A)*: Meta-analyses of existing data from interventional and clinical studies on age-related macular degeneration should be**

performed to provide age-specific and age-stratified data regarding type, timing of therapy, and visual and functional outcome.

Ophth 31 (Level B): **All interventional studies of age-related macular degeneration should include demonstration of improvement in function as well as in visual acuity.**

New Research Addressing These Questions: Significant impairment in vision-specific health-related QOL (using the NEI-VFQ 25) was reported by ARMD patients seen at a low-vision clinic who were treated with various low-vision techniques.[56] In an uncontrolled study, Khan et al concluded that the overall management of ARMD should include counseling, prescription of appropriate devices, and training.[57]

Modification of These Questions in Light of New Research: These recent studies do not impact the agenda items; studies addressing these questions are therefore still needed.

Glaucoma

See *New Frontiers*, pp. 190–191.

Ophth 32 (Level A): **Interventional studies are needed to determine if the type and timing of treatments of glaucoma alter efficacy and if efficacy in elderly patients improves functional outcome.**

Ophth 33 (Level A): **Interventional studies are needed to determine the cost-effectiveness and durability of stabilization or improvement of vision in elderly glaucoma patents.**

Ophth 34 (Level A): **Interventional studies should be performed to determine if preventive measures or screening for glaucoma in older persons is effective and improves functional outcome.**

Ophth 35 (Level B): **Observational studies are needed to determine if treatment efficacy and functional outcome for glaucoma therapy differ by age.**

Ophth 36 (Level B): **Meta-analyses of existing data from interventional and clinical studies on surgical and medical treatment for glaucoma should be performed to provide age-specific and age-stratified data on functional outcome.**

New Research Addressing This Question: Two major clinical trials published recently on glaucoma management tended to show higher risks for progression among older glaucoma patients.[58,59] However, interpreting these findings is complicated by the fact that glaucoma tends to be relatively slowly progressive, and shorter life expectancy may limit the impact of glaucoma in older persons. One report based on the case notes of glaucoma patients from a blind registry in Fife, Scotland, reported that poor adherence with treatment was noted in 26%, and that 24% were demented. The average age at registration was 78 years.[60]

Modification of These Questions in Light of New Research: Additional interventional studies demonstrating improvement in functional outcomes are still needed.

Diabetic Retinopathy

See *New Frontiers*, pp. 191–192.

> ***Ophth 37 (Level B)*: Observational studies should be performed to determine the functional impact of diabetic retinopathy on the health-related quality of life of older diabetic patients.**

> ***Ophth 38 (Level A)*: Interventional studies are needed to determine whether specific preventive strategies (eg, tight diabetic control measures or diabetic retinopathy screening programs) and treatment measures improve functional outcomes in older diabetic patients.**

> ***Ophth 39 (Level B)*: Observational studies are needed to determine if the age of the patient, age at onset of diagnosis, and age at initiation of treatment are important factors in functional outcome in diabetic retinopathy.**

> ***Ophth 40 (Level A)*: Meta-analyses of data from existing and future interventional studies on the treatment of diabetes, including diabetic control, laser treatment for proliferative diabetic retinopathy and diabetic macular edema, and surgical treatment, should be performed to provide age-specific and age-stratified data on functional outcome.**

New Research Addressing These Questions: No new research addressing these questions has come to light since the publication of *New Frontiers.*

Modification of These Questions in Light of New Research: These items should remain unchanged on the research agenda, as findings from research addressing them will contribute to improved ophthalmologic care of older adults.

LOW VISION

See *New Frontiers*, p. 193.

> ***Ophth 41 (Level A)*: Interventional studies should be performed in elderly persons to determine if the types and visual outcome effectiveness of low-vision therapies are important factors in functional outcomes.**

New Research Addressing This Question: One group has initiated a randomized trial of visual impairment interventions for nursing home residents. The study proposes to determine the physical and social function of nursing home residents with and without visual loss to determine the impact of vision rehabilitation service versus usual care, and to determine the cost-effectiveness of the interventional program.[61] A separate study of 71 persons reported on the impact of an interdisciplinary low-vision service on the QOL of low-vision patients. The provision of low-vision services was found to lead to a significant reduction in anxiety about deterioration of vision, home safety, and coping with everyday life. These authors concluded that low-vision service resulted in improvements in many areas of vision-related QOL.[62] An observational study of new referrals to a low-vision clinic (N = 168) documented improvement in function after evaluation and treatment.

Before low-vision intervention, 77% were unable to read N8 newsprint, whereas following low-vision services, 88% were able to read N8 or smaller text.[63] In an institutionalized cohort of 284 older persons, de Winter et al reported a 31% prevalence of binocular low vision.[64]

One large randomized controlled clinical trial of 226 patients with ARMD compared extended low-vision rehabilitation (including home visits along with hospital-based low-vision treatment) and standard hospital-based treatment. No benefit of additional home visits was found in this study, and the authors caution clinicians of the need for testing of low-vision therapies before implementing them widely.[65]

The Agency for Healthcare Research and Quality issued a Technology Assessment report on vision rehabilitation for older persons with low vision or blindness. The aims of this extensive project included the following: first, to estimate the number of elderly persons with visual loss that might benefit from low-vision rehabilitation services, and second, to systematically review the evidence for the effectiveness of vision rehabilitation services. In assessing effectiveness, the authors considered outcomes, including disability and function, activities of daily living, psychosocial status, and quality of life. The report concluded that comprehensive vision rehabilitation programs benefit individuals, but that the evidence supporting this statement is weak because of poor methodology in the research. Other conclusions were that optic devices and visual aids improve reading performance, that the efficacy of orientation and mobility training has yet to be demonstrated by a well-designed study using validated instruments, and that no evidence-based recommendation could be made regarding adaptive techniques training or group intervention programs.[66]

Modification of This Question in Light of New Research: Although much of the work to date is promising, more research to demonstrate functional improvement is still needed.

NEW HORIZONS IN GERIATRIC OPHTHALMOLOGY

Visual Loss and Falls

The following agenda item should be added to the research agenda to complement Ophth 5 as newer primary and secondary outcome assessments emerge for falls preventive measures; these assessments will be better than relying solely upon epidemiologic studies with falling as the primary outcome measure.

> *Ophth 42 (Level B)*: **Interventional studies (eg, low-vision rehabilitation) to improve visual functioning in elderly patients should be performed to assess improvements in mechanics of gait, stair negotiation, posture, and balance to reduce falls risk.**

Visual Loss and Mortality

Prior studies have shown an association of visual loss with increased mortality. More recently, McCarty et al reported on predictors of mortality in the 5-year follow-up of the Melbourne Visual Impairment Project (VIP), a population-based study of 3271 persons aged 40 years and older as of 1992, when the baseline study was done. Best corrected visual acuity lower than 6/12 was found to be associated with a significantly higher risk of mortality.[67]

Ophth 43 (Levels B, A): **Observational studies are recommended to determine the impact of visual loss on mortality in the elderly age group, and interventional studies might then follow, to demonstrate the reduction of mortality rates after specific visual interventions.**

VISUAL LOSS AND INSTITUTIONAL RESIDENCE

One study assessed the risk of institutionalization associated with visual impairment. Using national interview data, these authors concluded that visual handicap is associated with institutional admission.[68] In a large cohort study from Australia, older persons with visual impairment (both correctable and not correctable) were found to have about twice the rate of nursing home admission than those with good vision.[69] The study by Sloan et al also found self-reported declines in vision to be associated with increased probability of nursing home residence.[29]

Ophth 44 (Levels B, A): **Observational studies are recommended to determine the impact of visual loss on institutionalization in the elderly age group, and interventional studies might then follow, to demonstrate the reduction of institutionalization rates after specific visual interventions.**

REFERENCES

1. Lee AG, Coleman AL. Geriatric ophthalmology. In Solomon DH, LoCicero J, 3rd, Rosenthal RA (eds): New Frontiers in Geriatrics Research: An Agenda for Surgical and Related Medical Specialties. New York: American Geriatrics Society, 2004, pp. 177-202 (online at http://www.frycomm.com/ags/rasp).
2. Dandona R, Dandona L, Srinivas M, et al. Planning low vision services in India: a population-based perspective. Ophthalmology 2002;109:1871-1878.
3. Evans JR, Fletcher AE, Wormald RP, et al. Prevalence of visual impairment in people aged 75 years and older in Britain: results from the MRC trial of assessment and management of older people in the community. Br J Ophthalmol 2002;86:795-800.
4. Munoz B, West SK, Rubin GS, et al. Causes of blindness and visual impairment in a population of older Americans: The Salisbury Eye Evaluation Study. Arch Ophthalmol 2000;118:819-825.
5. Rodriguez J, Sanchez R, Munoz B, et al. Causes of blindness and visual impairment in a population-based sample of U.S. Hispanics. Ophthalmology 2002;109:737-743.
6. VanNewkirk MR, Weih L, McCarty CA, Taylor HR. Cause-specific prevalence of bilateral visual impairment in Victoria, Australia: the Visual Impairment Project. Ophthalmology 2001;108:960-967.
7. Hyman L, Wu SY, Connell AM, et al. Prevalence and causes of visual impairment in The Barbados Eye Study. Ophthalmology 2001;108:1751-1756.
8. Pascolini D, Mariotti SP, Pokharel GP, et al. 2002 global update of available data on visual impairment: a compilation of population-based prevalence studies. Ophthalmic Epidemiol 2004;11:67-115.

9. van der Pols JC, Bates CJ, McGraw PV, et al. Visual acuity measurements in a national sample of British elderly people. Br J Ophthalmol 2000;84:165-170.
10. Congdon N, O'Colmain B, Klaver CC, et al. Causes and prevalence of visual impairment among adults in the United States. Arch Ophthalmol 2004;122:477-485.
11. Iwano M, Nomura H, Ando F, et al. Visual acuity in a community-dwelling Japanese population and factors associated with visual impairment. Jpn J Ophthalmol 2004;48:37-43.
12. Vongphanit J, Mitchell P, Wang JJ. Prevalence and progression of myopic retinopathy in an older population. Ophthalmology 2002;109:704-711.
13. Younan C, Mitchell P, Cumming RG, et al. Myopia and incident cataract and cataract surgery: the Blue Mountains Eye Study. Invest Ophthalmol Vis Sci 2002;43:3625-3632.
14. Michon JJ, Lau J, Chan WS, Ellwein LB. Prevalence of visual impairment, blindness, and cataract surgery in the Hong Kong elderly. Br J Ophthalmol 2002;86:133-139.
15. Hsu WM, Cheng CY, Liu JH, et al. Prevalence and causes of visual impairment in an elderly Chinese population in Taiwan: the Shihpai Eye Study. Ophthalmology 2004;111:62-69.
16. Massof RW, Rubin GS. Visual function assessment questionnaires. Surv Ophthalmol 2001;45:531-548.
17. Mangione CM, Lee PP, Pitts J, et al. Psychometric properties of the National Eye Institute Visual Function Questionnaire (NEI-VFQ). NEI-VFQ Field Test Investigators. Arch Ophthalmol 1998;116:1496-1504.
18. Mangione CM, Lee PP, Gutierrez PR, et al. Development of the 25-item National Eye Institute Visual Function Questionnaire. Arch Ophthalmol 2001;119:1050-1058.
19. Clemons TE, Chew EY, Bressler SB, McBee W. National Eye Institute Visual Function Questionnaire in the Age-Related Eye Disease Study (AREDS): AREDS Report No. 10. Arch Ophthalmol 2003;121:211-217.
20. Lindblad AS, Clemons TE. Responsiveness of the National Eye Institute Visual Function Questionnaire to progression to advanced age-related macular degeneration, vision loss, and lens opacity: AREDS Report no. 14. Arch Ophthalmol 2005;123:1207-1214.
21. Cole SR, Beck RW, Moke PS, et al. The National Eye Institute Visual Function Questionnaire: experience of the ONTT. Optic Neuritis Treatment Trial. Invest Ophthalmol Vis Sci 2000;41:1017-1021.
22. Klein R, Moss SE, Klein BE, et al. The NEI-VFQ-25 in people with long-term type 1 diabetes mellitus: the Wisconsin Epidemiologic Study of Diabetic Retinopathy. Arch Ophthalmol 2001;119:733-740.
23. Schiffman RM, Jacobsen G, Whitcup SM. Visual functioning and general health status in patients with uveitis. Arch Ophthalmol 2001;119:841-849.
24. Sharma S, Brown GC, Brown MM, et al. Converting visual acuity to utilities. Can J Ophthalmol 2000;35:267-272.
25. Jampel HD. Glaucoma patients' assessment of their visual function and quality of life. Trans Am Ophthalmol Soc 2001;99:301-317.
26. Brown GC, Brown MM, Sharma S, et al. The reproducibility of ophthalmic utility values. Trans Am Ophthalmol Soc 2001;99:199-203; discussion 203-194.
27. Steinberg EP, Tielsch JM, Schein OD, et al. The VF-14: an index of functional impairment in patients with cataract. Arch Ophthalmol 1994;112:630-638.
28. Tsai SY, Chi LY, Cheng CY, et al. The impact of visual impairment and use of eye services on health-related quality of life among the elderly in Taiwan: the Shihpai Eye Study. Qual Life Res 2004;13:1415-1424.
29. Sloan FA, Ostermann J, Brown DS, Lee PP. Effects of changes in self-reported vision on cognitive, affective, and functional status and living arrangements among the elderly. Am J Ophthalmol 2005;140:618-627.

30. Stelmack J. Quality of life of low-vision patients and outcomes of low-vision rehabilitation. Optom Vis Sci 2001;78:335-342.
31. Lord SR, Menz HB. Visual contributions to postural stability in older adults. Gerontology 2000;46:306-310.
32. Lord SR, Dayhew J, Howland A. Multifocal glasses impair edge-contrast sensitivity and depth perception and increase the risk of falls in older people. J Am Geriatr Soc 2002;50:1760-1766.
33. Lord SR, Dayhew J. Visual risk factors for falls in older people. J Am Geriatr Soc 2001;49:508-515.
34. de Boer MR, Pluijm SM, Lips P, et al. Different aspects of visual impairment as risk factors for falls and fractures in older men and women. J Bone Miner Res 2004;19:1539-1547.
35. Ivers RQ, Cumming RG, Mitchell P, et al. Visual risk factors for hip fracture in older people. J Am Geriatr Soc 2003;51:356-363.
36. Buckley JG, Heasley KJ, Twigg P, Elliott DB. The effects of blurred vision on the mechanics of landing during stepping down by the elderly. Gait Posture 2005;21:65-71.
37. Startzell JK, Owens DA, Mulfinger LM, Cavanagh PR. Stair negotiation in older people: a review. J Am Geriatr Soc 2000;48:567-580.
38. Campbell AJ, Robertson MC, La Grow SJ, et al. Randomised controlled trial of prevention of falls in people aged > or =75 with severe visual impairment: the VIP trial. BMJ 2005;331:817.
39. Coleman AL, Stone K, Ewing SK, et al. Higher risk of multiple falls among elderly women who lose visual acuity. Ophthalmology 2004;111:857-862.
40. Tromp AM, Pluijm SM, Smit JH, et al. Fall-risk screening test: a prospective study on predictors for falls in community-dwelling elderly. J Clin Epidemiol 2001;54:837-844.
41. Abdelhafiz AH, Austin CA. Visual factors should be assessed in older people presenting with falls or hip fracture. Age Ageing 2003;32:26-30.
42. Lin MY, Gutierrez PR, Stone KL, et al. Vision impairment and combined vision and hearing impairment predict cognitive and functional decline in older women. J Am Geriatr Soc 2004;52:1996-2002.
43. Heine C, Browning CJ. Communication and psychosocial consequences of sensory loss in older adults: overview and rehabilitation directions. Disabil Rehabil 2002;24:763-773.
44. Bazargan M, Baker RS, Bazargan SH. Sensory impairments and subjective well-being among aged African American persons. J Gerontol B Psychol Sci Soc Sci 2001;56:P268-P278.
45. Wallhagen MI, Strawbridge WJ, Shema SJ, et al. Comparative impact of hearing and vision impairment on subsequent functioning. J Am Geriatr Soc 2001;49:1086-1092.
46. Galaria, II, Casten RJ, Rovner BW. Development of a shorter version of the geriatric depression scale for visually impaired older patients. Int Psychogeriatr 2000;12:435-443.
47. Horowitz A, Reinhardt JP, Boerner K. The effect of rehabilitation on depression among visually disabled older adults. Aging Ment Health 2005;9:563-570.
48. Brody BL, Roch-Levecq AC, Gamst AC, et al. Self-management of age-related macular degeneration and quality of life: a randomized controlled trial. Arch Ophthalmol 2002;120:1477-1483.
49. Reyes-Ortiz CA, Kuo YF, DiNuzzo AR, et al. Near vision impairment predicts cognitive decline: data from the Hispanic Established Populations for Epidemiologic Studies of the Elderly. J Am Geriatr Soc 2005;53:681-686.
50. Anstey KJ, Luszcz MA, Sanchez L. Two-year decline in vision but not hearing is associated with memory decline in very old adults in a population-based sample. Gerontology 2001;47:289-293.
51. Park WL, Mayer RS, Moghimi C, et al. Rehabilitation of hospital inpatients with visual impairments and disabilities from systemic illness. Arch Phys Med Rehabil 2005;86:79-81.

52. Friedman DS, Munoz B, Roche KB, et al. Poor uptake of cataract surgery in nursing home residents: the Salisbury Eye Evaluation in Nursing Home Groups study. Arch Ophthalmol 2005;123:1581-1587.
53. Buch H, Vinding T, La Cour M, et al. Prevalence and causes of visual impairment and blindness among 9980 Scandinavian adults: the Copenhagen City Eye Study. Ophthalmology 2004;111:53-61.
54. Tamura H, Tsukamoto H, Mukai S, et al. Improvement in cognitive impairment after cataract surgery in elderly patients. J Cataract Refract Surg 2004;30:598-602.
55. Lundstrom M, Stenevi U, Thorburn W. Cataract surgery in the very elderly. J Cataract Refract Surg 2000;26:408-414.
56. Scilley K, DeCarlo DK, Wells J, Owsley C. Vision-specific health-related quality of life in age-related maculopathy patients presenting for low vision services. Ophthalmic Epidemiol 2004;11:131-146.
57. Khan SA, Das T, Kumar SM, Nutheti R. Low vision rehabilitation in patients with age-related macular degeneration at a tertiary eye care centre in southern India. Clin Experiment Ophthalmol 2002;30:404-410.
58. Kass MA, Heuer DK, Higginbotham EJ, et al. The Ocular Hypertension Treatment Study: a randomized trial determines that topical ocular hypotensive medication delays or prevents the onset of primary open-angle glaucoma. Arch Ophthalmol 2002;120:701-713; discussion 829-730.
59. Heijl A, Leske MC, Bengtsson B, et al. Reduction of intraocular pressure and glaucoma progression: results from the Early Manifest Glaucoma Trial. Arch Ophthalmol 2002;120:1268-1279.
60. Sinclair A, Hinds A, Sanders R. Ten years of glaucoma blindness in Fife 1990-99 and the implications for ophthalmology, optometry and rehabilitation services. Ophthalmic Physiol Opt 2004;24:313-318.
61. West SK, Friedman D, Munoz B, et al. A randomized trial of visual impairment interventions for nursing home residents: study design, baseline characteristics and visual loss. Ophthalmic Epidemiol 2003;10:193-209.
62. Hinds A, Sinclair A, Park J, et al. Impact of an interdisciplinary low vision service on the quality of life of low vision patients. Br J Ophthalmol 2003;87:1391-1396.
63. Margrain TH. Helping blind and partially sighted people to read: the effectiveness of low vision aids. Br J Ophthalmol 2000;84:919-921.
64. de Winter LJ, Hoyng CB, Froeling PG, et al. Prevalence of remediable disability due to low vision among institutionalised elderly people. Gerontology 2004;50:96-101.
65. Reeves BC, Harper RA, Russell WB. Enhanced low vision rehabilitation for people with age related macular degeneration: a randomised controlled trial. Br J Ophthalmol 2004;88:1443-1449.
66. Vision rehabilitation for elderly individuals with low vision or blindness. Rockville, MD: ARHQ Technology Assessment Program; 2004 (online at: http://www.cms.hhs.gov/CoverageGenInfo/Downloads/RTCvisionrehab.pdf).
67. McCarty CA, Nanjan MB, Taylor HR. Vision impairment predicts 5 year mortality. Br J Ophthalmol 2001;85:322-326.
68. Brezin AP, Lafuma A, Fagnani F, et al. Prevalence and burden of self-reported blindness and low vision for individuals living in institutions: a nationwide survey. Health Qual Life Outcomes 2005;3:27.
69. Wang JJ, Mitchell P, Cumming RG, Smith W. Visual impairment and nursing home placement in older Australians: the Blue Mountains Eye Study. Ophthalmic Epidemiol 2003;10:3-13.

8

GERIATRIC OTOLARYNGOLOGY

*Michael M. Johns, MD; Sarah Wise, MD; Steven M. Parnes, MD**

Otolaryngology—head and neck surgery—is an important and diverse specialty. Otolaryngologists care for people with a wide variety of problems, ranging from quality-of-life–impairing communication disorders to life-threatening diseases of the head and neck. Commensurate with changing demographics of Western society, it is not surprising that up to one third of patients seen by the average otolaryngologist are aged 65 or over. Advances in public health and medicine have led to increased life expectancy and, with this increase, a growing emphasis on quality of life for older persons.

Pediatric otolaryngology has become a distinct subspecialty within the field, but geriatric otolaryngology has not; despite its importance, research, education, and clinical focus in geriatric otolaryngology has been lacking. The principles of geriatric medicine and issues of concern specific to elderly otolaryngologic patients have not been widely applied in otolaryngology. Furthermore, a significant portion of the literature dealing with geriatric issues in otolaryngology consists of case reports and uncontrolled case series. This review updates the chapter by Hinrich Staecker in *New Frontiers in Geriatrics Research*, which was the first comprehensive review outlining a research agenda in geriatric otolaryngology.[1] The purpose of this follow-up is to update the review of current knowledge in geriatric otolaryngology, to identify the extent to which the Key Questions defined in *New Frontiers* have been answered, and to further define the basic and clinical information needed for the future advancement of geriatric otolaryngology.

The original three Key Questions in otolaryngology from *New Frontiers* are listed below. This update identifies research that has addressed these questions in the interval since the initial publication and then expands upon these questions in light of the new research.

> ***Otolaryn KQ1*: How can research be used to improve hearing-related quality of life for elderly persons?**
>
> ***Otolaryn KQ2*: Can disorders of the peripheral vestibular system be accurately recognized and their causes determined, and does targeted treatment benefit elderly patients with balance disorders or dizziness?**
>
> ***Otolaryn KQ3*: Does standard management of head and neck cancer compromise quality of life in the elderly patient to a greater degree than in the younger patient?**

See also the subsection on new Key Questions in the section New Horizons in Geriatric Otolaryngology, at the end of the chapter.

---

* Johns: Assistant Professor of Otolaryngology, Director of Emory Voice Center, Emory University School of Medicine, Atlanta, GA; Wise: Assistant Professor of Otolaryngology, Emory University School of Medicine, Atlanta, GA; Parnes: Professor and Head, Department of Otolaryngology, Albany Medical College, Albany, NY.

METHODS

A comprehensive literature search was conducted on the National Library of Medicine's PubMed database. The initial review by Staecker covered the time period from 1980 to April 2001. [1] This follow-up review adds publications from April 2001 through October 2005. The search strategy combined various terms for otolaryngology: *hearing, balance, head and neck cancer, swallowing, allergy, sinusitis, voice, larynx, smell,* and *olfaction.* Individual hits were refined by the use of the "related articles" button. Otolaryngology textbooks with chapters on geriatrics were reviewed, and their bibliographies were added to the database. Additional requirements were either that the publication be a review, clinical trial, randomized controlled trial, or meta-analysis, and that terms for risk or age factors be present as title words or MeSH headings. Terms denoting age were *age factors, age, aging, elderly, geriatric, gerontologic, older,* or *octogenarian, nonagenarian,* or *centenarian.* Relevant reports were organized by subspecialty and reviewed, focusing on the extent to which Key Questions in *New Frontiers* were answered and new Key Questions were raised.

PROGRESS IN DISORDERS OF THE AUDITORY SYSTEM

For a new agenda item, see the subsection on disorders of the auditory system in New Horizons in Geriatric Otolaryngology, at the end of the chapter.

EPIDEMIOLOGY

See *New Frontiers,* pp. 203–204.

DISEASES OF THE PINNA AND EXTERNAL AUDITORY CANAL

See *New Frontiers,* p. 204.

DISEASES OF THE TYMPANIC MEMBRANE AND MIDDLE EAR

See *New Frontiers,* pp. 204–205.

***Otolaryn 1 (Levels A, B)*: Randomized controlled trials or prospective cohort studies of otosclerosis patients are needed to compare the effects of surgery or amplification on function and quality of life.**

New Research Addressing This Question: In the interval since publication of *New Frontiers*, no randomized or prospective studies have been performed to answer this question. A retrospective study of older adults helps shed light on this topic. [2] The authors note "that stapedioplasty offers greater improvement in quality of life for selected adults aged 60 and older than for younger adults. The operation also appears to be as safe for adults aged 60 and older as for younger adults. Stapedioplasty provides subjects with satisfactory social hearing level (hearing capacity sufficient for normal social relations) and slows the progression of otosclerosis. Providing older patients with good auditory functionality improves their state of health, quality of life, and cognitive processes." Furthermore, a retrospective study on patients of all ages (including older adults) suggests that amplification using a bone-anchored hearing aid improves function and quality of life in these patients.[3] Evidence has been published indicating that stapes surgery for otosclerosis in elderly adults is as safe and at least as effective as that in younger adults.[2,4–7] Additionally, geriatric patients may derive more quality-of-life benefit from otosclerosis surgery than younger patients.[2]

Modification of This Question in Light of New Research: This question should remain on the research agenda unmodified.

Otolaryn 2 (Level B): **Patients with unilateral hearing loss of any cause should be compared with those who have bilateral hearing loss in an observational study, either at a single time or longitudinally to assess functional and quality-of-life outcomes.**

New Research Addressing This Question: These studies have yet to be performed. The marginal quality-of-life and functional decrements that may occur in unilateral versus bilateral hearing loss remain unclear.

Modification of This Question in Light of New Research: This question should remain on the research agenda unmodified.

Otolaryn 3 (Level A): **The effects of bilateral surgery should be compared with those of unilateral surgery in randomized controlled trials or prospective cohort studies of elderly patients with otosclerosis.**

New Research Addressing This Question: The additional value of operating on the second ear in geriatric otosclerosis patients is not clear. However, evidence suggests an adequate degree of safety associated with bilateral surgery in both the young and elderly population.[8]

Modification of This Question in Light of New Research: This question should remain on the research agenda unmodified.

Otolaryn 4 (Level B): **In order to better define the contribution in older people of eustachian tube dysfunction to hearing loss, an observational study, at a single time or longitudinally, should be carried out in which audiogram and tympanogram findings are correlated with symptoms and signs of eustachian tube dysfunction.**

New Research Addressing This Question: Eustachian tube dysfunction has been described in older as well as younger patients, but new information has been published that demonstrates no greater incidence of eustachian tube dysfunction, related hearing loss, or middle ear pathology in older adults than in younger adults.[9] Additionally, over a 5-year span in aged adults, little change occurs in middle ear mechanics.[10] These clinical studies are in contrast to previously published work, which found functional compliance to change with aging, which affects the overall function of the eustachian tube.[11]

Modification of This Question in Light of New Research: This question has been addressed and can be dropped from the research agenda. Eustachian tube function does not appear to lead to change dramatically or lead to increased pathology in the elderly population.

Otolaryn 5 (Levels, B, A): **If a strong correlation between eustachian tube dysfunction and hearing loss is found (see Otolaryn 4), interventions to improve eustachian tube dysfunction should be tested in preliminary studies and ultimately in a randomized controlled trial to determine if improving eustachian tube function improves hearing in older people with and without presbycusis.**

New Research Addressing This Question: See previous section, where new research is described that refutes this strong correlation.

Modification of This Question in Light of New Research: This question becomes unnecessary as a result of new research, and the item can be dropped from the research agenda.

PRESBYCUSIS OR SENSORINEURAL HEARING LOSS

See *New Frontiers,* pp. 205–206.

Impact of Presbycusis on Quality of Life

See *New Frontiers,* pp. 206–207.

Inheritance of Presbycusis

See *New Frontiers,* p. 207.

The Impact of Hearing Loss on Dementia

See *New Frontiers,* pp. 207–208.

Treatment of Presbycusis

See *New Frontiers,* p. 208.

Neurotology

See *New Frontiers,* pp. 208–209.

Otolaryn 6 (Level B): **An instrument that would test hearing in small groups set in a noisy environment needs to be developed and validated. Such an instrument would be helpful in all the following recommended studies.**

New Research Addressing This Question: This instrument remains to be developed.

Modification of This Question in Light of New Research: This question should remain on the research agenda unmodified.

Otolaryn 7 (Levels B, A): **There is a need for a definitive test of the widely accepted belief that bilateral hearing aids are better than unilateral aids. This could be done by prospective cohort study or by randomized controlled trial. Such studies are needed both for implantable and external-ear hearing aids. Outcome measures**

should include hearing, speech discrimination, quality of life, and cost-benefit analysis. In the case of unilateral implantation, the unoperated ear can serve as an additional control regarding hearing.

New Research Addressing This Question: The value of hearing restoration for both ears versus only one remains unclear. No studies have been performed that shed light on this important question.

Modification of This Question in Light of New Research: This question should remain on the research agenda unmodified.

Otolaryn 8 (Level B): **The value of unilateral and bilateral implantable hearing aids needs to be assessed. A preliminary evaluation would require only measures of hearing and quality of life in the preoperative period with removable hearing aids in use, comparing these with similar measures taken after unilateral or bilateral implantation.**

New Research Addressing This Question: This research has yet to be performed.

Modification of This Question in Light of New Research: This question should remain on the research agenda unmodified.

Otolaryn 9 (Level B): **Studies of elderly patients with profound sensorineural hearing loss are needed that resemble trials for moderate to severe hearing loss in the same age group. The economic benefits of cochlear implantation in the geriatric population is beginning to be defined. Prospective observational studies are now needed that will take into account issues such as loss of independence and cost-benefit ratios.**

New Research Addressing This Question: Prospective observational studies to address this question have not been published. However, carefully designed retrospective outcomes studies demonstrate favorable cost-benefit ratios and functional results for cochlear implantation in the older adult. [12]

Modification of Question in Light of New Research: The magnitude of the problem of presbyacusis warrants the prospective studies that were originally suggested in *New Frontiers*. This question should remain on the research agenda unmodified.

Otolaryn 10 (Level B): **An observational study comparing temporal bone pathology, pertinent molecular markers, and audiometric data would significantly aid our understanding of age-related hearing loss.**

New Research Addressing This Question: Recent studies are beginning to define deficits in addition to the previously described degeneration of the auditory hair cells, auditory neurons, and stria vascularis. Schuknecht and Gacek classified presbycusis on the basis of histologic criteria. In their review of the subject, they reported that the four diagnostic criteria of age-related hearing loss (sensory cell degeneration, neural degeneration, strial atrophy, and cochlear conductive loss) held up in a review of 21 cases that met the clinical diagnosis of presbycusis. Of note was the observation that most cases seemed to have a mixed pathologic pattern.[13] More recent analysis of temporal bone specimens has shown a high incidence of mutations of mitochondrial DNA within the peripheral auditory system.[14]

Although hearing loss is a known and nearly ubiquitous phenomenon of aging, the factors associated with the age of onset, progression, and severity of hearing loss remain unknown. Increasing evidence suggests, however, that genetic makeup is an important factor.[15,16]

Modification of This Question in Light of New Research: Although much work continues in this important area, understanding of age-related hearing loss is far from complete. Ongoing studies to answer this question are needed, and the question should remain on the research agenda unmodified.

> *Otolaryn 11 (Level B)*: **Research has linked hearing loss with reduced quality of life, loss of independence, and depression. Observational studies are needed that would correlate patient-based outcomes measures and degree of hearing loss. These data should be used to develop guidelines for otolaryngologists to consider in obtaining geriatric consultation for at-risk patients.**

New Research Addressing This Question: New research, interestingly, demonstrates that elderly persons significantly underestimate the degree of their hearing loss and that, despite having significant deterioration in hearing thresholds over a 10-year period, they fail to notice worsening hearing. This research highlights the importance of education regarding hearing screening and rehabilitation. This is particularly important in light of evidence that suggests that hearing rehabilitation may be associated with improved cognitive function over time, although this is controversial.[17,18]

Modification of This Question in Light of New Research: Although new research highlights the need for increased education of both older persons and their physicians regarding the prevalence and impact of presbycusis, it is still not clear what effect hearing loss has on the older person's independence, depression, and other general outcomes. Therefore, this question should remain on the research agenda unmodified.

> *Otolaryn 12 (Level B)*: **Studies have defined impaired central auditory processing and identified its importance in aging. Central auditory testing is currently performed only in tertiary care centers and takes up to half a day for a single patient. Briefer test panels need to be developed and validated to aid the screening of older patients. This can be carried out as an observational trial for hypothesis generation.**

New Research Addressing This Question: No significant progress has been made to address this question.

Modification of This Question in Light of New Research: This question should remain on the research agenda unmodified.

PROGRESS IN DISORDERS OF THE VESTIBULAR SYSTEM

See *New Frontiers,* p. 210. For a new agenda item, see the subsection on disorders of the vestibular system in New Horizons in Geriatric Otolaryngology, at the end of the chapter.

HISTOLOGIC STUDIES

See *New Frontiers,* p. 210.

ETIOLOGY OF DIZZINESS

See *New Frontiers,* pp. 210–211.

DEVELOPMENTS IN VESTIBULAR TESTING

See *New Frontiers,* p. 211.

TREATMENT OF AGE-RELATED BALANCE PROBLEMS

See *New Frontiers,* pp. 211–212.

Otolaryn 13 (Level B): **The available literature supports the idea that vestibular disease is commonly misdiagnosed. An observational study is needed to determine how different practitioners evaluate and treat the chief complaint of dizziness that is assumed to be of vestibular or undefined origin. This study should also determine the prevalence of the use of medications such as meclizine and the prevalence of physical therapy referral. Findings should then be used to develop best practice guidelines.**

New Research Addressing This Question: New research into this important area is lacking, and the questions posed remain unaddressed.

Modification of This Question in Light of New Research: This question should remain on the research agenda unmodified.

Otolaryn 14 (Level A): **Currently, several patient-based outcomes questionnaires for vestibular disorders are available. Vestibular testing can consist of a combination of very different test modalities, including electronystagmography, rotary chair testing, testing of positional nystagmus, and posturography. A prospective randomized controlled study is needed to define which modality or combination of modalities is optimal for evaluating the elderly patient and determining level of vestibular system impairment and impact on quality of life.**

New Research Addressing This Question: No new research has been published to help sort out this complicated problem.

Modification of This Question in Light of New Research: This question should remain on the research agenda unmodified.

Otolaryn 15 (Level B): **Currently, no data exist correlating aging, vestibular function, and vestibular system histopathology. A collection of temporal bones of different aged patients with vestibular test results is needed to achieve a level of understanding similar to that we have for the auditory system.**

New Research Addressing This Question: This database remains to be generated, although its importance cannot be underestimated.

Modification of This Question in Light of New Research: This question should remain on the research agenda unmodified.

PROGRESS IN DISORDERS OF THE NOSE AND SINUSES

For a new agenda item, see the subsection on the aesthetics of the aging nose in New Horizons in Geriatric Otolaryngology, at the end of the chapter.

SMELL

See *New Frontiers,* pp. 212–213. For new agenda items, see also the subsection on smell in New Horizons in Geriatric Otolaryngology, at the end of the chapter.

SINUSITIS AND NASAL DISCHARGE

See *New Frontiers,* p. 213. For a new agenda item, see the subsection on sinusitis and nasal discharge in New Horizons in Geriatric Otolaryngology, at the end of the chapter.

Otolaryn 16 (Level B): **An observational study is needed to define the incidence of sinusitis in older people and to learn whether diagnostic and treatment approaches to the elderly patient are different. Most studies of sinusitis give an average age but have not assessed their data in terms of age cohorts. If age-related differences are identified, risk-factor assessment (elderly versus nonelderly) will have to be carried out by means of prospective cohort studies.**

New Research Addressing This Question: The fundamental question raised remains. The incidence of sinusitis in the population of elderly community-dwelling persons remains unclear. Whether older people are more or less prone to sinusitis and whether diagnostic and treatment approaches are the same as for younger patients remain unknown.

Rhinosinusitis is extremely common in the United States. Rhinosinusitis affects 16% of the adult population annually and has vast economic consequences. [19] The true prevalence of rhinosinusitis in the elderly population has not been studied and remains to be determined. However, given the increased incidence of comorbidities in older adults, medical and surgical therapies for rhinosinusitis may have significant implications in the elderly patient. Patients with rhinosinusitis are often treated with extended courses of antibiotics and steroids, and surgical therapy is recommended in selected patients. Colclasure et al compared 56 patients over the age of 60 who underwent endoscopic sinus surgery with a general adult population undergoing the same surgical procedure. These authors identified no major complications in the elderly cohort. Additionally, postoperative subjective and objective improvement was found to be consistent with reports of the same measures in the general adult population. The authors concluded that endoscopic sinus surgery is safe and effective in the elderly population.[20]

Some new information regarding the etiology and potential risk factors of sinonasal inflammatory disease in general has been published (see next section).

Modification of This Question in light of New Research: The core question seeking the differences in the incidence and prevalence of sinonasal disease in the geriatric patient remains. This question should remain on the research agenda unmodified.

> *Otolaryn 17 (Level B)*: **Depending on the outcome of the research recommended in Otolaryn 16, a prospective study on the risk factors for sinusitis in the elderly person is needed. This would examine the incidence of allergic and nonallergic rhinitis, as well as the environmental factors that predispose the older person to sinusitis.**

New Research Addressing This Question: Many elderly patients report symptoms of rhinitis (ie, an inflamed, irritated, or runny nose). Although there are many potential causes of rhinitis, seasonal and environmental allergies are present in older persons and should be considered in differential diagnoses. Some recent publications have addressed the diagnosis and treatment of allergy in the elderly patient. Crawford et al assessed allergic disease in the older person by studying 132 adult men. These authors found that the prevalence of rhinitis remained stable in the elderly age group. However, skin test reactivity and mean total serum IgE did decline among elderly subjects with rhinitis in comparison with younger subjects. This implies that although rhinitis is prevalent in older patients, nonallergic causes of rhinitis should also be considered in these patients.[21] King and Lockey also noted that because of atrophic or sun-damaged skin in elderly patients, skin-prick allergy testing in this population must be performed and interpreted with caution.[22]

Antihistamines are often used to treat allergy symptoms. However, first-generation H_1-antihistamine therapy must be used with caution in the elderly patient. These antihistamines may produce significant side effects in older persons because of the physiologic changes of normal aging, as well as drug-drug or drug-disease interactions.[23] The newer, nonsedating antihistamines appear to be safe and effective alternatives to earlier-generation antihistamines for treating older patients.

The use of injection immunotherapy in elderly patients has been debated. Asero evaluated specific injection immunotherapy to birch and ragweed in 39 elderly allergic patients, who were compared with 37 elderly control patients who refused to undergo immunotherapy. The patients who underwent immunotherapy had significantly reduced symptoms and significantly reduced use of oral antihistamines after 1 to 5 years of immunotherapy than the control patients. The author concluded that injection immunotherapy is an effective option in healthy elderly persons whose symptoms are not controlled symptomatically by medication therapy.[24]

Modification of This Question in Light of New Research: The agenda item should remain on the research agenda unchanged because the risk factors for the development of rhinosinusitis in the elderly population remain.

PROGRESS IN DISORDERS OF SWALLOWING

See *New Frontiers,* pp. 213–215.

***Otolaryn 18 (Level B)*: Currently, there is no consensus on the optimal evaluation of the dysphagia patient. A comparison of functional endoscopic evaluation of swallowing with modified barium swallow is needed to evaluate swallowing function and outcome of therapy in patients with dysphagia. Specificity and sensitivity should be determined, and cost-benefit analysis should be carried out.**

New Research Addressing This Question: Dysphagia is likely the most significant medical condition affecting the geriatric otolaryngic patient. The incidence of aspiration pneumonia is on the rise in comparison with other types of pneumonia, and pneumonia is the fifth leading cause of death in persons aged 65 and over. [25,26] Dysphagia is common in the elderly age group, with prevalence estimates ranging from 15% to 50%, depending on the population studied. [25] Although significant advances in geriatric dysphagia research have occurred since publication of *New Frontiers*, important questions remain in our understanding of this condition.

Swallowing is a complex function that depends on precise neurosensory and neuromuscular function of the upper aerodigestive tract. Age-related changes, such as sarcopenia, reduced laryngopharyngeal sensation, and diminished oral and pharyngeal coordination, make elderly persons at least prone to dysphagia, if not themselves causing the dysphagia. In a study of normal volunteers (N = 80) divided into four age cohorts, liquid and semisolid swallows were studied with manometry and videofluoroscopy. Total swallowing time and time to initiation of oropharyngeal swallowing were found to be prolonged in advanced age in this and surface electromyographic studies. [27] Upper esophageal sphincter pressure, peak pressure, and rate of bolus propagation do not appear to be affected by age above 65. [28] Other studies at least partially contradict these data, showing an overall slowing of pharyngeal swallowing time but also confirming an impairment in the opening of the upper esophageal sphincter. [29]

The high rate of dysphagia in the geriatric age group is likely related to these changes compounded by common geriatric conditions, such as Parkinson's disease, stroke, xerostomia, and frailty. Xerostomia is a common geriatric otolaryngic complaint that may significantly contribute to dysphagia. The incidence of this problem is estimated to be as high as 1 in 5 elderly noninstitutionalized adults. Whether xerostomia is a natural change with aging is controversial, with evidence for both sides of the argument. [30–35] However, xerostomia is a common side effect of many prescription and nonprescription medications. Astor et al observed that medication (particularly anticholinergics and antipsychotics) and systemic illness are probably the most common causes of xerostomia. [36] Furthermore, Sjögren's syndrome may be underdiagnosed in patients complaining of xerostomia. In an analysis of 100 consecutive patients aged 60 years and over presenting at a xerostomia clinic, 60% were found to have salivary gland hypofunction. Of these, two thirds were found to suffer from Sjögren's syndrome. [37]

Modification of This Question in Light of New Research: Important questions remain with respect to geriatric dysphagia. The true prevalence of this problem in the community-dwelling older population still needs to be determined, and level A studies are needed. Its impact on quality of life and overall nutritional status also need to be studied. New agenda items are therefore proposed; see the subsection on disorders of swallowing in New Horizons in Geriatric Otolaryngology, at the end of the chapter.

PROGRESS IN DISORDERS OF THE LARYNX

For new agenda items, see the subsection on disorders of the larynx in New Horizons in Geriatric Otolaryngology, at the end of the chapter.

VOICE

See *New Frontiers,* pp. 215–216.

Otolaryn 19 (Levels B, A): **An epidemiologic study of the true incidence and etiology of age-related voice disorders is needed. For this purpose, a normal population (ie, not referred or otherwise selected patients) needs to be identified and screened for voice disorders. New surgical methods of treatment should be explored. Prospective randomized studies comparing conservative with surgical treatment for presbylarynges would follow.**

New Research Addressing This Question: One commonly underdiagnosed area of health concern among the geriatric population is dysphonia. Despite the crucial role that phonation plays in communication, the prevalence of geriatric dysphonia has been ill characterized. The most widely reported figure of 12% vocal dysfunction in the elderly age group has, in fact, been erroneously disseminated for two decades.[38–42] A new study by Golub et al has set out to answer the first part of question Otolaryn 19, namely, the prevalence of dysphonia in the geriatric population. The authors screened over 100 persons in a community independent-living facility and demonstrated that the prevalence of perceived dysphonia in this population was 20%. Furthermore, moderate to severe quality-of-life impairment resulting from their dysphonia was found in 13%.[43] This study highlights the significant problem of dysphonia in the aging population and reinforces the need for further research in this area.

The major differential diagnosis of vocal symptoms in the geriatric population includes unilateral vocal fold paralysis, benign and malignant vocal fold lesions, inflammatory conditions (laryngopharyngeal reflux), neurologic disease (vocal tremor, Parkinson's disease, stroke, spasmodic dysphonia), and age-related dysphonia.[44] Age-related dysphonia, or presbylarynges, is generally regarded as a diagnosis of exclusion to be made only after thorough medical and speech evaluation. One study found it to be the cause of dysphonia in only 4% of such dysphonic patients.[45] Another found it to be much more common, however, and cited it as the cause of symptoms in 30%.[38]

Although its incidence may be uncertain, the impact of age-related dysphonia is well known. Patients may complain of vocal fatigue, an inability to project their voice, and an inability to be heard over noise. Such limitations on oral communication may lead to social withdrawal and depression. Surgical treatments for age-related dysphonia, such as injection laryngoplasty and laryngeal framework surgery, are limited by their invasive nature and uncertain efficacy. Behavioral intervention (voice therapy) is a safer alternative but is limited by the requirement for multiple visits. A new study by Berg et al demonstrates the efficacy of voice therapy in presbyphonia in a case-control study. Individuals with presbyphonia undergoing voice therapy were found to have significant voice-related quality-of-life improvement over that seen in control participants.[46]

Modification of This Question in Light of New Research: Even though work defining the prevalence of geriatric dysphonia has been performed, the incidence and causes remain unclear. Voice therapy appears to be effective for presbyphonia. The efficacy of surgical therapy (injection augmentation, laryngeal framework surgery) for this problem remains unclear. Studies comparing voice therapy and surgical treatments are warranted. The agenda item should remain on the research agenda unchanged.

MALIGNANCIES

See *New Frontiers,* p. 216.

PROGRESS IN HEAD AND NECK CANCER

See *New Frontiers,* pp. 216–218.

> *Otolaryn 20 (Level B)*: **We need to understand better the present practice regarding head and neck cancer care. For this purpose, we recommend a prospective, multi-institutional study of a cohort of older patients with head and neck cancer. Observations would include comorbidity, functional status, advance directives, and physician recommendations, followed by description of the perioperative and postoperative course, complications, recovery, and rehabilitation. The outcome would be a regression-based model of preoperative, perioperative, and postoperative risk factors predicting outcomes, as well as a description of present practice.**

New Research Addressing This Question: Much new research has been performed to shed light on the many elements of this question. A number of retrospective studies have examined the effect of age on surgical and survival outcomes in head and neck cancer patients, with varied results. To date, there have been no prospective randomized trials that evaluate surgical, survival, or quality-of-life issues resulting from head and neck malignancies in elderly patients. Some authors have reviewed treatment considerations relevant to older patients with head and neck cancer and offered general guidelines for treating this age group. Genden et al encourage strong consideration of comorbid conditions in the elderly patient with head and neck cancer when selecting a treatment strategy.[47] Similarly, Bernardi et al advise that treatment of head and neck malignancies in the elderly patient should take into account the physiologic age of the patient in addition to tumor characteristics.[48] Finally, Gillani and Grunberg specifically note that conditions such as cardiovascular disease and chronic obstructive pulmonary disease increase in incidence and severity with cumulative tobacco exposure, as do head and neck malignancies. Cardiovascular disease and chronic obstructive pulmonary disease may complicate both surgical and chemoradiotherapeutic cancer treatment regimens. However, with careful planning, head and neck cancer treatment strategies can be formulated for elderly patients that retain the same efficacy as therapies for younger patients.[49]

Differentiated thyroid carcinoma affects adults of all age ranges. However, in older persons with thyroid carcinoma, poorer prognostic features are often present, such as follicular or Hürthle cell subtypes, extrathyroidal extension, and metastases. [50] van Tol et al encourage therapy to include total thyroidectomy with node dissection and radioiodine ablation. These authors note that treatment of persistent, recurrent, or metastatic disease must be based on disease stage and not denied on the basis of age. [50]

Administration of chemotherapy in older patients must be considered carefully, given its potential systemic toxicities in a patient population with an increased prevalence of comorbidities. Argiris et al compared response and toxicity in elderly and younger patients undergoing palliative chemotherapy for head and neck cancer. Although they found objective response rates and median survival time of the two groups to be similar, they found the elderly patients to have significantly increased incidence of nephrotoxicity, thrombocytopenia, and diarrhea with palliative chemotherapy regimens. [51] Because of the increased toxicity of chemotherapy in older persons, trials of head and neck chemotherapy regimens specifically designed for elderly patients or patients with medical complications have recently been performed. [52] In addition, Gebbia et al have reported a prospective study of the use of recombinant human erythropoietin in elderly patients undergoing chemotherapy with carboplatin and 5-fluorouracil for the treatment of head and neck cancer. Patients treated with recombinant human erythropoietin were found to have a statistically significant decrease in transfusion requirements for chemotherapy-related anemia in comparison with patients who did not receive erythropoietin. Patients who received erythropoietin also had improved quality of life. [53]

Although there has been some clinical research progress in the treatment of head and neck cancer in elderly patients, no large-scale prospective randomized trials of outcomes and toxicities of head and neck cancer treatment in this age group have been performed. It is important to recognize that, on the basis largely of retrospective studies, it is thought that fit elderly individuals can usually tolerate surgical and radiation therapies typically performed for head and neck tumor resection. With regard to chemotherapeutic protocols, outcomes in younger and older patients are also equivalent. However, the toxicities of chemotherapy appear to be increased in the elderly patient. Prospective randomized trials are still needed to determine definitively the effect of surgery, radiation, and chemotherapy for the treatment of head and neck cancer in the elderly age group.

Modification of This Question in Light of New Research: The agenda item should remain on the research agenda unchanged.

> *Otolaryn 21 (Level B)*: **We need to know the outcomes to be expected in older patients with head and neck cancer who are surgical candidates. A prospective multi-institutional study is needed that measures functional status, quality of life, social functioning, and depression as outcomes. Preoperative data should be compared with follow-up data for 1 to 3 years. Observations should be stratified by the scope of the surgery performed.**

New Research Addressing This Question: Although the specific question above remains unanswered, new research does address elements of it. Authors have reviewed treatment considerations relevant to older patients with head and neck cancer and offered general guidelines for treating this age group. See the discussion of Otolaryn 20 for descriptions of the relevant research.[47–49]

Modification of This Question in Light of New Research: The agenda item should remain on the research agenda unchanged.

Otolaryn 22 (Level A): **Depending on the outcome of the study recommended in Otolaryn 21, a prospective, possibly randomized controlled study comparing different surgical approaches for individual cancers (eg, tongue, pharynx) should be designed and performed.**

New Research Addressing This Question: More and more patients with head and neck cancer are being treated primarily with organ preservation–based protocols (chemotherapy plus radiation therapy). See the discussion of Otolaryn 20 for descriptions of the relevant research[51–53] and comments that follow about the need for further research.

Modification of This Question in Light of New Research: Despite changing trends in head and neck cancer treatment away from primary surgical therapy, surgery will always play a role in certain situations. Keeping in mind the significant consequences of both medical and surgical therapy for head and neck cancer, the question stands, but may be modified. Outcomes studies (levels A, B) are needed comparing minimally invasive surgical techniques with lower morbidity and standard surgical extirpations in the geriatric population.

Otolaryn 23 (Level B): **The wealth of data emerging from molecular biology studies of head and neck cancer need to be explored in terms of age. Prospective observational studies are needed to determine if the markers and molecular genetics of head and neck cancer are different in the elderly persons and if this impacts treatment decisions.**

New Research Addressing This Question: Much research is ongoing in this new frontier of head and neck cancer research. No studies to date have been published identifying molecular markers, and genetics differ in the geriatric and the younger patient. Regardless, molecular predictors of response to therapy will be forthcoming and will change the care of all patients with head and neck cancer.

Modification of This Question in Light of New Research: The agenda item should remain on the research agenda unchanged.

NEW HORIZONS IN GERIATRIC OTOLARYNGOLOGY

NEW KEY QUESTIONS IN GERIATRIC OTOLARYNGOLOGY

Otolaryn KQ4: **Diseases in the otolaryngic arena commonly present diagnostic challenges for primary care physicians. These challenges are often magnified by the hearing and communicative difficulties**

of older persons. Research is needed to develop simple high-yield diagnostic tools that the primary care practitioner can use to detect otolaryngic diseases.

Hypothesis-generating studies: Studies of the diagnostic accuracy of otolaryngic history and physical examination in the primary care setting are necessary to determine areas of deficiency in otolaryngic diagnosis by primary care physicians. These could be preliminarily performed with large-scale retrospective reviews of reasons for primary care referral of elderly patients to otolaryngologists, comparing rationale for referral with the ultimate diagnosis following otolaryngologic evaluation.

Hypothesis-testing studies: Once the most common reasons for otolaryngologic referral and missed diagnosis of the elderly patient are identified, outcomes research studies of simple diagnostic tests for use by the primary care physician may be developed.

***Otolaryn KQ5*: Multiple medical comorbidities among older persons often increase the medical and surgical risk for older otolaryngology patients. Research is needed to determine whether the use of minimally invasive diagnostic and therapeutic techniques in the geriatric patient decreases the medical and surgical morbidity in this age group.**

Hypothesis-testing studies: Many minimally invasive diagnostic and therapeutic strategies have been developed and implemented in recent years. Investigation into the use of minimally invasive techniques for diagnosis and therapy in the elderly age group is necessary. The indications, complications, and postprocedure morbidity of minimally invasive techniques should be compared with traditional diagnostic and therapeutic strategies to determine the potential benefit of using minimally invasive techniques in treating otolaryngologic disorders in the elderly patient.

***Otolaryn KQ6*: Laboratory investigation and application of stem cell and other biological therapy for restoration of special sense and communication organs may provide elderly persons with olfactory, gustatory, and hearing rehabilitation without the use of external devices. Research is needed to determine whether stem cell therapy is a viable alternative for rehabilitation of the special senses in the elderly patient.**

Hypothesis-generating and -testing studies: Laboratory research into the possibility of stem cell engineering for special sense rehabilitation is necessary as a first step and would likely be performed initially by tissue-culture methodology. Animal models incorporating engineered special sense organs from stem cell propagation, with subsequent tests of organ function, would follow this. Ultimately, the feasibility of human implantation of special sense organs engineered from stem cells would be considered.

***Otolaryn KQ7*: Hearing aids have been used for many years for rehabilitation of failing auditory nerves or presbycusis. As patients age, nerves of swallowing and communicative organs also begin to have decreased function. Research is needed to determine whether advances in engineering solutions can assist in rehabilitation of failing swallowing or communicative organ function in the elderly person.**

Hypothesis-testing studies: The safety and feasibility of implantable devices for assistance in speaking and swallowing should be assessed in small-scale trials. Provided that implantable devices to assist the elderly person in speaking and swallowing function are proven feasible and safe, larger cohort studies are necessary to assess quality-of-life issues and long-term complications that appear to be associated with these devices. Newer devices should be compared with standard therapies, such as vocal cord injection or implants for speaking therapy and dietary changes or gastrostomy tube placement for swallowing difficulties.

DISORDERS OF THE AUDITORY SYSTEM

Cerumen impaction can have a significant effect on the hearing of elderly patients. In a random sampling of hospitalized elderly patients over a 1-year period, 30% were found to have cerumen impaction. Improved hearing was obtained in 75% of ears that underwent removal of cerumen.[54] Furthermore, a recent randomized controlled study suggests that cerumen impactions can be prevented by weekly administration by the patient of topical lipolotion.[55] Further hypothesis-testing research is needed on simple patient-based methods to prevent and treat cerumen impactions.

Otolaryn 24 (Level A): **Large-scale hypothesis-testing studies on the effectiveness of patient-based remedies to prevent and treat cerumen impaction are needed.**

DISORDERS OF THE VESTIBULAR SYSTEM

With increasing national emphasis on falls in the elderly age group, the role of vestibular rehabilitation in fall-prone patients is gaining importance. Vestibular rehabilitation is rehabilitation therapy for dizziness and balance and can be more generally referred to as *balance therapy.* Many health insurance companies do not pay for vestibular rehabilitation, citing this therapy as unproven. Further investigations into the efficacy of therapy are needed to support its role in treating the geriatric dizzy patient.

Otolaryn 25 (Level A): **Outcomes studies of vestibular therapy using controlled designs are needed to demonstrate the effectiveness of this therapeutic modality.**

DISORDERS OF THE NOSE AND SINUSES

Smell

Previous research has shown that olfactory sensitivity in older persons is diminished.[56,57] However, the true prevalence of olfactory disturbance in the elderly age group has been documented only recently. In 2002, Murphy et al reported results of olfactory testing as measured by the San Diego Odor Identification Test in 2491 persons aged 53 to 97 years. The mean prevalence of olfactory impairment found in this study was 24.5%. Olfactory impairment was noted to increase with age, with 62.5% of participants aged 80 to 97 exhibiting disturbance of olfaction. Additionally, self-report of olfactory disturbance in this study sample was low (9.5%), and olfactory disturbance self-report decreased in accuracy with increasing age.[58] The high prevalence of olfactory disturbance among older persons may have considerable impact on appetite, nutritional choices, and energy consumption, leading to adverse effects on protein and micronutrient intake and potential nutritional deficiencies. [59]

Since publication of *New Frontiers*, a substantial amount of research in the realm of olfactory changes with aging has been published. This recent literature encompasses olfactory loss in both normal aging and in various disease states. Wang et al used functional magnetic resonance imaging (fMRI) technology to assess age-related changes in the central olfactory system, comparing 11 young and 8 elderly participants; these authors found significantly reduced University of Pennsylvania Smell Identification Test (UPSIT) scores in the elderly group, as well as reduced volume and intensity of olfactory brain structure fMRI signal. [60] Another study, performed by Suzuki et al, comparing 6 young with 6 elderly participants using fMRI olfactory brain imaging also found decreased activation of olfactory areas in the elderly participants. [61] Finally, an investigation of cerebellar odor processing revealed significantly decreased fMRI activation of two out of three cerebellar odor processing areas in 10 aged participants in comparison with 10 young controls. [62]

Decreased olfactory sensitivity has been previously reported in individuals with Alzheimer's disease (AD). [63] Armed with this knowledge, researchers and clinicians have recently begun to explore the utility of olfactory testing in the diagnosis of elderly patients with cognitive impairments. Early diagnosis of AD allows early treatment of this devastating disease from both a medical and psychosocial standpoint. Devanand et al studied the predictive ability for eventual diagnosis of AD of deficiencies in olfactory identification in patients with mild cognitive impairment. In this study, 90 patients with mild cognitive impairment and 45 healthy control persons were given the UPSIT at baseline and followed for eventual development of AD. Patients with low olfaction scores exhibited greater likelihood for development of AD than the other patients. Furthermore, time to AD development was predicted by the combination of low olfaction scores and the lack of awareness of olfactory deficit. [64] Peters et al evaluated olfaction in 14 AD patients, 8 mild cognitive impairment patients, and 8 healthy control participants via olfactory event-related potential measurement. Seven patients with AD and 4 mild cognitive impairment patients demonstrated no olfactory event-related potentials, whereas all control participants showed discernible responses. [65] Finally, Schiffman et al studied olfaction in 33 patients at risk for development of AD because of multigenerational evidence of disease, comparing them with 32 control participants. The results supported the above findings that individuals at risk for AD development exhibit worse performance on olfactory measures than those not at risk. [66]

Olfactory testing has also been evaluated as a possible tool for early detection of cognitive decline in persons at genetic risk for AD. Wang et al studied olfactory identification in 28 persons with and mild cognitive impairment who exhibited the apolipoprotein E epsilon-4 (apoE4) allele, a predictor of early cognitive decline in AD, comparing their performance with that of 30 control persons. ApoE4-positive patients identified significantly fewer odors on the Cross-Cultural Smell Identification Test than did control persons. This suggests that the decreased olfactory identification in mild cognitive impairment may predict AD development. [67] Suzuki et al also found that among AD patients, those positive for apoE4 alleles had a stronger correlation between the Mini-Mental State Examination scores and Picture-Smell Identification Test scores than those without the apoE4 allele. [68]

In addition to early diagnosis of AD, differentiation between AD and other causes of dementia is important from a treatment perspective. Duff et al used the Pocket Smell Test to evaluate patients in three groups of 20, one group with AD, one with vascular dementia, and one with major depression. Significantly lower Pocket Smell Test scores were found in patients with AD than in patients with either vascular dementia or major depression. [69] This differentiation between AD and vascular dementia via olfactory testing was not supported by Gray et al in a 2001 study reporting that patients with vascular dementia and AD were found to have similar olfactory impairment. [70]

Gilbert et al assessed odor recognition memory in patients with AD and Lewy body variant (LBV) of AD confirmed by pathologic diagnosis, comparing them with healthy control persons. Olfactory recognition memory was found to be impaired in LBV and AD, with LBV patients exhibiting more impairment than AD patients on olfactory remote memory tasks. Odor memory tasks may be helpful in differentiating LBV and AD. [71] In addition to the utilization of odor recognition memory tasks for differentiation of LBV and AD, Westervelt et al have shown that odor identification testing can also be used to differentiate between these two entities, with LBV patients showing significantly lower odor identification ability than AD patients. [72]

Olfactory testing research has also been applied to the identification of Parkinson's disease (PD) and the differentiation among variants of PD. Among patients with PD, 70% to 90% exhibit olfactory impairment independently of disease severity and duration. [73] Double et al used the University of Pennsylvania 12-item Brief Smell Identification Test to test 49 nondemented PD patients and 52 control participants. Abnormal olfaction was exhibited by 82% of the PD patients but only 23% of the control participants. Five of the 12 Brief Smell Identification Test odors discriminated PD patients from controls. [73] Olfactory testing research has sought to evaluate the utility of olfactory impairment testing in diagnosing presymptomatic PD, as in AD. Sommer et al combined olfactory tests with substantia nigra transcranial sonography and single photon emission computed tomography (SPECT) imaging in patients with olfactory disturbance but without evidence of PD. These tests revealed abnormal substantia nigra findings in some patients, although the eventual development of PD will require longitudinal follow-up. [74] Research in olfactory testing has also revealed its utility in the differentiation between idiopathic and nonidiopathic PD, as well as between PD and vascular Parkinsonism. [75,76]

Otolaryn 26 (Level B): **New evidence has revealed the high prevalence of olfactory disturbance in elderly persons. However, self-recognition of olfactory impairment among older persons is low. Observational studies assessing the impact of olfactory impairment on the quality of life, safety, and health care of the elderly person are needed.**

Otolaryn 27 (Level A): **Basic science investigation of the biological mechanism of olfactory loss in the elderly person and potential mechanisms for preventing olfactory loss should be undertaken.**

Otolaryn 28 (Level A): **Large randomized controlled clinical trials of the utility of olfaction testing in the early detection and subtype differentiation of diseases affecting the geriatric patient (ie, Alzheimer's disease and Parkinson's disease) are necessary. Such trials will allow the establishment of parameters for further referral of elderly patients to specialists who diagnose and treat these entities. Addi-**

tionally, establishment of simple olfactory testing and parameters to evaluate early abnormal cognitive function will allow implementation of such tests in the primary care arena.

Aesthetics of the Aging Nose

Aesthetic surgical procedures are performed commonly and have gained popular acceptance in recent years. Functional and cosmetic rhinoplasties are increasingly being performed in older persons. The physical changes of the aging nose must be recognized if appropriate surgical procedures for elderly patients are to be performed. Vacher et al performed a fresh cadaver study on 40 subjects older than 70 years to examine external nasal characteristics. These investigators identified thin skin, muscular infiltration by subcutaneous fat, and involution of nasal tip muscles in the elderly noses. [77] In a 2004 review, Rohrich et al addressed a multitude of factors that should be considered when planning and executing rhinoplasty in the aging patient. Some of the factors include diminished skin elasticity and dermal thinning, as well as an increase in the density of sebaceous glands of the nasal tip, which may ultimately give way to the development of rhinophyma. As the external nose ages, the cartilaginous framework may become attenuated and fragmented, leading to drooping of the tip and relative elongation and convexity of the nasal dorsum. In addition, with loss of dentition, the maxillary alveolar bone becomes hypoplastic, which adds to the appearance of a relatively longer nose. Along with aesthetic concerns, loss of cartilaginous support in the nasal tip may produce symptomatic nasal airway obstruction by redistributing nasal airflow. Rohrich et al suggested that alteration of the external bony nasal framework in older individuals should be undertaken with caution because of the fragile nature of aged bones. [78] Thus, although rhinoplasty may be safely performed in the elderly patient, the anatomic and physiologic changes that commonly occur in the aging nose should be known and observed by the surgeon.

Otolaryn 29 (Level B): **Observational studies are warranted assessing the effect of loss of nasal function on quality of life for older adults. Outcomes studies investigating the results of rejuvenation therapy for the aging nose would follow.**

Sinusitis and Nasal Discharge

The basic physiology of nasal and sinus function in the elderly person still remains to be elucidated.

Otolaryn 30 (Level B): **The presence of an age-related alteration in mucociliary function or in the sinonasal inflammatory cascade should be investigated to assess the potential for an increased incidence of sinonasal disease in elderly patients.**

DISORDERS OF SWALLOWING

Novel treatment strategies, such as surface electrical stimulation therapy, are being promoted. However, little high-grade evidence exists as to the value of these therapies over traditional swallowing therapy. Hypothesis-generating and hypothesis-testing studies are needed to identify and develop the future treatment strategies for this difficult and important problem.

Otolaryn 31 (Level B): **Observational studies are needed to determine the prevalence of dysphagia among community-dwelling older persons, along with the quality-of-life and nutritional impairments that may result from this condition.**

Otolaryn 32 (Level A): **Hypothesis-testing studies (case-control and randomized controlled studies) are needed to determine the outcomes of traditional swallowing therapy and augmented swallowing therapy (ie, surface electrical stimulation).**

Otolaryn 33 (Level D): **Hypothesis-generating studies (basic bench and translational research studies) are needed to identify bioengineering-based and tissue-engineering–based treatment strategies for restoring neurosensory and neuromotor functional impairments in the older person with dysphagia.**

DISORDERS OF THE LARYNX

Although the clinical information and strategies outlined in the section Progress in Disorders of the Larynx are important areas for new research, future novel diagnostic and therapeutic strategies will ultimately rest upon foundations in basic science. The basic physiologic changes in the aging larynx are not completely understood.

Otolaryn 34 (Level B): **Further basic science investigation (bench research in animal models or controlled functional imaging studies) into the pathophysiology of presbyphonia is needed, with particular emphasis on changes in the central neuromuscular control of the aged larynx.**

Otolaryn 35 (Level B): **To serve the related agenda item Otolaryn 34, further development of an animal model (bench research) to study age-related voice change and regenerative strategies is needed.**

Otolaryn 36 (Levels D, B): **Hypothesis-generating and -testing studies are needed to identify and test novel strategies to treat the aging larynx (such as stem cell and bioengineered solutions). These would initially be performed in an animal model and then followed with controlled studies in human subjects.**

REFERENCES

1. Staecker H. Geriatric otolaryngology. In Solomon DH, LoCicero J, 3rd, Rosenthal RA (eds): New Frontiers in Geriatrics Research: An Agenda for Surgical and Related Medical Specialties. New York: American Geriatrics Society, 2004, pp. 203-224 (online at http://www.frycomm.com/ags/rasp).
2. Salvinelli F, Casale M, Trivelli M, et al. Otosclerosis and stapedioplasty in older adults. J Am Geriatr Soc 2002;50:1396-1400.
3. Gillett D, Fairley JW, Chandrashaker TS, et al. Bone-anchored hearing aids: results of the first eight years of a programme in a district general hospital, assessed by the Glasgow benefit inventory. J Laryngol Otol 2006;120:537-542.

4. Meyer TA, Lambert PR. Primary and revision stapedectomy in elderly patients. Curr Opin Otolaryngol Head Neck Surg 2004;12:387-392.
5. Ayache D, Corre A, Van Prooyen S, Elbaz P. Surgical treatment of otosclerosis in elderly patients. Otolaryngol Head Neck Surg 2003;129:674-677.
6. Salvinelli F, Casale M, Di Peco V, et al. Stapes surgery in relation to age. Clin Otolaryngol Allied Sci 2003;28:520-523.
7. Albera R, Giordano L, Rosso P, et al. Surgery of otosclerosis in the elderly. Aging (Milano) 2001;13:8-10.
8. Albrechet Ch G, Fonseca AS, Porto P, Bernardes GC. "Second ear" stapedotomy: is it safe? Acta Otorhinolaryngol Belg 2004;58:109-111.
9. Stenklev NC, Vik O, Laukli E. The aging ear: an otomicroscopic and tympanometric study. Acta Otolaryngol 2004;124:69-76.
10. Wiley TL, Nondahl DM, Cruickshanks KJ, Tweed TS. Five-year changes in middle ear function for older adults. J Am Acad Audiol 2005;16:129-139.
11. Kaneko A, Hosoda Y, Doi T, et al. Tubal compliance–changes with age and in tubal malfunction. Auris Nasus Larynx 2001;28:121-124.
12. Francis HW, Chee N, Yeagle J, et al. Impact of cochlear implants on the functional health status of older adults. Laryngoscope 2002;112:1482-1488.
13. Schuknecht HF, Gacek MR. Cochlear pathology in presbycusis. Ann Otol Rhinol Laryngol 1993;102:1-16.
14. Fischel-Ghodsian N, Bykhovskaya Y, Taylor K, et al. Temporal bone analysis of patients with presbycusis reveals high frequency of mitochondrial mutations. Hear Res 1997;110:147-154.
15. Keithley EM, Canto C, Zheng QY, et al. Age-related hearing loss and the ahl locus in mice. Hear Res 2004;188:21-28.
16. Johnson KR, Zheng QY, Erway LC. A major gene affecting age-related hearing loss is common to at least ten inbred strains of mice. Genomics 2000;70:171-180.
17. Cacciatore F, Napoli C, Abete P, et al. Quality of life determinants and hearing function in an elderly population: Osservatorio Geriatrico Campano Study Group. Gerontology 1999;45:323-328.
18. van Hooren SA, Anteunis LJ, Valentijn SA, et al. Does cognitive function in older adults with hearing impairment improve by hearing aid use? Int J Audiol 2005;44:265-271.
19. Anand VK. Epidemiology and economic impact of rhinosinusitis. Ann Otol Rhinol Laryngol Suppl 2004;193:3-5.
20. Colclasure JC, Gross CW, Kountakis SE. Endoscopic sinus surgery in patients older than sixty. Otolaryngol Head Neck Surg 2004;131:946-949.
21. Crawford WW, Gowda VC, Klaustermeyer WB. Age effects on objective measures of atopy in adult asthma and rhinitis. Allergy Asthma Proc 2004;25:175-179.
22. King MJ, Lockey RF. Allergen prick-puncture skin testing in the elderly. Drugs Aging 2003;20:1011-1017.
23. Kaliner MA. H_1-antihistamines in the elderly. Clin Allergy Immunol 2002;17:465-481.
24. Asero R. Efficacy of injection immunotherapy with ragweed and birch pollen in elderly patients. Int Arch Allergy Immunol 2004;135:332-335.
25. Robbins J. The current state of clinical geriatric dysphagia research. J Rehab Res Dev 2002;39:vii.
26. Baine WB, Yu W, Summe JP. Epidemiologic trends in the hospitalization of elderly Medicare patients for pneumonia, 1991-1998. Am J Public Health 2001;91:1121-1123.
27. Vaiman M, Eviatar E, Segal S. Surface electromyographic studies of swallowing in normal subjects: a review of 440 adults. Report 1. Quantitative data: timing measures. Otolaryngol Head Neck Surg 2004;131:548-555.

28. Robbins J, Hamilton JW, Lof GL, Kempster GB. Oropharyngeal swallowing in normal adults of different ages. Gastroenterology 1992;103:823-829.
29. McKee GJ, Johnston BT, McBride GB, Primrose WJ. Does age or sex affect pharyngeal swallowing? Clin Otolaryngol Allied Sci 1998;23:100-106.
30. Scott J. A morphometric study of age changes in the histology of the ducts of human submandibular salivary glands. Arch Oral Biol 1977;22:243-249.
31. Fischer D, Ship JA. Effect of age on variability of parotid salivary gland flow rates over time. Age Ageing 1999;28:557-561.
32. Ship JA, Fischer DJ. The relationship between dehydration and parotid salivary gland function in young and older healthy adults. J Gerontol A Biol Sci Med Sci 1997;52:M310-M319.
33. Shugars DC, Watkins CA, Cowen HJ. Salivary concentration of secretory leukocyte protease inhibitor, an antimicrobial protein, is decreased with advanced age. Gerontology 2001;47:246-253.
34. Wu AJ, Atkinson JC, Fox PC, et al. Cross-sectional and longitudinal analyses of stimulated parotid salivary constituents in healthy, different-aged subjects. J Gerontol 1993;48:M219-M224.
35. Lopez-Jornet MP, Bermejo-Fenoll A. Is there an age-dependent decrease in resting secretion of saliva of healthy persons? A study of 1493 subjects. Braz Dent J 1994;5:93-98.
36. Astor FC, Hanft KL, Ciocon JO. Xerostomia: a prevalent condition in the elderly. Ear Nose Throat J 1999;78:476-479.
37. Longman LP, Higham SM, Rai K, et al. Salivary gland hypofunction in elderly patients attending a xerostomia clinic. Gerodontology 1995;12:67-72.
38. Hagen P, Lyons GD, Nuss DW. Dysphonia in the elderly: diagnosis and management of age-related voice changes. South Med J 1996;89:204-207.
39. Shindo ML, Hanson DG. Geriatric voice and laryngeal dysfunction. Otolaryngol Clin North Am 1990;23:1035-1044.
40. Ward PH, Colton R, McConnell F, et al. Aging of the voice and swallowing. Otolaryngol Head Neck Surg 1989;100:283-286.
41. Von Leden HV, Alessi DM. The aging voice. In Benninger M, Jacobson B, Johnson A (eds): Vocal Arts Medicine: The Care and Prevention of Professional Voice Disorders. New York: Stuttgart, 1994, pp. 169-280.
42. Morrison MD, Gore-Hickman P. Voice disorders in the elderly. J Otolaryngol 1986;15:231-234.
43. Golub JS, Chen PH, Otto KJ, et al. Prevalence of perceived dysphonia in a geriatric population. J Am Geriatr Soc 2006;54:1736-1739.
44. Lundy DS, Silva C, Casiano RR, et al. Cause of hoarseness in elderly patients. Otolaryngol Head Neck Surg 1998;118:481-485.
45. Woo P, Casper J, Colton R, Brewer D. Dysphonia in the aging: physiology versus disease. Laryngoscope 1992;102:139-144.
46. Berg EE, Hapner E, Klein A, Johns MM, 3rd. Voice therapy improves quality of life in age-related dysphonia: a case-control study. J Voice 2006;Oct 24:(Epub ahead of print).
47. Genden EM, Rinaldo A, Shaha AR, et al. Treatment considerations for head and neck cancer in the elderly. J Laryngol Otol 2005;119:169-174.
48. Bernardi D, Barzan L, Franchin G, et al. Treatment of head and neck cancer in elderly patients: state of the art and guidelines. Crit Rev Oncol Hematol 2005;53:71-80.
49. Gillani AA, Grunberg SM. Aerorespiratory tract cancer in older patients. Semin Oncol 2004;31:220-233.
50. van Tol KM, de Vries EG, Dullaart RP, Links TP. Differentiated thyroid carcinoma in the elderly. Crit Rev Oncol Hematol 2001;38:79-91.

51. Argiris A, Li Y, Murphy BA, et al. Outcome of elderly patients with recurrent or metastatic head and neck cancer treated with cisplatin-based chemotherapy. J Clin Oncol 2004;22:262-268.
52. Kodaira T, Fuwa N, Furutani K, et al. Phase I trial of weekly docetaxel and concurrent radiotherapy for head and neck cancer in elderly patients or patients with complications. Jpn J Clin Oncol 2005;35:173-176.
53. Gebbia V, Di Marco P, Citarrella P. Systemic chemotherapy in elderly patients with locally advanced and/or inoperable squamous cell carcinoma of the head and neck: impact of anemia and role of recombinant human erythropoietin. Crit Rev Oncol Hematol 2003;48:S49-S55.
54. Lewis-Cullinan C, Janken JK. Effect of cerumen removal on the hearing ability of geriatric patients. J Adv Nurs 1990;15:594-600.
55. Saloranta K, Westermarck T. Prevention of cerumen impaction by treatment of ear canal skin: a pilot randomized controlled study. Clin Otolaryngol 2005;30:112-114.
56. Doty RL, Shaman P, Applebaum SL, et al. Smell identification ability: changes with age. Science 1984;226:1441-1443.
57. Deems DA, Doty RL. Age-related changes in the phenyl ethyl alcohol odor detection threshold. Trans Pa Acad Ophthalmol Otolaryngol 1987;39:646-650.
58. Murphy C, Schubert CR, Cruickshanks KJ, et al. Prevalence of olfactory impairment in older adults. JAMA 2002;288:2307-2312.
59. Schiffman SS, Graham BG. Taste and smell perception affect appetite and immunity in the elderly. Eur J Clin Nutr 2000;54 Suppl 3:S54-S63.
60. Wang J, Eslinger PJ, Smith MB, Yang QX. Functional magnetic resonance imaging study of human olfaction and normal aging. J Gerontol A Biol Sci Med Sci 2005;60:510-514.
61. Suzuki Y, Critchley HD, Suckling J, et al. Functional magnetic resonance imaging of odor identification: the effect of aging. J Gerontol A Biol Sci Med Sci 2001;56:M756-M760.
62. Ferdon S, Murphy C. The cerebellum and olfaction in the aging brain: a functional magnetic resonance imaging study. Neuroimage 2003;20:12-21.
63. Nordin S, Monsch AU, Murphy C. Unawareness of smell loss in normal aging and Alzheimer's disease: discrepancy between self-reported and diagnosed smell sensitivity. J Gerontol B Psychol Sci Soc Sci 1995;50:P187-P192.
64. Devanand DP, Michaels-Marston KS, Liu X, et al. Olfactory deficits in patients with mild cognitive impairment predict Alzheimer's disease at follow-up. Am J Psychiatry 2000;157:1399-1405.
65. Peters JM, Hummel T, Kratzsch T, et al. Olfactory function in mild cognitive impairment and Alzheimer's disease: an investigation using psychophysical and electrophysiological techniques. Am J Psychiatry 2003;160:1995-2002.
66. Schiffman SS, Graham BG, Sattely-Miller EA, et al. Taste, smell and neuropsychological performance of individuals at familial risk for Alzheimer's disease. Neurobiol Aging 2002;23:397-404.
67. Wang QS, Tian L, Huang YL, et al. Olfactory identification and apolipoprotein E epsilon 4 allele in mild cognitive impairment. Brain Res 2002;951:77-81.
68. Suzuki Y, Yamamoto S, Umegaki H, et al. Smell identification test as an indicator for cognitive impairment in Alzheimer's disease. Int J Geriatr Psychiatry 2004;19:727-733.
69. Duff K, McCaffrey RJ, Solomon GS. The Pocket Smell Test: successfully discriminating probable Alzheimer's dementia from vascular dementia and major depression. J Neuropsychiatry Clin Neurosci 2002;14:197-201.
70. Gray AJ, Staples V, Murren K, et al. Olfactory identification is impaired in clinic-based patients with vascular dementia and senile dementia of Alzheimer type. Int J Geriatr Psychiatry 2001;16:513-517.

71. Gilbert PE, Barr PJ, Murphy C. Differences in olfactory and visual memory in patients with pathologically confirmed Alzheimer's disease and the Lewy body variant of Alzheimer's disease. J Int Neuropsychol Soc 2004;10:835-842.
72. Westervelt HJ, Stern RA, Tremont G. Odor identification deficits in diffuse Lewy body disease. Cogn Behav Neurol 2003;16:93-99.
73. Double KL, Rowe DB, Hayes M, et al. Identifying the pattern of olfactory deficits in Parkinson disease using the brief smell identification test. Arch Neurol 2003;60:545-549.
74. Sommer U, Hummel T, Cormann K, et al. Detection of presymptomatic Parkinson's disease: combining smell tests, transcranial sonography, and SPECT. Mov Disord 2004;19:1196-1202.
75. Muller A, Mungersdorf M, Reichmann H, et al. Olfactory function in Parkinsonian syndromes. J Clin Neurosci 2002;9:521-524.
76. Katzenschlager R, Zijlmans J, Evans A, et al. Olfactory function distinguishes vascular parkinsonism from Parkinson's disease. J Neurol Neurosurg Psychiatry 2004;75:1749-1752.
77. Vacher C, Accioli J, Lezy JP. Surgical anatomy of the nose in the elderly: value of conservative rhinoplasty by transoral route. Surg Radiol Anat 2002;24:140-146.
78. Rohrich RJ, Hollier LH, Jr., Janis JE, Kim J. Rhinoplasty with advancing age. Plast Reconstr Surg 2004;114:1936-1944.

9

GERIATRIC GYNECOLOGY

*Erin Duecy, MD; Morton A. Stenchever, MD**

Geriatric gynecology is a rapidly expanding field. In the United States, the percentage of women aged 65 years and older is projected to increase significantly in coming decades.[1] The number of older women seeking both routine and acute gynecologic care, as well as surgical interventions, can be expected to rise dramatically. We must learn how the gynecologic needs of younger and older women differ and then re-evaluate the gynecologic care we have routinely offered in the past to determine outcomes and benefits in this older population of women. With rapidly changing technology and advances in gynecologic care, we must determine which interventions are appropriate and beneficial, identify unmet needs, and allocate resources accordingly. This chapter assesses the progress made in geriatric gynecology research since the publication of *New Frontiers in Geriatrics Research*[2] and proposes areas requiring future investigation.

The three Key Questions in gynecology identified in *New Frontiers* are quoted below. Progress made in answering these questions is outlined in this review. However, important areas of geriatric gynecology remain open for investigation; two new topics with new items for the research agenda are proposed (see the section New Horizons in Geriatric Gynecology, at the end of this chapter).

> ***Gyn KQ1*: How can the immediate and long-term functional impact of gynecologic surgery on older women be improved?**
>
> ***Gyn KQ2*: How can normal urogenital function be maintained in aging and age-related conditions?**
>
> ***Gyn KQ3*: Which older women should be encouraged to initiate or continue estrogen replacement or other hormonal therapy?**

METHODS

The MEDLINE database was searched via PubMed of the National Library of Medicine. All publications from 1 January 2001 to 31 December 2005 were included. The search was limited by the following specifications: English language, human female subjects, and subject age 65 years or greater. The search strategy combined the MeSH terms for gynecologic surgical procedures, hormone replacement therapy, cervical cancer and cervical cancer screening, breast cancer and breast cancer screening, ovarian cancers and ovarian cancer screening, pelvic organ prolapse, and postmenopausal osteoporosis with terms for age factors, risk factors, perioperative care, perioperative complications (including the specific terms *delirium, electrolyte imbalance, falls, deconditioning, urinary incontinence, functional loss*), comorbidity, outcome, quality of life, prognosis, recovery, length of stay, and discharge planning. All articles identified by the search specifications were reviewed,

* Duecy: Assistant Professor, Department of Obstetrics and Gynecology, University of Rochester Medical Center, Rochester, NY; Stenchever: Professor and Chairman Emeritus, Department of Obstetrics and Gynecology, University of Washington School of Medicine, Seattle, WA.

and those containing information pertinent to the research questions were selected for inclusion in this review.

PROGRESS IN GERIATRIC GYNECOLOGY RESEARCH

PERIOPERATIVE MANAGEMENT FOR GYNECOLOGIC SURGERY

See *New Frontiers,* pp. 225–227.

Gyn 1 (Level B): **Prospective observational studies should be undertaken to discover the magnitude and severity of common geriatric perioperative complications of gynecologic surgery, eg, delirium, electrolyte imbalance, falls, deconditioning, urinary incontinence, functional loss, and discharge to rehabilitation or long-term-care facilities.**

New Research Addressing This Question: No prospective observational studies designed to investigate common geriatric perioperative complications specifically after gynecologic surgeries were identified. One retrospective study of 62 women aged 80 years and older undergoing gynecologic surgery found that 14% experienced perioperative complications. Three percent had mental status changes consistent with delirium. There were no perioperative deaths. Mean hospital stay was 3.6 days, and 3% of the patients were discharged to a skilled nursing facility.[3] Two prospective studies from the Second International Study of Postoperative Cognitive Dysfunction included elderly (60 years and older) women undergoing gynecologic surgeries.[4,5] The incidence of long-term postoperative cognitive dysfunction was not higher after major noncardiac surgery in patients randomized to general anesthesia than in those randomized to regional anesthesia. However, the results did suggest a possible increase in early postoperative cognitive dysfunction in those receiving general anesthesia.[4] For patients undergoing minor surgery under general anesthesia, age 70 years and older plus inpatient surgery were risk factors for postoperative cognitive dysfunction.[5] In another study, men and women (mean age 73) undergoing cystoscopy or hysteroscopy were found to have a higher rate of cognitive dysfunction 24 hours after surgery than age-matched control persons not undergoing surgery.[6] Among all inpatient falls reported over 13 weeks at an academic hospital, half were found to be elimination-related.[7]

Modification of This Question in Light of New Research: This question remains inadequately addressed and should remain on the research agenda. Prospective observational studies designed to investigate common geriatric complications specifically after gynecologic surgery are still needed.

Gyn 2 (Level B): **Observational studies are needed to establish the risk factors for geriatric perioperative complications of gynecologic surgery, eg, delirium, electrolyte imbalance, falls, deconditioning, urinary incontinence, functional loss, and discharge to rehabilitation or long-term-care facilities.**

New Research Addressing This Question: No observational studies designed to identify risk factors for geriatric perioperative complications specifically after gynecologic surgery were identified. In a prospective study that included women (mean age 67) undergoing gynecologic surgery, age above 70, previous delirium, and pre-existing cognitive impairment were found to be predictive of postoperative delirium.[8]

Modification of This Question in Light of New Research: This question remains inadequately addressed, and studies are still needed to identify risk factors for geriatric perioperative complications after gynecologic surgery. The question should remain on the research agenda.

Gyn 3 (Level B): **All gynecologic surgery studies that evaluate or describe outcomes, morbidity, or mortality should describe comorbidities, functional status, cognitive status, and estrogen status of elderly women participants.**

New Research Addressing This Question: Most recent gynecologic surgery studies have included description of the comorbidities of their subjects. However, estrogen status is less often included (unless a focus of the study), and studies describing functional and cognitive status were not identified.

Modification of This Question in Light of New Research: Future gynecologic surgery studies that evaluate or describe outcomes, morbidity, or mortality should describe functional status, cognitive status, and estrogen status of elderly women subjects. Description of estrogen status should include both menopausal status and use of hormone replacement therapies.

Gyn 4 (Level B): **The results from existing and future gynecologic surgery studies should be stratified by age, even when statistical power is low, to facilitate systematic reviews of gynecologic surgery outcomes.**

New Research Addressing This Question: Few large observational or randomized gynecologic surgery studies have been published. Because of the difficulties of surgical randomization and objective evaluation, most published studies are descriptive and rarely large enough to permit meaningful stratification. The VALUE study evaluating more than 37,000 women undergoing hysterectomy did stratify results according to age group, with the oldest stratum aged 60 years and older.[9]

Modification of This Question in Light of New Research: Results from gynecologic surgery studies should be stratified by age. Stratification should be standardized, using defined age groups to facilitate comparisons between studies. A standard scheme of 5-year strata is recommended, ie, age 65 to 69, 70 to 74, 75 to 79, etc. For smaller studies or as an additional analysis in larger studies, comparison of age groups 65 to 79 and age 80 and older will help identify differences that may exist in the very elderly population.

Gyn 5 (Level B): **Prospective observational studies are needed to compare the quality-of-life and functional outcomes of surgical and nonsurgical management of gynecologic conditions.**

New Research Addressing This Question: Only one study designed to compare quality-of-life outcomes between surgical and nonsurgical management of a gynecologic condition was identified. In a prospective study of women (aged 30 to 75 years) undergoing either prophylactic salpingo-oophorectomy or gynecologic screening for high risk for hereditary ovarian cancer, no significant difference in general quality of life was found between the groups. Women undergoing prophylactic surgery had fewer condition-specific worries and a more favorable cancer risk perception, but also had significantly more endocrine symptoms and worse sexual function.[10]

Modification of This Question in Light of New Research: This question remains inadequately addressed, and studies comparing outcomes of surgical and nonsurgical management of gynecologic conditions are still needed. To improve study validity and facilitate comparisons, studies should employ standardized validated instruments for evaluation of quality-of-life and functional outcomes.

> *Gyn 6 (Level A)*: **Randomized controlled trials are needed to determine which interventions in elderly women are effective in reducing geriatric surgical risks, eg, delirium, electrolyte imbalance, falls, deconditioning, urinary incontinence, functional loss, and discharge to rehabilitation or long-term-care facilities.**

New Research Addressing This Question: No studies were identified.

Modification of This Question in Light of New Research: No modification of this question is recommended.

> *Gyn 7 (Level A)*: **Randomized controlled trials are needed to determine whether pre- and postoperative local estrogen therapy improves surgical outcomes in a variety of gynecologic conditions.**

New Research Addressing This Question: No studies were identified.

Modification of This Question in Light of New Research: No modification of this question is recommended.

> *Gyn 8 (Level A)*: **Randomized controlled trials are needed to determine whether discontinuation of estrogen replacement therapy improves perioperative morbidity in elderly women.**

New Research Addressing This Question: No randomized controlled trials were identified. In one case-control study of women undergoing joint arthroplasty, no association was found between perioperative hormone replacement therapy and the incidence of postoperative venous thromboembolism.[11]

Modification of This Question in Light of New Research: This question has been inadequately addressed, and studies evaluating discontinuation of estrogen replacement therapy in the perioperative period are still needed. Because of the low incidence of postoperative vascular complications in elderly women undergoing gynecologic surgery and the decreasing prevalence of the use of hormone replacement therapy, multicenter studies may be required to answer this question.

> *Gyn 9 (Level D)*: **Observational studies are needed to compare quality-of-life outcomes of different surgical techniques for gynecologic conditions, eg, urinary incontinence and pelvic organ prolapse.**

New Research Addressing This Question: No studies comparing different surgical techniques and using quality-of-life measurements as the primary outcome were identified. However, many studies now include quality of life as a secondary outcome. Six studies comparing various incontinence surgeries included quality-of-life data: suprapubic arch sling versus tension-free vaginal tape (TVT), [12] TVT versus pubovaginal sling, [13,14] periurethral versus transurethral collagen injections, [15] Burch versus laparoscopic colposuspension methods, [16] and Burch urethropexy versus TVT. [17] Quality-of-life outcomes were similar in all the comparisons in these studies except for two: improved subjective cure rates were better for open and laparoscopic colposuspensions utilizing suture placement than for laparoscopic mesh colposuspension, [16] and better for TVT than for Burch colposuspension. [17] One study on pelvic organ prolapse surgery included quality-of-life data in the comparison of abdominal sacral colpopexy and vaginal sacrospinous ligament suspension and found that both procedures improved postoperative quality of life. [18]

Modification of This Question in Light of New Research: The majority of gynecologic surgery studies are designed to evaluate a single procedure as treatment of a gynecologic condition and are commonly retrospective or descriptive. Studies are still needed comparing different procedures as treatment for the same gynecologic condition, especially for new surgical procedures. All studies evaluating outcomes of different surgical techniques should include quality-of-life data. To improve study validity and facilitate comparisons, studies should employ standardized validated instruments for evaluating quality-of-life outcomes.

> *Gyn 10 (Level D)*: **Observational studies should be performed to determine patient and condition characteristics that are associated with improvement in quality of life after surgical treatment.**

New Research Addressing This Question: No studies were identified.

Modification of This Question in Light of New Research: No modification of this question is recommended.

> *Gyn 11 (Level D)*: **Guidelines for selecting candidates for gynecologic surgery from among older institutionalized populations on the basis of quality-of-life benefits should be prepared and validated.**

New Research Addressing This Question: No guidelines have been presented or validated.

Modification of This Question in Light of New Research: Before guidelines for the selection of patients can be established, observational studies must be performed describing both objective and quality-of-life outcomes of gynecologic surgery in older institutionalized women.

> *Gyn 12 (Level D)*: **As medical care changes and improves, descriptive and observational studies should be performed to compare the risks of gynecologic surgery that are associated with age alone and those that are associated with comorbidities.**

New Research Addressing This Question: No studies were identified.

Modification of This Question in Light of New Research: Though many studies do describe comorbidities present in the study population (see Gyn 3), this is often provided solely to describe the study population. Few studies are adequately powered to provide meaningful data regarding the effect of these comorbidities on outcomes. The question should remain unmodified on the research agenda.

UROGENITAL HEALTH

Pelvic Organ Prolapse

See *New Frontiers,* pp. 228–230. For new agenda items under this topic, see the section New Horizons in Geriatric Gynecology at the end of the chapter.

***Gyn 13 (Level B)*: Observational studies are needed to define long-term quality-of-life outcomes of nonoperative management of pelvic organ prolapse.**

New Research Addressing This Question: No studies were identified.

Modification of This Question in Light of New Research: No modification of this question is recommended.

***Gyn 14 (Level B)*: Observational studies are needed to define long-term quality-of-life outcomes of operative management of pelvic organ prolapse.**

New Research Addressing This Question: Observational studies evaluating surgical outcomes now more commonly include quality-of-life measures as a secondary outcome and more commonly use validated quality-of-life measures. Three studies included only postoperative quality-of-life data but described favorable quality-of-life results after vaginal paravaginal defect repair [19] and abdominal sacrocolpopexy. [20,21] Three years after high uterosacral ligament suspension, women were found to have had improvement in each component of a quality-of-life survey. [22] Quality of life was improved 24 months after cadaveric prolapse repair for treatment of cystocele and stress urinary incontinence. [23] Posterior colporrhaphy with graft augmentation was found to be associated with improved quality of life at 1 year postoperatively. [24] Two studies focused specifically on quality of life after prolapse repair in elderly women. After anterior vaginal wall surgery, women (mean age 70, range 6 to-88) reported improvement over preoperative values in all quality-of-life components. [25] Age-stratified results confirmed improvement in women aged 65 to 70 years, 71 to 79, and 80 or older. Cystocele repair in women (mean age 83, range 80 to 93) resulted in improved quality-of-life scores at 21 months. [26]

Modification of This Question in Light of New Research: All studies describing outcomes of surgical treatment of pelvic organ prolapse should include both preoperative and postoperative assessment of quality of life by the use of standardized, validated instruments. Long-term (5 years or longer) data on quality-of-life outcomes are still needed.

***Gyn 15 (Level B)*: Observational studies are needed to determine the patient factors, device factors, and management factors that are associated with successful long-term pessary use.**

New Research Addressing This Question: Two studies were identified evaluating factors associated with long-term pessary use. Of women (mean age 65 years, range 29 to 90) treated with a pessary for pelvic organ prolapse or urinary incontinence, 60% were found to have continued to use the pessary over the long term (median 147 days).[27] Another study found continued use to be significantly more likely in women being treated for prolapse and in those who were sexually active. After successful fitting and initial satisfaction at 2 months, 73% of women (mean age 71, range 40 to 92) continued to use a pessary at 1 year. Continued pessary use was found to be associated with older age and poor surgical risk, and decision to proceed with surgical repair to be associated with sexual activity, stress incontinence, stage III to IV posterior wall prolapse, and desire for surgery at first visit. Age 65 years or older was the best age cut-off to predict continued pessary use.[28]

Several studies have evaluated short-term outcomes of pessary use as treatment of pelvic organ prolapse and provide data important to an understanding of which women are more likely to use a pessary successfully. In women with pelvic organ prolapse (mean age 70, range 24 to 92), a ring or Gellhorn pessary was successfully fitted in 73%. Unsuccessful fitting was associated with vaginal length 6 cm or less and introitus 4 fingerbreadths or larger. In a 2-month follow-up of the women successfully fitted with a pessary, 92% of the women were satisfied with use of the pessary.[28] Vaginal bulge, pressure, discharge, and splinting were all significantly decreased with pessary use. In women with urinary symptoms prior to pessary placement, urinary symptoms were improved, but in those without baseline urinary symptoms, de novo stress incontinence occurred in 21%.[29] Continued pessary use at 3 weeks after successful fitting was not associated with prolapse stage or compartment and was lower in women with history of hysterectomy or prolapse surgery.[30]

Modification of This Question in Light of New Research: Studies have adequately described factors associated with successful pessary fitting and both short- and medium-term use. Observational studies are needed to determine the impact of pessary type on treatment of different degrees of prolapse, prolapse in different vaginal compartments, or for different combinations of prolapse. Observational studies are needed to describe factors associated with long-term (more than 1 year) and very long-term (more than 5 years) use of pessaries.

> *Gyn 16 (Level B)*: **Pessaries (or other devices) should be developed for use in conservative management of pelvic organ prolapse in women with poor introital support and in whom currently available pessaries are not retained.**

New Research Addressing This Question: No studies were identified.

Modification of This Question in Light of New Research: No modification of this question is recommended.

> *Gyn 17 (Level B)*: **Basic science and clinical studies should be performed to delineate the pathophysiology of pelvic organ prolapse, particularly the way that genetic tissue factors confer risk.**

New Research Addressing This Question: Multiple studies in this area have been published or are under way. They are discussed here in three groups: those focused on pelvic tissue alterations, those focused on anatomic changes, and those focused on genetics.

Six studies addressed smooth muscle alterations. Three studies found the fractional area of smooth muscle in vaginal cuff specimens and round ligament tissue to be smaller from women with pelvic organ prolapse than from those without prolapse.[31–33] Caldesmon, a protein involved in regulation of smooth muscle contractility, was found to be increased in vaginal muscularis from women with prolapse.[34] No difference was found in smooth muscle content of the arcus tendineus fasciae pelvis of premenopausal or postmenopausal women with anterior vaginal prolapse.[35] Comparison of myofibroblasts from vaginal tissue of women with and without prolapse found those from women with prolapse to be significantly less contractile.[36]

Three studies assessed elastin or elastolytic activity and prolapse: In periurethral vaginal tissue biopsies from women with urinary incontinence or prolapse or both, alpha-1 antitrypsin mRNA and protein levels were found to be significantly decreased. Elastolytic and proteolytic enzyme activity were not different between the groups.[37] The elastin content of the arcus tendineus fasciae pelvic in women with anterior wall prolapse was not found to be different premenopausal and postmenopausal women.[35] Biomechanical assessment of anterior vaginal wall specimens from premenopausal and postmenopausal women with symptomatic prolapse demonstrated a higher elastic modulus in and increased stiffness of the tissue in the postmenopausal women.[38]

Several studies focused on the role of collagen in pelvic organ prolapse. Collagen type I was decreased in arcus tendineus fasciae pelvic of unestrogenized menopausal women with anterior vaginal wall prolapse.[35] Another found the cervical collagen content of 14 women with pelvic organ prolapse (with or without stress urinary incontinence) to be significantly lower than in 17 control subjects.[39] The collagen type III content of paravaginal and uterosacral tissue was not found to differ in women with and without prolapse.[40] Other researchers found women with stress incontinence and pelvic organ prolapse to have increased collagen breakdown in comparison with women in the control group.[41] One study comparing women with and without uterine prolapse found that those with prolapse had decreased collagen content of the parametrial tissue; however, no differences in collagen content at the vaginal apex were found.[42] In parametrial tissue samples of women with and without prolapse, collagen type I content was found to be the same in both groups, but the collagen type I fiber of women with prolapse was shorter and thinner.[43]

One study of other tissue components found total glycosaminoglycans, chondroitin sulfate, dermatan sulphate, and heparin sulfate to be decreased in vaginal tissue of postmenopausal women with stage 2 or 3 prolapse.[44]

A number of studies examined hormone levels and receptors in prolapse. One such study found levels of androstene-3 beta, 16 beta, 17 beta-triol (5-AT), 11 beta-hydroxy, and 17 beta-estradiol to be increased in postmenopausal women with prolapse, but tetrahydrocortisone to be increased in women without prolapse.[45] The percentage of cells expressing estrogen receptor-α, estrogen receptor-β, androgen receptor, and progesterone receptor was found to be higher in cardinal ligament samples from women with prolapse.[46] In a study comparing premenopausal women with and without prolapse, serum estradiol levels and ligament estrogen receptor levels were found to be significantly lower in cardinal and uterosacral ligament and blood samples from those with prolapse. There was no difference in serum or tissue levels between postmenopausal women with and without prolapse.[47] Analysis of uterosacral ligaments from 45 women revealed decreased numbers of estrogen and progesterone receptors in the ligaments of postmenopausal women; however, this change did not correlate with changes in ligament resilience.[48]

The role of anatomic alterations in pelvic organ prolapse was the focus of four studies. One such study, using color thickness mapping with magnetic resonance imaging, found women without prolapse to have bilaterally thicker and bulkier puborectalis muscles.[49] In a second magnetic resonance imaging study of women with varying stages of prolapse, changes in levator ani morphology were found to be independent of prolapse stage and were not identified in all women with prolapse. The levator hiatus was wider with increasing prolapse stage, suggesting changes in puborectalis function.[50] In another study, magnetic resonance imaging measurements indicated that women with prolapse at least 2 cm beyond the introitus had larger vaginal perimeter and cross-sectional area than women in the control group. These researchers saw no difference in vaginal thickness.[51] In a case-control study of women with and without pelvic floor disorders who underwent magnetic resonance imaging of the pelvis, wider transverse pelvic inlet and shorter obstetrical conjugate were found to be associated with pelvic floor dysfunction.[52]

Three studies have addressed the role of genetics in pelvic organ prolapse. In a study of nulliparous white twins and their sisters (ages 18 to 24), the majority (59%) of the variance in bladder neck descent as seen on ultrasound was found to be due to genetic factors.[53] In the same population, the association of pelvic organ and elbow mobility was also found to be mediated by common genes.[54] Analysis of gene expression in pubococcygeus muscle specimens from women with and without prolapse identified 280 genes that were underexpressed and 500 genes that were overexpressed in women with prolapse. Differential gene expression was seen in genes related to actin, myosin, and extracellular matrix proteins.[55]

Modification of This Question in Light of New Research: Many studies in the basic science of pelvic organ prolapse are ongoing, research attention which promises results that could impact clinical management. When and if genetic pathways are clearly delineated that predispose a woman to the development of pelvic organ prolapse, studies will be needed to identify and quantify the contribution of environmental factors on the expression of these genetic susceptibilities.

Gyn 18 (Level B): **Therapies to retard the progression of pelvic organ prolapse by targeting the pathophysiologic tissue factors should be developed.**

New Research Addressing This Question: No studies were identified.

Modification of This Question in Light of New Research: No modification of this question is recommended.

Gyn 19 (Level B): **Long-term observational studies are needed to determine the relative contributions of routes of delivery (cesarean section, operative vaginal, spontaneous vaginal) to the development of pelvic organ prolapse.**

New Research Addressing This Question: No long-term studies evaluating the relative contributions of delivery route on development of pelvic organ prolapse were identified.

Studies evaluating pelvic organ prolapse in the immediate postpartum period are available. Pelvic organ prolapse quantification (POP-Q) measurements were significantly different in women after vaginal delivery and nulliparous women who constituted the control group. Differences were seen in Aa, Ba, TVL, and GH after spontaneous delivery and in Aa, Ab, Ap, Bp, D, TVL, and GH after vacuum-assisted delivery. [56] In another study, nulliparous pregnant women who underwent POP-Q staging before and after delivery were found to have POP-Q stage that was higher in the third trimester and postpartum than during the first trimester. Postpartum POP-Q stage was higher after vaginal delivery than after cesarean delivery. [57] In a study of nulliparous pregnant women who underwent prolapse evaluation at 36 weeks gestation and 6 weeks postpartum, 32% who underwent spontaneous vaginal delivery and 35% who underwent cesarean section during active labor were found to have developed prolapse beyond that seen at 36 weeks. [58]

Modification of This Question in Light of New Research: Pelvic organ prolapse may develop during pregnancy and delivery. However, no data are available from studies evaluating regression or progression of pregnancy and delivery-related prolapse and its relationship to the development of symptomatic prolapse later in life. This question therefore should remain unmodified on the research agenda.

***Gyn 20 (Level B)*: Observational studies are needed to determine the condition-specific functional impact of surgery for incontinence and pelvic organ prolapse in elderly women, including sexual function.**

New Research Addressing This Question: No studies were identified.

Modification of This Question in Light of New Research: No modification of this question is recommended.

***Gyn 21 (Level A)*: Long-term randomized controlled trials are needed to determine whether estrogen use, local or systemic, confers benefit or risk for the progression of pelvic organ prolapse.**

New Research Addressing This Question: One randomized, double-blind, placebo-controlled study of the effect of systemic estrogen on the progression of pelvic organ prolapse was identified. Women with similar stages of prolapse were randomized to 0.625 mg of conjugated equine estrogen, 20 mg of tamoxifen, 60 mg of raloxifene, or placebo for 20 weeks. After treatment, 75% of women receiving raloxifene, 60% receiving tamoxifen, 22% receiving estrogen, and 18% receiving placebo were found to have increases in prolapse on repeat examination. The changes in the raloxifene and tamoxifen groups were significant. However, only one subject had a large enough change in POP-Q measurements to increase the prolapse stage. [59] An analysis of three randomized, controlled, long-term trials of raloxifene found no evidence of increased rates of surgery for prolapse in women receiving the medication. [60]

Modification of This Question in Light of New Research: Even though short-term use of selective estrogen receptor modulators may be associated with greater progression of prolapse than the use of estrogen or placebo, these changes do not appear to be clinically significant. Long-term studies and studies evaluating the effect of local estrogen are still needed. This question should remain unmodified on the research agenda.

Gyn 22 (Level A): **Randomized controlled trials are needed to determine whether pre- and postoperative local estrogen therapy improves outcomes of pelvic organ prolapse surgery.**

New Research Addressing This Question: No studies were identified.

Modification of This Question in Light of New Research: No modification of this question is recommended.

Gyn 23 (Level A): **Long-term randomized controlled trials are needed to determine whether selective estrogen receptor modulator use confers benefit or risk for the progression of pelvic organ prolapse.**

New Research Addressing This Question: As discussed in Gyn 21, women randomized to a 20-week course of raloxifene or tamoxifen had significantly greater progression of prolapse than women receiving estrogen or placebo.[59] However, changes appeared to be subclinical, and in an analysis of three randomized, controlled, long-term trials of raloxifene, there was no evidence of increased rates of surgery for prolapse in women receiving the medication.[61] In a randomized controlled trial of women aged 65 years or older that was stopped after 10 months because of adverse events, women randomized to levormeloxifene for the treatment of osteoporosis were found to have significantly increased pelvic organ prolapse in comparison with women on placebo (7% versus 2%). However, the method of prolapse quantification was not identified, and data on degree of prolapse or development of symptomatic prolapse were not presented.[60]

Modification of This Question in Light of New Research: The question has been inadequately addressed and should remain unmodified on the research agenda.

Gyn 24 (Level C): **Randomized controlled trials should be performed to determine whether pessary use in early stages of pelvic organ prolapse retards progression.**

New Research Addressing This Question: No randomized controlled trials evaluating whether pessary use retards progression of pelvic organ prolapse were identified, but one observational study has been published. Women (mean age 75 years, range 62 to 83) who used a pessary for at least 1 year were evaluated for progression of prolapse. After 1 year, there was a significantly significant improvement in prolapse stage: 4 women were improved and no women were worse. However, prolapse evaluation after 1 year may have been compromised, as one third of the women did not remove their pessary at least 48 hours prior to examination.[62]

Modification of This Question in Light of New Research: The question has been inadequately addressed and should remain unmodified on the research agenda.

Gyn 25 (Levels D, C): **Long-term observational trials are needed to obtain indications as to whether pelvic floor muscle exercises retard the progression of pelvic organ prolapse; subsequently, these hypotheses need to be tested through randomized controlled trials.**

New Research Addressing This Question: One observational study was identified evaluating pelvic floor exercise in women age 60 or older to prevent progression of pelvic organ prolapse. After 24 months, 27.3% of women who were trained in pelvic floor muscle exercise and followed a daily regimen showed progression of prolapse, in comparison with 72.2% of women in the control group. The difference in prolapse progression rate was significant only in women with severe prolapse.[63] No randomized controlled trials have evaluated pelvic floor muscle exercises as a treatment to retard progression of pelvic organ prolapse.

Modification of This Question in Light of New Research: The question has been inadequately addressed and should remain unmodified on the research agenda.

Gyn 26 (Level D): **Longitudinal observational studies are needed to define the natural history of untreated pelvic organ prolapse.**

New Research Addressing This Question: Two studies on the natural history of pelvic organ prolapse were identified, one in pregnant women and one in postmenopausal women. In nulliparous pregnant women (mean age 21.7 years, range 18 to 38) who underwent POP-Q evaluation during their pregnancy, the majority had stage 1 prolapse and none had prolapse beyond stage 2. Comparisons of POP-Q measurements were not significantly different between the first and second or the second and third trimesters. However, significant differences were seen between the first and third trimesters, with an increase in POP-Q stage observed. The most important changes occurred at point Aa. No data were presented on further changes or resolution after delivery.[64] In the second study, 31.8% of women (mean age 64.9 years, range 50 to 79) enrolled in the Women's Health Initiative were found to have some degree of pelvic organ prolapse at baseline. The annual incidence rate was 9.3 per 100 women-years for cystocele, 5.7 for rectocele, and 1.5 for uterine prolapse. Annual progression rate for grade 1 prolapse to grade 2 or 3 (per 100 women-years) was 9.5 for cystocele, 13.5 for rectocele, and 1.9 for uterine prolapse. Progression rates for grade 0 to grade 2 or 3 were 1.2 for cystocele, 1.4 for rectocele, and .06 for uterine prolapse. No subjects progressed to grade 4 prolapse in any compartment. Annual regression rates for grade 2 or 3 prolapse to grade 0 were 9.3 for cystocele, 3.3 for rectocele, and 0 for uterine prolapse.[65]

Modification of This Question in Light of New Research: The Women's Health Initiative provides data on both progression and regression of prolapse in postmenopausal women over the course of 2 to 8 years. However, an unvalidated descriptive method of prolapse evaluation was used, and no data on development or regression of prolapse-related symptoms were provided. Without data regarding prolapse-related symptoms and correlation with stage of prolapse, the clinical relevance of the findings is unclear. Future studies describing the progression and regression of pelvic organ prolapse should describe prolapse by using a validated reproducible system such as the POP-Q and collect data regarding associated symptoms by using standardized questionnaires.

Gyn 27 (Level D): **Observational studies are needed to determine the incidence of hydronephrosis in pelvic organ prolapse.**

New Research Addressing This Question: No studies were identified.

Modification of This Question in Light of New Research: No modification of this question is recommended.

Gyn 28 (Level D): **Observational studies are needed to determine modifiable risk factors for pelvic organ prolapse other than childbirth.**

New Research Addressing This Question: In a cross-sectional analysis of women enrolled in the Women's Health Initiative, potentially modifiable risk factors (excluding childbirth) identified for prolapse were waist circumference greater than 88 cm, overweight (body mass index or BMI 25 to 30), obesity (BMI greater than 30), and constipation.[66] A case-control study of women with stage III or IV prolapse identified age, weight of largest vaginal delivery, hysterectomy, and previous prolapse surgery as risk factors for severe prolapse.[67] Of these, only history of hysterectomy may be potentially modifiable, as alternative treatments for conditions traditionally treated with hysterectomy are developed. In this study, BMI was not found to be a significant risk factor. In the Pelvic Organ Support Study, potentially modifiable risk factors for prolapse were overweight and obesity.[68] A second analysis of this study found straining at stool to be significantly associated with anterior vaginal wall prolapse and perineal descent.[69] A case-control study of women with prolapse (84% with stage III or IV) found the risk for constipation to be higher in women with prolapse, although this may be at least partially explained by lower fiber intake in that group.[70]

Modification of This Question in Light of New Research: This question has been adequately addressed and can be dropped from the research agenda.

Vulvovaginal Conditions

See *New Frontiers,* pp. 232–233.

> *Gyn 29 (Level B)*: **Quality-of-life instruments targeting vulvovaginal symptoms need to be developed and validated.**

New Research Addressing This Question: The Female Sexual Function Index was used in assessing 42 women with vulvodynia and was found to be a valid measure of sexual function in this population of women.[71] The Functional Assessment of Cancer Therapy—Vulvar was used in assessing 20 women undergoing treatment of vulvar cancer and was found to be a reliable and valid measure of quality of life of women with vulvar cancer.[72] Studies regarding the development of instruments evaluating other aspects of quality of life in women with vulvovaginal conditions were not identified.

Modification of This Question in Light of New Research: Only two validated questionnaires have been developed, and their use is limited to very specific populations. The question has been inadequately addressed and should remain unmodified on the research agenda.

> *Gyn 30 (Level B)*: **Clinical studies, including studies of young castrates, are needed to determine the relative contributions of hypoestrinism, local environment, and aging to vulvovaginal symptoms.**

New Research Addressing This Question: No studies were identified.

Modification of This Question in Light of New Research: No modification of this question is recommended.

> *Gyn 31 (Level B, A)*: **Observational studies (and eventually randomized controlled trials) should be performed to determine what degree of quality-of-life improvement in frail older women can be attained by detection and treatment of vulvovaginal disorders.**

New Research Addressing This Question: Of women (mean age 42.1 years, range 18 to 84) evaluated at a vulvar specialty clinic, 66% reported an overall improvement in symptoms. In comparison with female norms in the United States, quality-of-life measures were found to be significantly lower in all three categories: general health, role physical, and role emotional; however, scores in all three categories were higher for women who were subjectively improved. Quality-of-life measures were not stratified by age. [73]

Modification of This Question in Light of New Research: The question has been inadequately addressed and should remain unmodified on the research agenda.

Gyn 32 (Level A): **Randomized controlled trials are needed to determine the impact of long-term local estrogen replacement therapy on the incidence and prevalence of urogenital symptoms.**

New Research Addressing This Question: Randomized trials of local estrogen for treatment of urogenital symptoms were identified, with study periods from 3 months to 1 year. In postmenopausal women randomized to 25 µg estradiol tablet or 1 g of conjugated estrogen cream for 12 weeks, estrogen cream was found to be superior in relieving vaginal dryness and dyspareunia, but both medications produced improvement in urogenital symptoms. [74] Postmenopausal women (mean age 53.4, range 40 to 64) treated with transdermal hormone therapy (17-β-estradiol plus medroxyprogesterone acetate) for 4 months plus either vaginal estriol or placebo had similar improvements in urinary symptoms after 4 months. However, women in the vaginal estriol group reached significant improvement in urinary complaints more quickly than women randomized to placebo. [75] Another study found that treatment of postmenopausal women with intravaginal estriol ovules for 6 months produced greater improvement of urogenital symptoms than placebo. [76] A study comparing 25 µg of micronized 17-β-estradiol for 12 months and placebo found symptomatic improvement of vaginal atrophy to be significantly higher in the treatment group. Women in the treatment group had significant improvements in vaginal dryness, itching or burning, recurrent vaginitis, dyspareunia, and atrophy. [77]

Modification of This Question in Light of New Research: Treatment of urogenital symptoms with estrogen appears to be superior to placebo. This question has been adequately addressed, and the question can be dropped from the research agenda.

Gyn 33 (Level A): **Randomized controlled trials are needed to determine the relative contributions of local estrogen and vehicle to improved urogenital symptoms.**

New Research Addressing This Question: No studies were identified.

Modification of This Question in Light of New Research: No modification of this question is recommended.

Gyn 34 (Level D): **Basic science and clinical investigations are needed to learn more about the causes of lichen sclerosus.**

New Research Addressing This Question: In a family with four of five siblings diagnosed with lichen sclerosus, the HLA-B08 and HLA-B18 alleles were identified in each of the affected children and were absent in the unaffected sibling, suggesting a possible genetic link. [78] Analysis of tissue samples from patients with lichen sclerosus have also suggested possible roles of oxidative stress, autoantibodies to extracellular matrix protein 1, antigen-mediated vasculitis, and alterations in cell-mediated immunity.[79–84] In one study, alterations in inter-α-trypsin inhibitor were found to cause accumulation of hyaluronic acid in the superficial dermis of persons with lichen sclerosus.[85] Differential distribution of transforming growth factor subtypes and collagens type I and III, elastin, and fibrillin have been identified in lichen sclerosus specimens.[86,87]

Modification of This Question in Light of New Research: Although a few studies have addressed this question, results are preliminary. The question has been inadequately addressed and should remain unmodified on the research agenda.

> *Gyn 35 (Level D)*: **Basic science and clinical investigations are needed to learn more about the age-related factors that increase susceptibility to vulvar cancer.**

New Research Addressing This Question: No studies were identified.

Modification of This Question in Light of New Research: No modification of this question is recommended.

> *Gyn 36 (Level D)*: **Observational studies should be performed to determine the profiles of susceptibility to vulvar cancer.**

New Research Addressing This Question: No studies were identified.

Modification of This Question in Light of New Research: No modification of this question is recommended.

> *Gyn 37 (Level C)*: **Randomized trials are needed to determine whether topical immune modulators (eg, imiquimod) reduce the incidence of vulvar cancer in vulnerable individuals.**

New Research Addressing This Question: No randomized trials were identified. Small observational studies have documented clinical improvement in vulvar intraepithelial neoplasia treated with topical imiquimod, although treatment may be limited by local side effects.[88–91] No studies evaluated its effect on progression to invasive disease.

Modification of This Question in Light of New Research: The question has been inadequately addressed and should remain unmodified on the research agenda.

> *Gyn 38 (Level D)*: **Observational studies are needed to determine the prevalence of untreated vulvovaginal symptoms in frail and institutionalized populations.**

New Research Addressing This Question: No studies were identified.

Modification of This Question in Light of New Research: No modification of this question is recommended.

Urinary Incontinence

Urinary incontinence in elderly persons is covered in the chapter on geriatric urology (see Chapter 10).

Sexuality

See *New Frontiers,* pp. 234–235. For new agenda items under this topic, see the section New Horizons in Geriatric Gynecology at the end of the chapter.

Gyn 39 (Level B): **Current investigations into the diverse causes of younger women's sexual dysfunction and its pathophysiology and management should be extended to include older women.**

New Research Addressing This Question: No information was identified concerning the extension of ongoing studies to include older women.

Modification of This Question in Light of New Research: No modification of the question is recommended.

Gyn 40 (Level B): **Observational studies are needed to determine the medication side effects that adversely affect specific aspects of sexual function in older women.**

New Research Addressing This Question: In one study, in postmenopausal women (aged 51 to 55 years) with hypertension, treatment with valsartan was found to significantly improve sexual desire, changes in behavior, and sexual fantasies, while treatment with atenolol resulted in worsened sexual desire and fantasies.[92]

Modification of This Question in Light of New Research: The question has been inadequately addressed and should remain unmodified on the research agenda.

Gyn 41 (Level B): **Observational studies are needed to define the adverse effects on older women's sexuality of specific medical conditions.**

New Research Addressing This Question: Searches of the literature addressing specific medical conditions were performed—hypertension, heart disease, diabetes mellitus, end-stage renal failure, stroke, breast cancer, and ovarian cancer—with the following results.

No studies evaluating the effects of hypertension on sexual function in older women were identified.

One study concerning heart disease was located. The medical outcomes study of the Heart and Estrogen/Progestin Replacement Study evaluated sexual function in 2763 women with a mean age of 67 years and known coronary disease. Of the women studied, 39% were sexually active and 65% reported at least one type of sexual dysfunction. No specific problems related to coronary artery disease were reported except that lack of chest discomfort was associated with being sexually active.[93]

No studies were identified evaluating sexual dysfunction in older women with diabetes mellitus.

Sexual dysfunction was found to be common in women undergoing routine hemodialysis for end-stage renal failure. Sexual dysfunction was associated with older age and depression, and women with lower sexual function scores also had poorer quality-of-life scores.[94]

Two small studies that included older women evaluated the effect of stroke on sexual function. Depressive symptoms, impaired activities of daily living or disability, age, and psychological aspects or relationship with partner were found to be associated with worse sexual function.[95,96]

Breast cancer and sexuality were the focus of two studies. In a cross-sectional analysis of data from a randomized controlled trial of nonhormonal treatments of menopause symptoms, relationship factors and body self-image were identified as major contributors to sexual functioning in women with a history of breast cancer. However, conditions more amenable to physician intervention included vaginal discomfort and urinary incontinence.[97] No studies addressing sexual function in women currently undergoing breast cancer treatment were identified, but one study found that women's satisfaction with their sexual life is significantly decreased after surgical treatment of breast cancer. Most women in this study reported their partner to be supportive and to have the same attitude toward them after surgery. Women who underwent modified mastectomy with adjuvant therapy had greater changes in body image than those who underwent lumpectomy with radiation.[98]

One study addressed sexual function in ovarian cancer patients. Of women up to age 75 currently undergoing treatment for epithelial ovarian cancer, 50% engaged in sexual activity within the preceding month. The women who were sexually active reported decreased sexual desire, vaginal dryness, and dyspareunia. Reasons for sexual inactivity were lack of interest, physical limitations making sex difficult, and fatigue. Women were more likely to be sexually active if they were younger, had positive body self-image, were farther out from diagnosis, and were not receiving active treatment.[99]

Modification of This Question in Light of New Research: The question has been inadequately addressed, especially for hypertension and diabetes, which are commonly present in older women. The question should remain unmodified on the research agenda.

Gyn 42 (Level B): Dose-effect cohort studies of optimal dosage, frequency, and route of administration are needed to learn more about androgen replacement in elderly women.

New Research Addressing This Question: Two studies have evaluated the pharmacokinetics of oral testosterone undecanoate in postmenopausal women. In the first, women received two doses of 20, 40, or 80 mg at 12-hour intervals, and serum testosterone levels were found to be dose proportional after oral administration of two doses.[100] The second study found the administration of testosterone with food to increase bioavailability.[101]

Treatment of postmenopausal women (mean age 55.3 years, range 45 to 70) with 10, 20, or 30 mg of testosterone as a 1% testosterone percutaneous gel daily for 2 weeks resulted in adequate serum levels at the 10 mg dose.[102] A second dose-effect trial evaluated the transdermal testosterone patch in women (mean age 50, range 24 to 70) at doses of 150 μg/day, 300 μg/day, or 450 μg/day twice a week for 24 weeks. Women receiving the 300 μg/day patch experienced higher increases in sexual desire and in frequency of sexual activity than women receiving placebo. There was no apparent treatment effect in the 150 μg/day group, and there was no difference between the 450 μg/day group and the 300 μg/day or placebo groups. There were no differences in adverse effects between any of the groups.[103]

Modification of This Question in Light of New Research: This question has been adequately addressed, and it can be dropped from the research agenda.

Gyn 43 (Level A): **Clinical trials are needed to determine the ability of androgen replacement in older women to enhance outcomes, including specific aspects of sexual function (eg, libido, orgasmic function).**

New Research Addressing This Question: Four studies investigating the effect of androgen replacement on sexual function were identified that enrolled women age 65 or older. Surgically postmenopausal women on estrogen replacement who also used the 300 μg/day testosterone patch for 24 weeks experienced significantly higher increases in sexual desire and in frequency of satisfying sexual activity than the women on placebo. [103] Women receiving esterified estrogen plus methyltestosterone (1.25mg/2.5mg) reported more frequent sexual activity and increased pleasure or orgasm than women receiving estrogen alone. [104] Postmenopausal women on estrogen plus progesterone replacement receiving oral testosterone supplements were found to have a significant improvement in sexual desire and satisfaction in comparison with those on unsupplemented hormone replacement. [105] Surgically menopausal women on estrogen replacement therapy with hypoactive sexual desire disorder treated with testosterone patch twice weekly were found to have increased sexual desire and satisfying sexual activity in comparison with women receiving placebo. [106] The addition of testosterone undecanoate to estrogen replacement therapy in postmenopausal women (aged 45 to 60) was found to improve enjoyment of sex, satisfaction with frequency of sexual activity, and interest in sex in comparison with estrogen alone. [107] Other outcomes associated with testosterone replacement therapy in older woman are reduction in total cholesterol, high-density lipoprotein, and triglyceride levels, reduction in plasma viscosity, increased total lean body mass, and decreased body fat percentage. [104,105,108] According to one study, the use of dehydroepiandrosterone in postmenopausal women does not increase muscle cross-sectional area, muscle strength, or muscle function. [109]

Modification of This Question in Light of New Research: The addition of androgen replacement to hormone replacement therapy in menopausal women appears to improve sexual function and may have other health benefits. This question has been adequately addressed and can be dropped from the research agenda.

Gyn 44 (Level A): **Randomized controlled trials should be performed to determine whether oral estrogen replacement adversely affects sexual function in older women, presumably by decreasing free testosterone levels, and whether this is avoided by the use of transdermal estrogen.**

New Research Addressing This Question: One study of the effects of oral and transdermal estrogen replacement therapy on sex hormone–binding globulin (SHBG) and free testosterone levels was identified; however, the mean age of participants was 45 years. SHBG levels were significantly higher than baseline in the group on oral estrogen replacement after 1 year, although levels were not different at 2 years from those at 1 year. There was no increase in SHBG levels in the transdermal group at either 1 or 2 years. Free testosterone levels were significantly higher in the transdermal group than in the oral group after 2 years of therapy. There were no outcomes regarding sexual function. [110] In a randomized, double-blind, placebo-controlled, cross-over study of 40 women, use of the transdermal estrogen patch for estrogen replacement was found to be associated with high variability in estrogen levels between women. Although there was an increase in levels of SHBG, there were no significant differences in androgen levels. [111]

Modification of This Question in Light of New Research: The question has been inadequately addressed and should remain unmodified on the research agenda.

Gyn 45 (Level D): **The emotional and physical components of the sexual response cycle in the older woman should be observed and defined in light of new and more sophisticated information about female sexuality.**

New Research Addressing This Question: In a study of 19 women, including 8 postmenopausal women, subjects underwent magnetic resonance imaging of the pelvis while watching erotic video. Changes observed in both pre- and postmenopausal women included increased width of vestibular bulb and labia minora and increased enhancement of the bulb, labia minora, and clitoris. Unlike premenopausal women, postmenopausal women did not show any enhancement of the vagina. There were no structural or enhancing changes in the labia majora, urethra, cervix, or rectum in either group. Blood flow changes were seen and were mainly the same in both pre-and postmenopausal women. [112]

Modification of This Question in Light of New Research: The question has been inadequately addressed and should remain unmodified on the research agenda.

Gyn 46 (Level D): **Pilot studies should be performed to determine educational strategies for partners of cognitively impaired patients that enable them to deal with sexuality issues.**

New Research Addressing This Question: No studies were identified.

Modification of This Question in Light of New Research: No modification of this question is recommended.

Gyn 47 (Level C): **Clinical trials should be undertaken to improve the treatment of dyspareunia secondary to urogenital atrophy in women unable to use estrogen products.**

New Research Addressing This Question: In one study, polycarbophil-based vaginal moisturizer treatment in postmenopausal women was found to have a positive effect on the vaginal maturation, as evidenced by increased mean cellular area; however, there were no differences in maturation value or index. [113] The only study identified on nonhormonal treatment of vaginal atrophy evaluated the effect of a soy-rich diet on the vaginal epithelium. In asymptomatic postmenopausal women under 60 years of age, both the hormone replacement and soy diet were found to increase vaginal maturation in comparison with the control group. Maturation indices were higher in the hormone replacement therapy group than in the diet group. [114]

Modification of This Question in Light of New Research: Though nonhormonal treatments may improve vaginal maturation index, no data are available indicating whether higher vaginal maturity index resulted in decreased dyspareunia. The question has been inadequately addressed and should remain unmodified on the research agenda.

PROGRESS IN ROUTINE CARE OF THE WELL ELDERLY WOMAN

CERVICAL CANCER SCREENING

See *New Frontiers,* pp. 236–239.

Gyn 48 (Level B): **Cost analysis should be performed to measure the comprehensive costs to the primary care provider of obtaining a Pap smear in an elderly woman and to compare these with current Medicare reimbursement.**

New Research Addressing This Question: Results from the Health and Retirement Study and the Asset and Health Dynamics Among the Oldest Old were combined to evaluate the cost of routine screening for cervical cancer in older women. The authors estimate that, in 2000, 3.7 million screening Pap smears were performed in women older than 70 years at a cost of $47 million. [115] No studies provided a measure of comprehensive costs to primary care providers for obtaining Pap smears in elderly women for comparison with reimbursement.

Modification of This Question in Light of New Research: The question has been inadequately addressed and should remain unmodified on the research agenda.

Gyn 49 (Level B): **As the baby boomers age, observational studies are needed to determine the cervical cancer incidence in a changing elderly population with different sexual risk factors and to compare this with previous incidence rates.**

New Research Addressing This Question: In women aged 65 to 69 years, the incidence of cervical invasive neoplasia grade 3 was 1.39 per 1000 person-years. [116] Data from nine population-based cancer registries in the U.S. Surveillance, Epidemiology, and End Results Program described trends in incidence rates of cervical cancer between 1976 and 2000. In situ squamous carcinoma of cervix (SCC) has steadily increased in women aged 55 years or older. In situ adenocarcinoma increased in white American women aged 55 to 74, but decreased after age 75. This same increase was not seen in black American women. Invasive SCC decreased in both white and black American women over this time interval. Invasive adenocarcinoma of the cervix increased with age in black American women but plateaued with age in white American women. [117] No studies have specifically focused on the incidence of cervical neoplasia and associated risk factors in elderly women.

Modification of This Question in Light of New Research: No modification of the question is recommended.

Gyn 50 (Level B): **Observational studies are needed to delineate all factors associated with the increased mortality rate of cervical cancer among elderly women.**

New Research Addressing This Question: Of women treated for invasive cervical carcinoma, those 70 years or older were significantly more likely to present with more advanced stage tumors and to have nonsquamous neoplasms. There were differences in treatment offered to older women, with older women more likely to receive primary radiotherapy, less likely to undergo surgical treatment, and nine times more likely to receive no treatment. The risk of death from cervical carcinoma was higher in women aged 70 or older.[118] Another study found that in women with invasive cervical cancer, 5-year survival rates for those aged 65 to 74 and 75 years or older (69% and 42%) were significantly lower than the 75% survival rate seen in women under age 65. Women aged 65 or older were more likely to present with advanced disease, including higher clinical stage, vaginal bleeding, and vaginal and parametrial involvement. Prognostic factors related to age were cervical gross appearance, clinical vaginal involvement, histologic grade, and microscopic cervical and parametrial involvement.[119] Other researchers found that women older than 60 years who were diagnosed with cervical cancer at an older age were more likely to die of their disease within 3 years than were younger women; however, this result was found no longer to be significant when controlled for stage at diagnosis.[120] Another study found that when cancer was diagnosed within 3 years of a normal Pap smear, women aged 60 or older were more likely to die within 3 years than women under 60. Significantly better survival in women aged 35 years or younger with adenocarcinoma of the cervix compared with women aged 65 or older was due to differing therapy; 90% of younger women but only 41% of older women underwent radical surgery. Twenty percent of older women had primary radiotherapy, and 6% had only palliative treatment.[121] Other researchers found that more than 16% of women aged 65 or older with stage IIB/IV received no treatment while 6% of those aged 50 or younger went untreated; 10.7% of women aged 65 or older were never staged.[122] Lower 5-year survival in women aged 65 or older was due to the presence of more advanced disease at diagnosis.[123] Women aged 70 or older were found to be more likely to have higher stage at diagnosis, less likely to undergo surgery, and more likely to receive primary radiotherapy or no treatment.[124]

Modification of This Question in Light of New Research: Observational studies indicate that higher cervical cancer mortality in elderly women may be attributable to more advanced disease at diagnosis, increased likelihood of having a nonsquamous lesion, and differences in treatment offered or accepted. This question has been adequately addressed and can be dropped from the research agenda.

> *Gyn 51 (Level A)*: **Clinical trials should be performed to determine whether strategies to improve cervical cancer screening in impoverished and minority elderly women result in decreased cervical cancer mortality, and which strategies are most cost-effective.**

New Research Addressing This Question: Only one study was identified describing the impact of a cervical cancer screening program on the incidence of cervical cancer. The Norwegian coordinated cervical cancer screening program was started in 1995; letters were sent to women without a screen in the previous 3 years rather than the usual practice of inviting all women to screening regardless of past screening. In the last 2 years of the program, cervical cancer incidence was 22% lower than in the period prior to the screening program. The proportion of women receiving Pap smears increased while overall number of Pap smears decreased, as the screening interval was increased to 3 years.[125] No studies were identified describing screening programs and their impact on cervical cancer incidence specifically targeted to low-income or minority women.

Modification of This Question in Light of New Research: The question has been inadequately addressed and should remain unmodified on the research agenda.

Gyn 52 (Level D): **Observational studies should be performed to determine the relationship of well-established risk factors (eg, multiple sex partners, history of human papilloma virus, cervical dysplasia, smoking, medical or viral immune suppression) to the incidence of cervical or vaginal cancer in elderly women.**

New Research Addressing This Question: No studies were identified.

Modification of This Question in Light of New Research: No modification of the question is recommended.

Gyn 53 (Level D): **Observational studies should be performed to determine whether early detection of cervical neoplasia confers quality-of-life benefits on frail elderly women.**

New Research Addressing This Question: One study found that women with primary gynecologic cancers did not have quality-of-life scores different from the expected age-specific mean values of a healthy population. Cervical carcinoma patients (up to age 83, but not stratified by age) had increase in quality-of-life scores for physical functioning, bodily pain, vitality, social functioning, and mental health associated with increasing age, while lower scores were associated with increasing age in women with ovarian and endometrial cancers. Women with progressive or recurrent cervical cancer had the lowest scores in all quality-of-life scales.[126]

Modification of This Question in Light of New Research: The question has been inadequately addressed and should remain unmodified on the research agenda.

Breast Cancer Screening

See *New Frontiers,* pp. 239–241.

Gyn 54 (Level B): **The results of existing and future mammography studies should be stratified by age, even when power is low, to facilitate systematic reviews of results in older women.**

New Research Addressing This Question: The data from five Swedish mammography trials have been stratified by age for analysis of long-term outcomes.[127]

Modification of This Question in Light of New Research: Large mammography studies have presented data stratified by age. Stratification should be standardized, using defined age groups to facilitate comparisons between studies. A standard scheme of 5-year strata is recommended, ie, age 65 to 69, 70 to 74, 75 to 79, etc. For smaller studies or as an additional analysis in larger studies, comparison of age groups 65 to 79 and age 80 and older will help identify differences that may exist in the very elderly population.

Gyn 55 (Level B): **Observational studies are needed to determine what functional impairments and comorbid conditions are associated with a lack of mammography benefit.**

New Research Addressing This Question: No observational studies were identified. Two large cross-sectional studies including women between 50 and 90 years of age have confirmed that overall rates of mammography decline with age; however, elderly women in subjectively poor health do not discontinue screening more often than healthy women.[115,128] In a third large cross-sectional study of women with a mean age of 79 years, the presence of medical comorbidities was not found to be associated with a decrease in screening, and both hypertension and the presence of multiple comorbidities were found to be associated with increased rates of screening.[129] Among community-living nursing home–eligible women (mean age 81), 17% experienced burden from screening mammography while only 0.9% may have received benefit from screening.[130]

Modification of This Question in Light of New Research: The question has been inadequately addressed and should remain unmodified on the research agenda.

> *Gyn 56 (Level B)*: **Guidelines using functional impairment and comorbid condition measures for discontinuation of mammography should be developed and validated.**

New Research Addressing This Question: No guidelines were identified.

Modification of This Question in Light of New Research: Before guidelines can be developed, studies are needed identifying which, if any, functional impairments and comorbid conditions are associated with lack of mammography benefit.

> *Gyn 57 (Level A)*: **Randomized controlled trials are needed to determine the impact of mammography on the quality of life and burden of disease in older women.**

New Research Addressing This Question: No studies were identified.

Modification of This Question in Light of New Research: No modification of this question is recommended.

> *Gyn 58 (Level A)*: **Clinical trials are needed to determine whether strategies to improve mammography screening rates among impoverished and minority elderly women result in decreased breast cancer mortality or burden of disease, and which strategies are most cost-effective.**

New Research Addressing This Question: No clinical trials were identified. Several studies have been published describing successful strategies for increasing mammography screening rates among low-income and minority women, but none were designed to link these strategies to improved outcomes.[131–136]

Modification of This Question in Light of New Research: The question has been inadequately addressed and should remain unmodified on the research agenda.

> *Gyn 59 (Level D)*: **Observational studies should be performed to determine whether the increase in mammographic density that is related to hormone replacement therapy increases breast cancer mortality or burden of disease in older women.**

New Research Addressing This Question: No studies were identified. The positive association between mammographic density and breast cancer has been confirmed in several studies that enrolled a substantial number of elderly women; however, none of the studies exclusively enrolled women over the age of 65 or included data on subsequent morbidity and mortality.[137–141] One study found that in older women (mean age 60 years), increased breast density was associated with worse prognostic factors (tumors of higher grade, larger size, and estrogen receptor [ER] negative status) than in women with fatty breast tissue. Subjects were not stratified by use of hormone replacement therapy.[142] Mammographic density has been found to be associated with both ER-positive and ER-negative tumors, suggesting that factors other than estrogen are involved.[143] Current hormone replacement therapy users are more likely to have false-negative screening mammograms than non-users, but the effect cannot be entirely attributed to the increase in breast tissue density seen with hormone replacement therapy use.[144]

Modification of This Question in Light of New Research: The question has been inadequately addressed and should remain unmodified on the research agenda.

> ***Gyn 60 (Level D)*: The concurrence and variability of mammogram interpretations by different radiologists in elderly women should be observed and defined.**

New Research Addressing This Question: Only one study was identified that investigated the interpretation of mammograms in women aged 50 to 69 years. The study found that rates of breast cancer detection were not related to the radiologist's mammography volume, but rates did increase when the facilities' overall mammography volume increased. False-positive rates were lower with increased volume.[145] No studies were identified that investigated concurrence and variability of mammogram interpretations by different radiologists. In one study of a general population of patients, accuracy in screening mammogram interpretation was found to be associated with interpretation by a recently trained radiologist, number of diagnostic breast imaging examinations at the facility, designation as a comprehensive breast diagnostic screening center or freestanding mammography center, and use of double reading.[146] Other researchers found no association between accuracy and years of experience or mammography volume.[147] However, higher accuracy was found in a separate study to be associated with more experience and higher focus on screening mammography rather than diagnostic mammography. Higher specificity was associated with greater experience, increased reading volume, and focus on screening rather than diagnostic mammography.[148]

Modification of This Question in Light of New Research: The question has been inadequately addressed and should remain unmodified on the research agenda.

PROGRESS IN ESTROGEN REPLACEMENT THERAPY

ESTROGEN REPLACEMENT AND CARDIOVASCULAR DISEASE

See *New Frontiers,* pp. 242–244.

> ***Gyn 61 (Level B)*: Basic science research, pilot studies, and observational trials are needed to determine which are the more sophisticated measures of potential cardiovascular benefits and risks associated with hormone replacement (eg, C-reactive protein levels, homocysteine levels, activated protein C deficiency, intestinal calcium absorption).**

New Research Addressing This Question: Several studies have described the effects of hormone replacement therapy on cardiovascular biomarkers, including increases in C-reactive protein (CRP), interleukin-6 (IL-6), and reductions in lipoprotein a and homocysteine.[149–155] However, the relationship between these types of markers and outcomes is less clear. In a subset of women enrolled in the Women's Health Initiative, CRP and IL-6 levels were found to predict incident cardiovascular events independently of use or non-use of hormone replacement therapy.[149] In the Women's Health Initiative Observational Study, postmenopausal hormone therapy was found to be associated with higher CRP, high-density lipoprotein, and triglyceride levels. Homocysteine levels were lower in hormone users, and no differences were seen in IL-6 or total cholesterol levels between users and non-users.[156] The Estrogen Replacement on Progression of Coronary Artery Atherosclerosis trial evaluated effects of hormone replacement therapy on CRP and IL-6 in women with coronary artery disease and demonstrated a significant increase in CRP but no change in IL-6 in women on either estrogen or estrogen plus progesterone therapy. The changes in CRP were not associated with progression of atherosclerosis.[157] Hormone replacement with conjugated equine estrogens plus medroxyprogesterone (0.625 mg/5 mg per day) was found not to be associated with elevated homocysteine levels.[158]

Modification of This Question in Light of New Research: The question has been inadequately addressed and should remain unmodified on the research agenda.

> *Gyn 62 (Level A)*: **Placebo-controlled randomized trials, starting with women who have been on hormone replacement therapy for more than 5 years, are needed to determine whether continuation, lowering the dose, or discontinuation confers more cardiovascular benefit for older women.**

New Research Addressing This Question: No studies have been published evaluating the effects of continuation, dose adjustment, or discontinuation after 5 years of therapy on cardiovascular disease.

Modification of This Question in Light of New Research: No modification of the question is recommended.

> *Gyn 63 (Level A)*: **Randomized controlled trials should be performed to determine the effect in elderly women of selective estrogen receptor modulators on primary cardiovascular endpoints, such as myocardial infarction, cardiac death, pulmonary embolism, and stroke.**

New Research Addressing This Question: In the Multiple Outcomes of Raloxifene Evaluation trial, 7705 postmenopausal women (mean age 67) were randomly assigned to raloxifene (60 mg/day or 120 mg/day) or placebo for 4 years. Overall, there was no significant difference in the number of coronary and cerebrovascular events between the groups.[159] In the subset of women with increased baseline cardiovascular risk, women taking raloxifene were found to have significantly fewer cardiovascular events than those taking placebo (relative risk [RR] 0.60, confidence interval [CI] 0.38 to 0.95). Raloxifene was associated with an overall increased risk of venous thromboembolism (RR 2.1, CI 1.2 to 3.8). The risk was higher in the raloxifene group for the first 2 years of treatment, but then decreased to the same rate as the placebo group.[160]

In a randomized controlled trial of 4175 postmenopausal women taking adjuvant tamoxifen for prevention of breast cancer recurrence, women who took tamoxifen for 5 years were found to have significantly reduced mortality from coronary heart disease than women taking the drug for only 2 years (RR 0.67, CI 0.47 to 0.94).[161] In a breast cancer prevention trial, 13,338 women were randomized to tamoxifen or placebo. No difference in cardiovascular mortality was found between the groups after 2 years of follow-up.[162]

Between 1998 and 2000, the Raloxifene Use for the Heart trial recruited 10,101 postmenopausal women (mean age 68 years) for randomization to raloxifene (60 mg/day) or placebo. Approximately half of the women had documented coronary heart disease, and the rest had multiple cardiovascular risk factors. The study was completed in December 2005.[163]

Modification of This Question in Light of New Research: Overall, the available data suggest potential cardiovascular benefit from the use of selective estrogen receptor modulators. However, there is increased risk of venous thromboembolism. Results of the Raloxifene Use for the Heart trial are pending. The question should remain unmodified on the research agenda.

Gyn 64 (Level A): **Randomized controlled trials should be performed to determine whether age modifies hormone effects on the cardiovascular system and cardiovascular risk factors (eg, platelet function, arterial distensibility, angiotensinogen levels, calcium absorption).**

New Research Addressing This Question: No studies were identified that directly addressed this question. In an autopsy study of coronary arteries from 46 postmenopausal and 10 premenopausal women, estrogen-treated postmenopausal women were found to have lower mean coronary calcium content and plaque area than untreated postmenopausal women. The effect of estrogen status on calcium content and plaque size was independent of age.[164] Current hormone replacement therapy has been found to be associated with significant reduction in coronary artery calcium content.[165]

Modification of This Question in Light of New Research: The question has been inadequately addressed and should remain unmodified on the research agenda.

Gyn 65 (Level B): **The results from existing and future studies of hormone replacement should be stratified by age, even when power is low, to facilitate systematic reviews.**

New Research Addressing This Question: Of the major randomized clinical trials investigating hormone replacement therapy and cardiovascular disease, only studies from the Women's Health Initiative included data stratified by age.[166,167]

Modification of This Question in Light of New Research: All hormone replacement studies should include data stratified by age. Stratification should be standardized, using defined age groups to facilitate comparisons between studies. A standard scheme of 5-year strata is recommended, ie, age 65 to 69, 70 to 74, 75 to 79, etc. For smaller studies or as an additional analysis in larger studies, comparison of age groups 65 to 79 and age 80 and older will help identify differences that may exist in the very elderly population.

Gyn 66 (Level C): **Randomized controlled trials are needed to determine whether aspirin eliminates the thrombogenic effect of estrogen in elderly women.**

New Research Addressing This Question: The Heart and Estrogen/Progestin Replacement Study of estrogen plus progestin for secondary prevention of coronary heart disease found no significant difference in coronary heart disease events among women taking aspirin.[168]

Modification of This Question in Light of New Research: The question has been inadequately addressed and should remain unmodified on the research agenda.

ESTROGEN REPLACEMENT THERAPY AND ALZHEIMER'S DISEASE

See *New Frontiers,* pp. 245–247.

Gyn 67 (Level B): **Basic science research and animal studies are needed to determine the differential effects of estrogen and estrogen-progestin replacement on cognition.**

New Research Addressing This Question: In rats, the administration of 17β-estradiol and progesterone, alone or in combination, potentiated the glutamate-mediated rise in intracellular calcium in rat hippocampal neurons. However, the administration of medroxyprogesterone acetate alone or with 17β-estradiol produced no effect or blocked the effect of 17β-estradiol, respectively.[169] In a water maze study of ovariectomized rats, both chronic estrogen and chronic estrogen plus progesterone replacement were found to prevent forgetting between tasks. The study results also suggested that future cognition studies should be conducted specifically on aged female animals.[170]

In a study of cynomolgus monkeys, treatment with conjugated equine estrogens plus medroxyprogesterone acetate for 2 years was found to be associated with reduced acetylcholine esterase activity in the basal forebrain in comparison with estrogen alone.[171]

Modification of This Question in Light of New Research: Estrogen and progesterone may have different effects on cognition, and effects may also depend on the type of progesterone administered. To increase the validity of results, future animal studies should be conducted specifically on aged female animals. The question has been inadequately addressed and should remain otherwise unmodified on the research agenda.

Gyn 68 (Level B): **Basic science research, animal studies, and observational studies are needed to determine which physiologic characteristics, if any, are associated with a benefit or detriment of long-term postmenopausal hormone use.**

New Research Addressing This Question: No studies were identified.

Modification of This Question in Light of New Research: No modification of this question is recommended.

Gyn 69 (Level B): **Basic science research is needed to reconcile and explain the discrepant findings of estrogen neuroprotection in the laboratory in comparison with cognitive detriment with estrogen-progestin in clinical experience.**

New Research Addressing This Question: No studies specifically designed to answer this question were identified. However, as discussed in Gyn 67, the choice of progestin may be important, and results of studies using different progestins may not be comparable.

Modification of This Question in Light of New Research: No modification of the question is recommended.

> ***Gyn 70 (Level B)*: Autopsy studies should be performed to determine the types of dementia most associated with postmenopausal hormone use.**

New Research Addressing This Question: No studies were identified.

Modification of This Question in Light of New Research: No modification of this question is recommended.

> ***Gyn 71 (Level B)*: Results from existing and future studies of hormone replacement and Alzheimer's disease should be stratified by age, even when power is low, to facilitate systematic reviews.**

New Research Addressing This Question: Two substudies from the Women's Health Initiative evaluating the effect of estrogen plus progestin on global cognitive function and the incidence of dementia and mild cognitive impairment provided data for three age groups: 65 to 69, 70 to 74, and 75 years and older. [172,173] Results for the Multiple Outcomes of Raloxifene Evaluation trial reported results of 3 years of raloxifene treatment in 7705 women with osteoporosis. The effects of treatment on cognitive function were reported for women 70 years or younger and women older than 70 years. [174]

Modification of This Question in Light of New Research: All study results should be stratified by age. Stratification should be standardized, using defined age groups to facilitate comparisons between studies. A standard scheme of 5-year strata is recommended, ie, age 65 to 69, 70 to 74, 75 to 79, etc. For smaller studies or as an additional analysis in larger studies, comparison of age groups 65 to 79 and age 80 and older will help identify differences that may exist in the very elderly population.

> ***Gyn 72 (Level A)*: Randomized controlled trials of long-term postmenopausal hormone users are needed to determine whether discontinuation or continuation into the 70s, 80s, and 90s affects cognition.**

New Research Addressing This Question: No studies specifically addressing continuation versus discontinuation in elderly women were identified; however, the results concerning cognition in two major long-term hormone replacement studies have been published.

In the Women's Health Initiative, 4532 women (aged 65 or older) were also enrolled in the estrogen plus progestin arm of the Women's Health Initiative Memory Study. All women were free of dementia at baseline and provided at least one follow-up cognitive function score before the study was ended. Mean follow-up was 4.2 years. There was a significant decline in Modified Mini-Mental Status Examination score in the treatment group in comparison with the placebo group (6.7% versus 4.8%, $P = .008$). [172] The hazard ratio for probable dementia in women in the estrogen plus progestin group was 2.05 (CI 1.21 to 3.48). However, there was no difference in development of mild cognitive impairment between the groups.[173] The authors of both reports concluded that estrogen plus progestin should not be used for prevention of cognitive impairment or dementia.[172,173]

In the Heart and Estrogen/Progestin Replacement Study, 1063 postmenopausal women (mean age 71 years) enrolled in the cognitive function substudy. After 4 years, women in the treatment group had significantly worse scores on the verbal fluency test than those in the placebo group ($P = .02$), but no other differences were seen between the two groups.[175]

Estrogen Replacement Therapy, Modified Estrogens, and Cancer

See *New Frontiers*, pp. 247–249.

Gyn 73 (Level B): **Cross-sectional or prospective cohort studies should be performed to determine the factors, whether breast cancer pathophysiology or other health factors, that are associated with the apparent lower mortality among women whose breast cancer is diagnosed during hormone replacement therapy use.**

New Research Addressing This Question: Women diagnosed with breast cancer while on hormone replacement therapy are more likely to present with smaller tumor size,[176–179] lower stage,[177–180] and lower grade.[179–181] In addition, women on hormone replacement are more likely to be diagnosed with lobular cancers.[176,180] There are no differences between users and non-users in tumor expression of c-erb B-2, p53, her 2-neu, or Ki67.[178,182] Some studies have reported no difference in hormone-receptor status between users and non-users,[176,180] while others have found more estrogen receptor–positive tumors in women on long-term hormone replacement[178] and more estrogen receptor– and progesterone receptor–positive tumors only in women on continuous combined hormone replacement.[177]

Three prospective cohort studies were identified describing prognostic factors in women on hormone replacement at the time of diagnosis. In the Malmo preventive cohort, women diagnosed with breast cancer while on hormone replacement were more likely to present with stage 1 tumors, lobular carcinomas, and tubular tumors. Hormone-receptor status was not different between user and non-users.[182] The Danish Nurses' study found women on hormone replacement more likely to be diagnosed with hormone receptor–positive cancer, invasive ductal carcinoma, and cancer of a low histologic grade than women who had never used hormone replacement.[183] In the Nurses' Health Study, women on hormone replacement were found to be more likely to develop hormone receptor–positive cancer than women who were non-users, and this effect increased with duration of hormone use. The association between hormone receptor–positive cancer and hormone replacement therapy was stronger in women on combined therapy than in women on estrogen alone.[184]

Data regarding differential prognostic factors in women diagnosed with breast cancer while on hormone replacement in the Women's Health Initiative are different from data seen in observational studies. Women in the estrogen plus progestin treatment arm diagnosed with breast cancer had larger tumor size, more frequent node invasion, and more advanced stage than those diagnosed while on placebo. There were no differences between groups in histology, grade, or hormone-receptor status.[185]

Modification of This Question in Light of New Research: Data on the characteristics of breast cancer diagnosed in women on hormone replacement therapy from observational trials and the Women's Health Initiative are quite different. This may be attributable to the different study populations. Further studies are needed to adequately answer this question. The question should remain unmodified on the research agenda.

Gyn 74 (Level B): **Observational studies are needed to determine what functional factors and comorbidities are associated with a lack of benefit of mammography or colon cancer screening, for the development of clinical guidelines.**

New Research Addressing This Question: No studies were identified.

Modification of This Question in Light of New Research: No modification of this question is recommended.

Gyn 75 (Level B): **The results from existing and future studies of estrogen, estrogen-progestin, and selective estrogen receptor modulator use should be stratified by age, even when power is low, to facilitate systematic reviews.**

New Research Addressing This Question: Results from the Women's Health Initiative study regarding the risk of colorectal cancer with estrogen or estrogen plus progestin versus placebo are provided with age stratification (ages 50 to 59, 60 to 69, 70 to 79). [167,186] Results from the Polyp Prevention Trial prospectively evaluating the association between hormone replacement therapy and adenoma recurrence were provided with age stratification (ages younger than 55, 55 to 62, 63 to 69, 70 and older). [187] Women's Health Initiative results regarding breast cancer and mammography in women randomized to estrogen plus progestin or placebo are presented with age-stratified data (ages 50 to 59, 60 to 69, 70 to 79). [185,188]

Modification of This Question in Light of New Research: All study results should be stratified by age. Stratification should be standardized, using defined age groups to facilitate comparisons between studies. A standard scheme of 5-year strata is recommended, ie, age 65 to 69, 70 to 74, 75 to 79, etc. For smaller studies or as an additional analysis in larger studies, comparison of age groups 65 to 79 and age 80 and older will help identify differences that may exist in the very elderly population.

Gyn 76 (Level A): **Randomized trials of continuous therapy since menopause are needed to determine the effects of estrogen and hormone replacement on breast and colon cancer incidence and mortality.**

New Research Addressing This Question: No studies were identified that enrolled only women continuously on hormone replacement therapy since menopause.

Modification of This Question in Light of New Research: The Kronos Early Estrogen Prevention trial study will be evaluating outcomes associated with hormone replacement therapy in postmenopausal women beginning within 3 years of menopause. [189] The study is expected to be completed in December 2010. The question should remain unmodified on the research agenda.

Gyn 77 (Level A): **Randomized trials are needed to determine the effects of long-term use of selective estrogen receptor modulators on breast and colon cancer incidence and mortality.**

New Research Addressing This Question: In the Breast Cancer Prevention Trial of the National Surgical Adjuvant Breast and Bowel Project P-1 Study, the risk of invasive breast cancer was found to be decreased in women on tamoxifen (RR 0.57, CI 0.46 to 0.70), as was the risk of noninvasive breast cancer (RR 0.63, CI 0.45 to 0.89). Of 288 women who developed breast cancer during this trial, 19% were found to have BRCA mutations.[190] Within this subset of women, tamoxifen reduced breast cancer in those with BRCA2 but not BRCA1 mutations.[191] In the Continuing Outcomes Relevant to Evista trial, raloxifene was found to significantly decrease the incidence of invasive breast cancer and estrogen receptor–positive invasive breast cancer in comparison with placebo. Hazard ratios were 0.34 (CI 0.22 to 0.50) and 0.24 (CI 0.15 to 0.40), respectively.[192] Results from the Multiple Outcomes of Raloxifene Evaluation trial found no difference in the incidence of colorectal cancer between treatment and placebo groups.[193]

Modification of This Question in Light of New Research: Use of selective estrogen receptor modulators appears to decrease the incidence of breast cancer, but data regarding the effect on breast cancer mortality are not available. The only randomized trial evaluating the effect on risk of colon cancer suggests no benefit. The question has been inadequately addressed and should remain unmodified on the research agenda.

Gyn 78 (Level D): **Basic science and observational trials are needed to determine the mechanisms by which estrogen reduces colon cancer incidence.**

New Research Addressing This Question: Estrogen receptor-beta (ERβ) is the predominant estrogen receptor expressed in human colon, and decreased levels of ERβ mRNA are associated with colon cancer in women.[194] Loss of ERβ expression is associated with advanced Dukes stage.[195] Differential expression of isoforms of ERβ may also be associated with differential effect on colorectal tumorigenesis. ERβ1 may be associated with microsatellite unstable colorectal cancer, a type characterized by mutations leading to failure of the mismatch repair system.[196] Microsatellite unstable colorectal cancer is associated with lack of estrogen and is more common in older women.[197] Polymorphisms of the ERβ gene may be associated with development of colorectal cancer.[198] Women who have two long alleles and are estrogen negative are at higher risk of colorectal cancer than women with short alleles and estrogen. The use of hormone replacement therapy reduces the risk of colon cancer in women with the R allele of the ERβ gene. Postmenopausal women with the R allele who did not take hormone replacement therapy were found to be at higher risk for developing colorectal cancer. Colon cancer risk was also increased in postmenopausal women not in hormone replacement therapy with $>$ 25 cytosine-adenine repeats of the ERβ gene.[199] Other investigations have implicated estrogen receptor–related receptor α,[198] acquired p53 mutations,[200] and insulin-like growth factor polymorphisms[201] in colorectal cancer in women.

Modification of This Question in Light of New Research: Data are available suggesting that genetic susceptibility to colon cancer may be modified by estrogen. Further studies are needed to confirm genetic sources of susceptibility and the impact of menopause and estrogen therapy. The question should remain unmodified on the research agenda.

Gyn 79 (Level C): **Randomized trials are needed to determine whether estrogen or estrogen-progestin replacement after breast cancer treatment affects recurrence and mortality.**

New Research Addressing This Question: Two randomized trials were identified. The Hormonal Replacement Therapy After Breast Cancer—Is It Safe? (HABITS) trial openly randomized women with a history of breast cancer to hormone replacement therapy or best treatment without hormones. After median follow-up of 2.1 years, the study was stopped when 26 women in the hormone therapy arm and 8 in the non-hormone group had breast cancer recurrences. The women who were enrolled will be followed for the originally intended 5 years after randomization. [202] In the Stockholm trial, postmenopausal women with a history of breast cancer were openly randomized to hormone therapy or no hormone therapy. After a median follow-up of 4.1 years, this trial was also stopped after analysis of the combined data from the Stockholm and HABITS trials revealed a significantly increased risk of cancer recurrence in women on hormone therapy. However, there was no significant increase in breast cancer recurrence specifically among hormone users enrolled in the Stockholm trial. [203] The difference in results may be due to the much higher percentage of women using tamoxifen in the Stockholm trial than in the HABITS trial (52% versus 21%).

Modification of This Question in Light of New Research: Data suggest that the use of hormone replacement therapy by women with a history of breast cancer may increase the risk of recurrence. However, this risk may be modified by the concurrent use of a selective estrogen receptor modulator. This question has been adequately addressed in its current form and can be dropped from the research agenda.

PROGRESS IN OSTEOPOROSIS

HORMONAL THERAPIES

See *New Frontiers,* pp. 250–251.

Gyn 80 (Level B): **Prospective cohort studies are needed to compare the quality-of-life outcomes of long-term estrogen, estrogen-progestin, selective estrogen receptor modulator, and bisphosphonate use.**

New Research Addressing This Question: In a randomized study comparing neridronate and no treatment for osteoporosis in women (aged 65 to 80), 12 months of treatment was found to improve quality of life (pain, general health perception, vitality, emotional functioning, and physical functioning). [204] No studies evaluating quality-of-life outcomes of long-term therapy with estrogen, estrogen-progestin, or selective estrogen receptor modulator therapy were identified.

Modification of This Question in Light of New Research: The question has been inadequately addressed and should remain unmodified on the research agenda.

Gyn 81 (Level B): **Observational and pilot studies are needed to determine whether hormone replacement therapy and selective estrogen receptor modulators act synergistically with other fracture-**

prevention interventions, such as physical therapy for balance and strength.

New Research Addressing This Question: In postmenopausal women (aged 40 to 65 years) randomized to weight-bearing and resistance exercise for 1 year, the combination of exercise and hormone replacement therapy was found to produce greater increases in bone mineral density than either alone.[205]

In elderly women (aged 75 to 87) on hormone replacement therapy, the addition of a supervised exercise program produced greater increases in lumbar spine bone mineral density than unsupervised exercise at home (3.5% versus 1.5%, $P = .048$).[206] There were no significant decreases in hip or total body bone mineral density. Postmenopausal women randomized to a supervised aerobic and weight-bearing exercise regimen three times a week had 1% increase in trochanteric bone mineral density; women who also used hormone replacement therapy had 1% to 2% increase in bone mineral density at the femoral neck, trochanter, and lumbar spine.[207]

Modification of This Question in Light of New Research: Combining hormone replacement therapy with a supervised exercise regimen increases bone mineral density more than hormone therapy alone or hormone therapy with unsupervised exercise. No studies investigating synergistic effects of selective estrogen receptor modulators with exercise or other interventions were identified. The question has been inadequately addressed and should remain unmodified on the research agenda.

Gyn 82 (Levels B, A): **Observational and eventually randomized trials are needed to determine whether low-dose estrogen replacement therapy initiated at menopause reduces hip, vertebral, and other osteoporotic fractures in advanced age.**

New Research Addressing This Question: Two randomized, double-blind, placebo-controlled trials of low-dose estrogen on bone mineral density were identified. Postmenopausal women randomized to 0.25 mg/day of micronized 17β-estradiol or placebo for 3 years were found to have increased bone density at the hip, spine, and total body as well as reduced bone turnover.[208] Postmenopausal women randomized to 0.014 mg/day of transdermal estradiol for 2 years were found to have increased bone mineral density and decreased bone turnover.[209]

Modification of This Question in Light of New Research: Low-dose estrogen therapy increases bone mineral density and decreases bone turnover, but no data are available regarding the reduction of fracture risk. Studies of the initiation of low-dose estrogen therapy specifically at menopause were not identified. The question has been inadequately addressed and should remain unmodified on the research agenda.

Gyn 83 (Level B): **Results from existing and future studies of hormone replacement to prevent or treat osteoporosis need to be stratified by age, even when power is low, to facilitate systematic reviews.**

New Research Addressing This Question: Results of the Women's Health Initiative trial pertaining to fracture and bone mineral density are presented with age stratification.[210] Results of the Million Women Study are also presented in an age-stratified manner.[211]

Modification of This Question in Light of New Research: All studies should include age stratification of data. Stratification should be standardized, using defined age groups to facilitate comparisons between studies. A standard scheme of 5-year strata is recommended, ie, age 65 to 69, 70 to 74, 75 to 79, etc. For smaller studies or as an additional analysis in larger studies, comparison of age groups 65 to 79 and age 80 and older will help identify differences that may exist in the very elderly population.

Gyn 84 (Level A): **Randomized trials are needed to determine the differences in overall quality of life with hormone replacement therapy, selective estrogen receptor modulators, and bisphosphonates.**

New Research Addressing This Question: No studies were identified.

Modification of This Question in Light of New Research: No modification of this question is recommended.

Gyn 85 (Level A): **A placebo-controlled randomized trial should be performed to determine whether bisphosphonates, hormone replacement therapy, or selective estrogen receptor modulators best reduce osteoporosis morbidity and mortality in frail and institutionalized elderly women, including data on overall cost, burden of care, and quality of life.**

New Research Addressing This Question: No studies were identified.

Modification of This Question in Light of New Research: No modification of this question is recommended.

Gyn 86 (Level A): **A randomized controlled trial should be performed to determine the fracture benefit of initiating selective estrogen receptor modulators after age 75 among both osteoporotic and osteopenic women.**

New Research Addressing This Question: No studies were identified.

Modification of This Question in Light of New Research: No modification of this question is recommended.

NONHORMONAL THERAPIES: CALCIUM AND VITAMIN D

See *New Frontiers,* pp. 252–253.

Gyn 87 (Level D): **Observational trials and pilot studies are needed to determine the importance of factors in adolescence, such as milk and carbonated beverage consumption, on peak bone mass and bone matrix.**

New Research Addressing This Question: In a study that assigned adolescent girls to calcium supplements or increased intake of dairy foods, both interventions were found to increase peak bone mass. Calcium increases volumetric bone density and dairy foods may also increase bone growth and periosteal bone expansion.[212] In adolescent girls, implementation of an exercise program has been found to be associated with increases in bone mineral density.[213–217] Daily intake of at least three servings of fruits and vegetables was found to be associated with increased bone area in early adolescent girls.[218]

Modification of This Question in Light of New Research: Early studies suggest that calcium supplementation, increased intake of dairy foods, diet including fruits and vegetables, and exercise may help in attaining maximum peak bone mass. No studies evaluated the effect of carbonated beverages. The question has been inadequately addressed and should remain unmodified on the research agenda.

Gyn 88 (Level D): **Observational studies are needed to define the costs and side effects associated with calcium and vitamin D supplementation.**

New Research Addressing This Question: Calcium supplementation has been associated with mild transient hypotensive effects in postmenopausal women (mean age 74),[219] increases in high-density lipoprotein cholesterol levels in postmenopausal women,[220] and no increased risk of calcium oxalate nephrolithiasis.[221,222] In the Randomised Evaluation of Calcium or Vitamin D trial of 5292 people (including 4481 women) aged 70 or older, compliance with calcium supplementation was significantly lower partly because of gastrointestinal symptoms. Serious adverse effects were rare and were not different between groups.[223] In a randomized cross-over study in postmenopausal women, three readily available calcium sources (calcium carbonate, encapsulated calcium carbonate, calcium citrate) were all shown to be readily absorbed and equally bioavailable. Cost-benefit analysis determined that the less expensive calcium carbonate products were cost-effective for universal supplementation while the calcium citrate product was not.[224]

Modification of This Question in Light of New Research: Adverse effects of calcium supplementation are rare. Compliance may be limited by gastrointestinal symptoms. Calcium carbonate supplementation is cost-effective. This question has been adequately addressed and can be dropped from the research agenda.

Gyn 89 (Level C): **Randomized trials are needed to determine the optimal time in a woman's life span to benefit from calcium supplementation.**

New Research Addressing This Question: Postmenarchal girls (mean age 14) with a diet low in calcium randomized to placebo or 1000 mg calcium daily supplementation were found to have greater increase in total body bone mineral density and spine bone mineral density on calcium. The effect was enhanced in girls who had onset of menarche more than 2 years before intervention.[225] Early adolescent girls receiving 1000 mg calcium supplementation daily were found to have significantly greater distal and proximal radius bone mineral density, total body bone mineral density, and metacarpal cortical indices at 4 years than those on placebo.[212] At 7 years, significant effects remained at the proximal radius and metacarpals.[226] Women aged 45 or older taking 500 mg calcium plus 200 IU vitamin D daily for 30 months were found to have significantly different changes in bone mineral density than those on placebo; placebo use resulted in loss of bone mineral density.[227]

Modification of This Question in Light of New Research: Calcium supplementation appears to be beneficial in both adolescent girls and women over the age of 45 years. The question has been inadequately addressed and should remain unmodified on the research agenda.

Gyn 90 (Level C): **Randomized trials should be performed to determine the best method of calcium supplementation to maximize absorption and minimize side effects.**

New Research Addressing This Question: In a four-period, three-way, randomized cross-over trial of calcium carbonate, calcium citrate, or placebo in postmenopausal women, all calcium sources were found to have been equally absorbed and bioavailable. Cost analysis favored the least expensive calcium supplement—calcium carbonate.[224] In a four-way cross-over study of placebo versus calcium as calcium carbonate, calcium citrate, or calcium formate in adult women, calcium formate was found to produce significantly higher levels of serum calcium.[228] Calcium-fortified orange juice, calcium carbonate supplements, and milk were found to have similar bioavailabilities in subjects older than 50 years.[229]

Modification of This Question in Light of New Research: Calcium carbonate is consistently identified as readily absorbed and bioavailable as well as the most cost-effective method of supplementation. Although these studies did not specifically address side effects, serious adverse effects from calcium supplementation are rare (see Gyn 88). This question has been adequately addressed and can be dropped from the research agenda.

Gyn 91 (Level C): **Randomized trials are needed to determine the best form of vitamin D supplementation.**

New Research Addressing This Question: No studies were identified.

Modification of This Question in Light of New Research: No modification of this question is recommended.

Nonhormonal Therapies: Bisphosphonates

See *New Frontiers,* pp. 253–254.

Gyn 92 (Level B): **Long-term observational studies are needed to obtain information about the efficacy, safety, and adverse effects of very long-term bisphosphonate use (30 to 40 years) for postmenopausal osteoporosis prevention and treatment.**

New Research Addressing This Question: There are no studies evaluating the very long-term use of bisphosphonates for postmenopausal osteoporosis. The majority of studies provide data for 3 to 5 years of use. In postmenopausal women with osteoporosis treated with risedronate for 3 years, one study found a significant decrease in bone formation rate reflecting decreased turnover in comparison with placebo, while bone mineralization remained normal. Treated women had formation of normal lamellar bone and normal osteoid thickness. Bone resorption was decreased with 58% and 47% reductions in mineralizing surface and activation frequency.[230] In another study, after 5 years of risedronate therapy or placebo, no significant histomorphometric differences were found between groups in structural or resorption parameters. Bone turnover was continuous in both groups, and lumbar spine bone mineral density was significantly increased in the risedronate group in comparison with the placebo group.[231]

After initial 5-year treatment with alendronate, a further 3 years of treatment was found to increase bone mineral density at the spine and to maintain it at the hip. In women taking placebo after 5 years of alendronate, bone mineral density and reduction in bone turnover was greater than at baseline.[232] Bisphosphonate suppression of bone formation is partially reversible with intermittent parathyroid hormone.[233] In a study of women who took alendronate for 10 years, the fracture rate observed between 6 and 10 years was similar to the rate in years 1 to 3. Prolonged treatment was not found to be associated with any loss of benefit, and the drug was well tolerated.[234]

A potential risk of suppression of bone turnover and accumulation of microdamage with long-term use of bisphosphonates has been described. In a case series of 8 postmenopausal women and 1 man (aged 49 to 76) with atraumatic nonvertebral fractures on alendronate therapy for 3 to 8 years, 6 of the patients had delayed healing for 3 months to 2 years after diagnosis. All 9 patients had decreased bone volume and suppression of bone formation, and 4 patients continued to have delayed healing after discontinuation of alendronate.[235] In women (aged 55 to 80) receiving ibandronate (orally or IV) for 3 years, no differences in yearly rate of progression or in the 3-year change in aortic calcification were found between intervention groups. Three-year changes in bone mineral density and simultaneous changes in aortic calcification were not correlated.[236]

Modification of This Question in Light of New Research: The maximum length of bisphosphonate therapy investigated was 10 years. The question should remain unmodified on the research agenda.

Gyn 93 (Level B): Medications that selectively reduce bone resorption without limiting bone formation should be developed.

New Research Addressing This Question: Isosorbide mononitrate is a precursor of nitric oxide, which is thought to mediate bone loss by decreasing osteoclast activity. In one study, postmenopausal women were randomly assigned to treatment with isosorbide mononitrate for 12 weeks or to placebo; significant increases in urine N-telopeptide and decreases in serum bone-specific alkaline phosphatase consistent with decreased bone resorption and increased bone formation were found in the treatment group. Women in the treatment group reported significantly more headaches, and 16 of them discontinued treatment because of headache but only 2 women in the placebo group did so.[237]

Modification of This Question in Light of New Research: Only one new medication was identified. The question has been inadequately addressed and should remain unmodified on the research agenda.

Gyn 94 (Level B): Medications that stimulate bone formation should be developed.

New Research Addressing This Question: Strontium ranelate is a compound of ranelic acid and two atoms of strontium that has been associated with stimulation of bone formation. In the Treatment of Peripheral Osteoporosis study, postmenopausal women were randomly assigned to either 2g/day strontium ranelate or placebo for 3 years. Treatment with strontium ranelate was shown to produce significant increase in bone mineral density at the femoral neck and hip and reduce the risk of nonvertebral fracture by 16%. There was no difference in adverse reactions between treatment and placebo groups.[238] The Strontium Ranelate for Treatment of Osteoporosis trial (Phase II) randomized postmenopausal women with osteoporosis and at least one previous vertebral fracture to 0.5g/day or 2g/day of strontium ranelate or placebo for 2 years. In the treatment groups, vertebral bone mineral density was significantly increased. Of the two doses studied, 2g/day of strontium ranelate produced the greatest increase in bone mineral density and was associated with a significant decrease in incidence of vertebral fractures. The higher dose of strontium ranelate produced a significant increase in serum bone-specific alkaline phosphatase and significantly decreased urinary excretion of N-telopeptide.[239] In a phase III trial, postmenopausal women with osteoporosis and at least one vertebral fracture were randomized to 2g/day of strontium ranelate or placebo for 3 years. In the treatment group, relative risk of vertebral fracture was 0.59 (CI 0.48 to 0.73). Lumbar bone mineral density was increased by 14.4% and 8.3% at the femoral neck. No differences in adverse effects between treatment and placebo were found.[240]

Modification of This Question in Light of New Research: Only one new medication was identified. In initial studies, strontium ranelate does appear to increase bone mineral density and decrease the risk of fracture. The question has been inadequately addressed and should remain unmodified on the research agenda.

Gyn 95 (Level A): **Randomized controlled trials are needed to determine the utility of bisphosphonates for osteoporosis benefit in healthy women.**

New Research Addressing This Question: One study found that healthy, early postmenopausal women taking 10 mg/day of alendronate for 6 years had significantly increased spine and hip bone mineral density and decreased incidence of fracture in comparison with those on placebo. Adverse effects were similar in treatment and placebo.[241] In the Fracture Intervention Trial subgroup analysis of postmenopausal women with osteopenia (but not osteoporosis) randomized to treatment with alendronate (5mg/day for 2 years, then 10 mg/day thereafter) found 60% and 43% decreases in risk of clinical and radiographic fracture, respectively, in comparison with placebo.[242]

Modification of This Question in Light of New Research: Alendronate therapy increases bone mineral density and decreases the risk of fracture in healthy women and women with osteopenia. This question has been adequately addressed and can be dropped from the research agenda.

Gyn 96 (Level A): **Randomized controlled trials should be performed to determine the additive effects, if any, of hormonal and nonhormonal osteoporosis therapies.**

New Research Addressing This Question: In postmenopausal women randomized in a 2 × 2 factorial design to hormone replacement therapy (conjugated equine estrogen 0.625 mg/day, with or without medroxyprogesterone 2.5 mg/day) and alendronate 10 mg/day, both agents, or neither for 3 years, those receiving combination therapy were found to have significantly higher femoral and vertebral bone mineral density than those receiving monotherapy.[243] In elderly women with normal bone density for their age, combination treatment with hormone replacement therapy and calcitriol was found to increase bone mineral density significantly more at the total hip and trochanter than did hormone replacement alone.[244] One study found that in postmenopausal women with osteoporosis, treatment with both teriparatide and raloxifene increased bone formation to the same degree as teriparatide alone, but that combination therapy produced greater decreases in bone resorption and increases in bone mineral density at the total hip than teriparatide alone.[245] In women with postmenopausal osteoporosis, therapy with parathyroid hormone and alendronate was not found to produce greater increases in bone mineral density at the spine than parathyroid hormone alone. The anabolic effects of parathyroid hormone were reduced with the co-administration of alendronate.[233]

Modification of This Question in Light of New Research: Hormone replacement therapy may act synergistically with bisphosphonates or calcitriol. Combining parathyroid hormone with a selective estrogen receptor modulator may have additive effects, and combination with a bisphosphonate may reduce the anabolic effects of parathyroid hormone alone. Further studies are needed to identify potentially adverse interactions of combination therapy as well as additive effects. The question should remain unmodified on the research agenda.

> ***Gyn 97 (Level D)*: Decision and cost-effectiveness analyses are needed to calculate whether health care dollars spent on medication, including evaluation and management of complications, would be better spent on physical and occupational therapy in frail elderly women.**

New Research Addressing This Question: No studies were identified.

Modification of This Question in Light of New Research: No modification of this question is recommended.

NEW HORIZONS IN GERIATRIC GYNECOLOGY

PELVIC ORGAN PROLAPSE

The true prevalence of pelvic organ prolapse is unknown, and our ability to determine this prevalence is limited by lack of a standard and clinically relevant definition of the condition. The International Continence Society currently defines pelvic organ prolapse as descent of stage I or greater, although the authors themselves noted the definition to be inadequate.[246] By this definition, baseline data from the Women's Health Initiative suggests that 60% of women over the age of 50 have pelvic organ prolapse.[66] Age-group prevalences included 28% of women aged 50 to 69, 47% aged 60 to 69, and 24% aged 70 to 79. Similarly, the Pelvic Organ Support Study found pelvic organ prolapse of some degree in 75% of women undergoing annual gynecologic examination. However, with use of a clinical definition of prolapse as leading edge at −0.5 cm or greater from the hymen, only 22% of subjects were classified as having prolapse.[68] Several studies have advocated the use of a clinically relevant definition of prolapse, with the disease state defined as leading edge of prolapse at the hymen or beyond.[247–250]

> ***Gyn 98 (Level B)*: A clinically relevant definition of pelvic organ prolapse should be established and used to determine the prevalence of pelvic organ prolapse in elderly women. Subsequent surgical outcome studies should use this definition to describe outcomes.**

> ***Gyn 99 (Level B)*: Gynecologic surgery studies describing the outcomes of surgical treatment of pelvic organ prolapse should include both preoperative and postoperative description of prolapse using the pelvic organ prolapse quantification (POP-Q) system to facilitate comparison of results.**

Gyn 100 (Level B): **Observational studies are needed to determine the risk factors for recurrence of pelvic organ prolapse after surgical treatment in elderly women.**

Several studies have been published describing the use of local anesthesia with sedation for pelvic organ prolapse surgery as an alternative to general or regional anesthesia.[251–255] Minimizing anesthesia in elderly women undergoing gynecologic surgeries may reduce perioperative morbidity such as nausea, vomiting, and cognitive changes. However, no studies directly comparing anesthesia type in this population were identified.

Gyn 101 (Level A): **Randomized controlled trials of general, regional, and local anesthesia for pelvic organ prolapse surgery in elderly women are needed to determine whether their rates of perioperative morbidity differ.**

SEXUALITY

The prevalence of sexual dysfunction among older women is unknown. Indeed, the definition of normal sexual function in older women remains elusive. Lack of knowledge concerning what is "normal" complicates investigations of prevalence and treatment interventions. In a prospective longitudinal study, sexual responsivity was found to be significantly decreased with time in both women transitioning through the perimenopausal period and in postmenopausal women. From the early to late perimenopausal periods, overall sexual functioning significantly decreases. From late perimenopause to menopause, there are decreases in overall sexual function, libido, and frequency of sexual activity, as well as increased vaginal dyspareunia.[256] However, sexual inactivity in older women is not always related to their own sexual dysfunction. In a study of community-dwelling women with pelvic floor disorders, the most commonly cited reason for sexual inactivity was a partner's physical ailment making sexual activity embarrassing or uncomfortable.[257]

Gyn 102 (Level B): **Observational studies are needed to describe normal sexual function and activity of elderly women and to provide a basis for developing a definition of sexual dysfunction that is appropriate for women in this age group.**

Gyn 103 (Level B): **Observational studies are needed to establish the prevalence of sexual dysfunction in elderly women.**

Gyn 104 (Level B): **Observational studies are needed to establish the effect of sexual dysfunction on the quality of life of elderly women.**

Gyn 105 (Level B): **Observational studies are needed to establish the effect of partners' sexual dysfunction on the quality of life of elderly women.**

REFERENCES

1. U.S. Census Bureau, Population Division. Population Projections Branch. March, 2004 (available online: http://www.census.gov/ipc/www/usinterimproj/).

2. Miller KL, Stenchever MA, Richter HE, et al. Geriatric gynecology. In Solomon DH, LoCicero J, 3rd, Rosenthal RA (eds): New Frontiers in Geriatrics Research: An Agenda for Surgical and Related Medical Specialties. New York: American Geriatrics Society, 2004, pp. 225-267 (online at http://www.frycomm.com/ags/rasp).
3. Parker DY, Burke JJ, 2nd, Gallup DG. Gynecological surgery in octogenarians and nonagenarians. Am J Obstet Gynecol 2004;190:1401-1403.
4. Rasmussen LS, Johnson T, Kuipers HM, et al. Does anaesthesia cause postoperative cognitive dysfunction? A randomised study of regional versus general anaesthesia in 438 elderly patients. Acta Anaesthesiol Scand 2003;47:260-266.
5. Canet J, Raeder J, Rasmussen LS, et al. Cognitive dysfunction after minor surgery in the elderly. Acta Anaesthesiol Scand 2003;47:1204-1210.
6. Rohan D, Buggy DJ, Crowley S, et al. Increased incidence of postoperative cognitive dysfunction 24 hr after minor surgery in the elderly. Can J Anaesth 2005;52:137-142.
7. Hitcho EB, Krauss MJ, Birge S, et al. Characteristics and circumstances of falls in a hospital setting: a prospective analysis. J Gen Intern Med 2004;19:732-739.
8. Litaker D, Locala J, Franco K, et al. Preoperative risk factors for postoperative delirium. Gen Hosp Psychiatry 2001;23:84-89.
9. McPherson K, Metcalfe MA, Herbert A, et al. Severe complications of hysterectomy: the VALUE study. BJOG 2004;111:688-694.
10. Madalinska JB, Hollenstein J, Bleiker E, et al. Quality-of-life effects of prophylactic salpingo-oophorectomy versus gynecologic screening among women at increased risk of hereditary ovarian cancer. J Clin Oncol 2005;23:6890-6898.
11. Hurbanek JG, Jaffer AK, Morra N, et al. Postmenopausal hormone replacement and venous thromboembolism following hip and knee arthroplasty. Thromb Haemost 2004;92:337-343.
12. Andonian S, Chen T, St-Denis B, Corcos J. Randomized clinical trial comparing suprapubic arch sling (SPARC) and tension-free vaginal tape (TVT): one-year results. Eur Urol 2005;47:537-541.
13. Hung MJ, Liu FS, Shen PS, et al. Analysis of two sling procedures using polypropylene mesh for treatment of stress urinary incontinence. Int J Gynaecol Obstet 2004;84:133-141.
14. Abdel-Fattah M, Barrington JW, Arunkalaivanan AS. Pelvicol pubovaginal sling versus tension-free vaginal tape for treatment of urodynamic stress incontinence: a prospective randomized three-year follow-up study. Eur Urol 2004;46:629-635.
15. Schulz JA, Nager CW, Stanton SL, Baessler K. Bulking agents for stress urinary incontinence: short-term results and complications in a randomized comparison of periurethral and transurethral injections. Int Urogynecol J Pelvic Floor Dysfunct 2004;15:261-265.
16. Ankardal M, Milsom I, Stjerndahl JH, Engh ME. A three-armed randomized trial comparing open Burch colposuspension using sutures with laparoscopic colposuspension using sutures and laparoscopic colposuspension using mesh and staples in women with stress urinary incontinence. Acta Obstet Gynecol Scand 2005;84:773-779.
17. Paraiso MF, Walters MD, Karram MM, Barber MD. Laparoscopic Burch colposuspension versus tension-free vaginal tape: a randomized trial. Obstet Gynecol 2004;104:1249-1258.
18. Maher CF, Qatawneh AM, Dwyer PL, et al. Abdominal sacral colpopexy or vaginal sacrospinous colpopexy for vaginal vault prolapse: a prospective randomized study. Am J Obstet Gynecol 2004;190:20-26.
19. Mallipeddi PK, Steele AC, Kohli N, Karram MM. Anatomic and functional outcome of vaginal paravaginal repair in the correction of anterior vaginal wall prolapse. Int Urogynecol J Pelvic Floor Dysfunct 2001;12:83-88.
20. Hilger WS, Poulson M, Norton PA. Long-term results of abdominal sacrocolpopexy. Am J Obstet Gynecol 2003;189:1606-1610; discussion 1610-1601.

21. Culligan PJ, Murphy M, Blackwell L, et al. Long-term success of abdominal sacral colpopexy using synthetic mesh. Am J Obstet Gynecol 2002;187:1473-1480; discussion 1481-1472.
22. Karram M, Goldwasser S, Kleeman S, et al. High uterosacral vaginal vault suspension with fascial reconstruction for vaginal repair of enterocele and vaginal vault prolapse. Am J Obstet Gynecol 2001;185:1339-1342; discussion 1342-1333.
23. Frederick RW, Leach GE. Cadaveric prolapse repair with sling: intermediate outcomes with 6 months to 5 years of followup. J Urol 2005;173:1229-1233.
24. Altman D, Lopez A, Gustafsson C, et al. Anatomical outcome and quality of life following posterior vaginal wall prolapse repair using collagen xenograft. Int Urogynecol J Pelvic Floor Dysfunct 2005;16:298-303.
25. Bukkapatnam R, Shah S, Raz S, Rodriguez L. Anterior vaginal wall surgery in elderly patients: outcomes and assessment. Urology 2005;65:1104-1108.
26. Carey JM, Leach GE. Transvaginal surgery in the octogenarian using cadaveric fascia for pelvic prolapse and stress incontinence: minimal one-year results compared to younger patients. Urology 2004;63:665-670.
27. Brincat C, Kenton K, Pat Fitzgerald M, Brubaker L. Sexual activity predicts continued pessary use. Am J Obstet Gynecol 2004;191:198-200.
28. Clemons JL, Aguilar VC, Sokol ER, et al. Patient characteristics that are associated with continued pessary use versus surgery after 1 year. Am J Obstet Gynecol 2004;191:159-164.
29. Clemons JL, Aguilar VC, Tillinghast TA, et al. Patient satisfaction and changes in prolapse and urinary symptoms in women who were fitted successfully with a pessary for pelvic organ prolapse. Am J Obstet Gynecol 2004;190:1025-1029.
30. Mutone MF, Terry C, Hale DS, Benson JT. Factors which influence the short-term success of pessary management of pelvic organ prolapse. Am J Obstet Gynecol 2005;193:89-94.
31. Boreham MK, Wai CY, Miller RT, et al. Morphometric analysis of smooth muscle in the anterior vaginal wall of women with pelvic organ prolapse. Am J Obstet Gynecol 2002;187:56-63.
32. Boreham MK, Wai CY, Miller RT, et al. Morphometric properties of the posterior vaginal wall in women with pelvic organ prolapse. Am J Obstet Gynecol 2002;187:1501-1508; discussion 1508-1509.
33. Ozdegirmenci O, Karslioglu Y, Dede S, et al. Smooth muscle fraction of the round ligament in women with pelvic organ prolapse: a computer-based morphometric analysis. Int Urogynecol J Pelvic Floor Dysfunct 2005;16:39-43; discussion 43.
34. Boreham MK, Miller RT, Schaffer JI, Word RA. Smooth muscle myosin heavy chain and caldesmon expression in the anterior vaginal wall of women with and without pelvic organ prolapse. Am J Obstet Gynecol 2001;185:944-952.
35. Moalli PA, Talarico LC, Sung VW, et al. Impact of menopause on collagen subtypes in the arcus tendineous fasciae pelvis. Am J Obstet Gynecol 2004;190:620-627.
36. Poncet S, Meyer S, Richard C, et al. The expression and function of the endothelin system in contractile properties of vaginal myofibroblasts of women with uterovaginal prolapse. Am J Obstet Gynecol 2005;192:426-432.
37. Chen B, Wen Y, Polan ML. Elastolytic activity in women with stress urinary incontinence and pelvic organ prolapse. Neurourol Urodyn 2004;23:119-126.
38. Goh JT. Biomechanical properties of prolapsed vaginal tissue in pre- and postmenopausal women. Int Urogynecol J Pelvic Floor Dysfunct 2002;13:76-79; discussion 79.
39. Wong MY, Harmanli OH, Agar M, et al. Collagen content of nonsupport tissue in pelvic organ prolapse and stress urinary incontinence. Am J Obstet Gynecol 2003;189:1597-1599; discussion 1599-1600.

40. Liapis A, Bakas P, Pafiti A, et al. Changes of collagen type III in female patients with genuine stress incontinence and pelvic floor prolapse. Eur J Obstet Gynecol Reprod Biol 2001;97:76-79.
41. Chen BH, Wen Y, Li H, Polan ML. Collagen metabolism and turnover in women with stress urinary incontinence and pelvic prolapse. Int Urogynecol J Pelvic Floor Dysfunct 2002;13:80-87; discussion 87.
42. Takano CC, Girao MJ, Sartori MG, et al. Analysis of collagen in parametrium and vaginal apex of women with and without uterine prolapse. Int Urogynecol J Pelvic Floor Dysfunct 2002;13:342-345; discussion 345.
43. Barbiero EC, Sartori MG, Girao MJ, et al. Analysis of type I collagen in the parametrium of women with and without uterine prolapse, according to hormonal status. Int Urogynecol J Pelvic Floor Dysfunct 2003;14:331-334; discussion 334.
44. Bezerra LR, Feldner PC, Jr., Kati LM, et al. Sulfated glycosaminoglycans of the vagina and perineal skin in pre- and postmenopausal women, according to genital prolapse stage. Int Urogynecol J Pelvic Floor Dysfunct 2004;15:266-271.
45. Bai SW, Jung BH, Chung BC, et al. Steroid hormone metabolism in women with pelvic organ prolapse. J Reprod Med 2002;47:303-308.
46. Ewies AA, Thompson J, Al-Azzawi F. Changes in gonadal steroid receptors in the cardinal ligaments of prolapsed uteri: immunohistomorphometric data. Hum Reprod 2004;19:1622-1628.
47. Lang JH, Zhu L, Sun ZJ, Chen J. Estrogen levels and estrogen receptors in patients with stress urinary incontinence and pelvic organ prolapse. Int J Gynaecol Obstet 2003;80:35-39.
48. Reay Jones NH, Healy JC, King LJ, et al. Pelvic connective tissue resilience decreases with vaginal delivery, menopause and uterine prolapse. Br J Surg 2003;90:466-472.
49. Hoyte L, Jakab M, Warfield SK, et al. Levator ani thickness variations in symptomatic and asymptomatic women using magnetic resonance-based 3-dimensional color mapping. Am J Obstet Gynecol 2004;191:856-861.
50. Singh K, Jakab M, Reid WM, et al. Three-dimensional magnetic resonance imaging assessment of levator ani morphologic features in different grades of prolapse. Am J Obstet Gynecol 2003;188:910-915.
51. Hsu Y, Chen L, Delancey JO, Ashton-Miller JA. Vaginal thickness, cross-sectional area, and perimeter in women with and those without prolapse. Obstet Gynecol 2005;105:1012-1017.
52. Handa VL, Pannu HK, Siddique S, et al. Architectural differences in the bony pelvis of women with and without pelvic floor disorders. Obstet Gynecol 2003;102:1283-1290.
53. Dietz HP, Hansell NK, Grace ME, et al. Bladder neck mobility is a heritable trait. BJOG 2005;112:334-339.
54. Hansell NK, Dietz HP, Treloar SA, et al. Genetic covariation of pelvic organ and elbow mobility in twins and their sisters. Twin Res 2004;7:254-260.
55. Visco AG, Yuan L. Differential gene expression in pubococcygeus muscle from patients with pelvic organ prolapse. Am J Obstet Gynecol 2003;189:102-112.
56. Dannecker C, Lienemann A, Fischer T, Anthuber C. Influence of spontaneous and instrumental vaginal delivery on objective measures of pelvic organ support: assessment with the pelvic organ prolapse quantification (POPQ) technique and functional cine magnetic resonance imaging. Eur J Obstet Gynecol Reprod Biol 2004;115:32-38.
57. O'Boyle AL, O'Boyle JD, Calhoun B, Davis GD. Pelvic organ support in pregnancy and postpartum. Int Urogynecol J Pelvic Floor Dysfunct 2005;16:69-72; discussion 72.
58. Sze EH, Sherard GB, 3rd, Dolezal JM. Pregnancy, labor, delivery, and pelvic organ prolapse. Obstet Gynecol 2002;100:981-986.
59. Vardy MD, Lindsay R, Scotti RJ, et al. Short-term urogenital effects of raloxifene, tamoxifen, and estrogen. Am J Obstet Gynecol 2003;189:81-88.

60. Goldstein SR, Nanavati N. Adverse events that are associated with the selective estrogen receptor modulator levormeloxifene in an aborted phase III osteoporosis treatment study. Am J Obstet Gynecol 2002;187:521-527.
61. Goldstein SR, Neven P, Zhou L, et al. Raloxifene effect on frequency of surgery for pelvic floor relaxation. Obstet Gynecol 2001;98:91-96.
62. Handa VL, Jones M. Do pessaries prevent the progression of pelvic organ prolapse? Int Urogynecol J Pelvic Floor Dysfunct 2002;13:349-351; discussion 352.
63. Piya-Anant M, Therasakvichya S, Leelaphatanadit C, Techatrisak K. Integrated health research program for the Thai elderly: prevalence of genital prolapse and effectiveness of pelvic floor exercise to prevent worsening of genital prolapse in elderly women. J Med Assoc Thai 2003;86:509-515.
64. O'Boyle AL, O'Boyle JD, Ricks RE, et al. The natural history of pelvic organ support in pregnancy. Int Urogynecol J Pelvic Floor Dysfunct 2003;14:46-49; discussion 49.
65. Handa VL, Garrett E, Hendrix S, et al. Progression and remission of pelvic organ prolapse: a longitudinal study of menopausal women. Am J Obstet Gynecol 2004;190:27-32.
66. Hendrix SL, Clark A, Nygaard I, et al. Pelvic organ prolapse in the Women's Health Initiative: gravity and gravidity. Am J Obstet Gynecol 2002;186:1160-1166.
67. Swift SE, Pound T, Dias JK. Case-control study of etiologic factors in the development of severe pelvic organ prolapse. Int Urogynecol J Pelvic Floor Dysfunct 2001;12:187-192.
68. Swift S, Woodman P, O'Boyle A, et al. Pelvic Organ Support Study (POSST): the distribution, clinical definition, and epidemiologic condition of pelvic organ support defects. Am J Obstet Gynecol 2005;192:795-806.
69. Kahn MA, Breitkopf CR, Valley MT, et al. Pelvic Organ Support Study (POSST) and bowel symptoms: straining at stool is associated with perineal and anterior vaginal descent in a general gynecologic population. Am J Obstet Gynecol 2005;192:1516-1522.
70. Arya LA, Novi JM, Shaunik A, et al. Pelvic organ prolapse, constipation, and dietary fiber intake in women: a case-control study. Am J Obstet Gynecol 2005;192:1687-1691.
71. Masheb RM, Lozano-Blanco C, Kohorn EI, et al. Assessing sexual function and dyspareunia with the Female Sexual Function Index (FSFI) in women with vulvodynia. J Sex Marital Ther 2004;30:315-324.
72. Janda M, Obermair A, Cella D, et al. The functional assessment of cancer-vulvar: reliability and validity. Gynecol Oncol 2005;97:568-575.
73. Jensen JT, Wilder K, Carr K, et al. Quality of life and sexual function after evaluation and treatment at a referral center for vulvovaginal disorders. Am J Obstet Gynecol 2003;188:1629-1635; discussion 1635-1627.
74. Manonai J, Theppisai U, Suthutvoravut S, et al. The effect of estradiol vaginal tablet and conjugated estrogen cream on urogenital symptoms in postmenopausal women: a comparative study. J Obstet Gynaecol Res 2001;27:255-260.
75. Palacios S, Castelo-Branco C, Cancelo MJ, Vazquez F. Low-dose, vaginally administered estrogens may enhance local benefits of systemic therapy in the treatment of urogenital atrophy in postmenopausal women on hormone therapy. Maturitas 2005;50:98-104.
76. Dessole S, Rubattu G, Ambrosini G, et al. Efficacy of low-dose intravaginal estriol on urogenital aging in postmenopausal women. Menopause 2004;11:49-56.
77. Simunic V, Banovic I, Ciglar S, et al. Local estrogen treatment in patients with urogenital symptoms. Int J Gynaecol Obstet 2003;82:187-197.
78. Senturk N, Aydin F, Birinci A, et al. Coexistence of HLA-B*08 and HLA-B*18 in four siblings with lichen sclerosus. Dermatology 2004;208:64-66.
79. Sander CS, Ali I, Dean D, et al. Oxidative stress is implicated in the pathogenesis of lichen sclerosus. Br J Dermatol 2004;151:627-635.

80. Chan I, Oyama N, Neill SM, et al. Characterization of IgG autoantibodies to extracellular matrix protein 1 in lichen sclerosus. Clin Exp Dermatol 2004;29:499-504.
81. Oyama N, Chan I, Neill SM, et al. Autoantibodies to extracellular matrix protein 1 in lichen sclerosus. Lancet 2003;362:118-123.
82. Regauer S, Liegl B, Reich O, Beham-Schmid C. Vasculitis in lichen sclerosus: an under recognized feature? Histopathology 2004;45:237-244.
83. Tchorzewski H, Rotsztejn H, Banasik M, et al. The involvement of immunoregulatory T cells in the pathogenesis of lichen sclerosus. Med Sci Monit 2005;11:CR39-CR43.
84. Gross T, Wagner A, Ugurel S, et al. Identification of TIA-1+ and granzyme B+ cytotoxic T cells in lichen sclerosus et atrophicus. Dermatology 2001;202:198-202.
85. Kuroda K, Fujimoto N, Tajima S. Abnormal accumulation of inter-alpha-trypsin inhibitor and hyaluronic acid in lichen sclerosus. J Cutan Pathol 2005;32:137-140.
86. Farrell AM, Dean D, Charnock M, Wojnarowska F. Distribution of transforming growth factor-beta isoforms TGF-beta 1, TGF-beta 2 and TGF-beta 3 and vascular endothelial growth factor in vulvar lichen sclerosus. J Reprod Med 2001;46:117-124.
87. Farrell AM, Dean D, Millard PR, et al. Alterations in fibrillin as well as collagens I and III and elastin occur in vulval lichen sclerosus. J Eur Acad Dermatol Venereol 2001;15:212-217.
88. van Seters M, Fons G, van Beurden M. Imiquimod in the treatment of multifocal vulvar intraepithelial neoplasia 2/3: results of a pilot study. J Reprod Med 2002;47:701-705.
89. Todd RW, Etherington IJ, Luesley DM. The effects of 5% imiquimod cream on high-grade vulval intraepithelial neoplasia. Gynecol Oncol 2002;85:67-70.
90. Wendling J, Saiag P, Berville-Levy S, et al. Treatment of undifferentiated vulvar intraepithelial neoplasia with 5% imiquimod cream: a prospective study of 12 cases. Arch Dermatol 2004;140:1220-1224.
91. Diaz-Arrastia C, Arany I, Robazetti SC, et al. Clinical and molecular responses in high-grade intraepithelial neoplasia treated with topical imiquimod 5%. Clin Cancer Res 2001;7:3031-3033.
92. Fogari R, Preti P, Zoppi A, et al. Effect of valsartan and atenolol on sexual behavior in hypertensive postmenopausal women. Am J Hypertens 2004;17:77-81.
93. Addis IB, Ireland CC, Vittinghoff E, et al. Sexual activity and function in postmenopausal women with heart disease. Obstet Gynecol 2005;106:121-127.
94. Peng YS, Chiang CK, Kao TW, et al. Sexual dysfunction in female hemodialysis patients: a multicenter study. Kidney Int 2005;68:760-765.
95. Giaquinto S, Buzzelli S, Di Francesco L, Nolfe G. Evaluation of sexual changes after stroke. J Clin Psychiatry 2003;64:302-307.
96. Kimura M, Murata Y, Shimoda K, Robinson RG. Sexual dysfunction following stroke. Compr Psychiatry 2001;42:217-222.
97. Greendale GA, Petersen L, Zibecchi L, Ganz PA. Factors related to sexual function in postmenopausal women with a history of breast cancer. Menopause 2001;8:111-119.
98. Bukovic D, Fajdic J, Hrgovic Z, et al. Sexual dysfunction in breast cancer survivors. Onkologie 2005;28:29-34.
99. Carmack Taylor CL, Basen-Engquist K, Shinn EH, Bodurka DC. Predictors of sexual functioning in ovarian cancer patients. J Clin Oncol 2004;22:881-889.
100. Houwing NS, Maris F, Schnabel PG, Bagchus WM. Pharmacokinetic study in women of three different doses of a new formulation of oral testosterone undecanoate, Andriol Testocaps. Pharmacotherapy 2003;23:1257-1265.
101. Bagchus WM, Hust R, Maris F, et al. Important effect of food on the bioavailability of oral testosterone undecanoate. Pharmacotherapy 2003;23:319-325.

102. Nathorst-Boos J, Jarkander-Rolff M, Carlstrom K, et al. Percutaneous administration of testosterone gel in postmenopausal women—a pharmacological study. Gynecol Endocrinol 2005;20:243-248.
103. Braunstein GD, Sundwall DA, Katz M, et al. Safety and efficacy of a testosterone patch for the treatment of hypoactive sexual desire disorder in surgically menopausal women: a randomized, placebo-controlled trial. Arch Intern Med 2005;165:1582-1589.
104. Dobs AS, Nguyen T, Pace C, Roberts CP. Differential effects of oral estrogen versus oral estrogen-androgen replacement therapy on body composition in postmenopausal women. J Clin Endocrinol Metab 2002;87:1509-1516.
105. Penotti M, Sironi L, Cannata L, et al. Effects of androgen supplementation of hormone replacement therapy on the vascular reactivity of cerebral arteries. Fertil Steril 2001;76:235-240.
106. Buster JE, Kingsberg SA, Aguirre O, et al. Testosterone patch for low sexual desire in surgically menopausal women: a randomized trial. Obstet Gynecol 2005;105:944-952.
107. Floter A, Nathorst-Boos J, Carlstrom K, von Schoultz B. Addition of testosterone to estrogen replacement therapy in oophorectomized women: effects on sexuality and well-being. Climacteric 2002;5:357-365.
108. Basaria S, Nguyen T, Rosenson RS, Dobs AS. Effect of methyl testosterone administration on plasma viscosity in postmenopausal women. Clin Endocrinol (Oxf) 2002;57:209-214.
109. Dayal M, Sammel MD, Zhao J, et al. Supplementation with DHEA: effect on muscle size, strength, quality of life, and lipids. J Womens Health (Larchmt) 2005;14:391-400.
110. Serin IS, Ozcelik B, Basbug M, et al. Long-term effects of continuous oral and transdermal estrogen replacement therapy on sex hormone binding globulin and free testosterone levels. Eur J Obstet Gynecol Reprod Biol 2001;99:222-225.
111. Kraemer GR, Kraemer RR, Ogden BW, et al. Variability of serum estrogens among postmenopausal women treated with the same transdermal estrogen therapy and the effect on androgens and sex hormone binding globulin. Fertil Steril 2003;79:534-542.
112. Suh DD, Yang CC, Cao Y, et al. MRI of female genital and pelvic organs during sexual arousal. J Psychosom Obstet Gynaecol 2004;25:153-162.
113. van der Laak JA, de Bie LM, de Leeuw H, et al. The effect of Replens on vaginal cytology in the treatment of postmenopausal atrophy: cytomorphology versus computerised cytometry. J Clin Pathol 2002;55:446-451.
114. Chiechi LM, Putignano G, Guerra V, et al. The effect of a soy rich diet on the vaginal epithelium in postmenopause: a randomized double blind trial. Maturitas 2003;45:241-246.
115. Ostbye T, Greenberg GN, Taylor DH, Jr., Lee AM. Screening mammography and Pap tests among older American women 1996-2000: results from the Health and Retirement Study (HRS) and Asset and Health Dynamics Among the Oldest Old (AHEAD). Ann Fam Med 2003;1:209-217.
116. Peto J, Gilham C, Deacon J, et al. Cervical HPV infection and neoplasia in a large population-based prospective study: the Manchester cohort. Br J Cancer 2004;91:942-953.
117. Wang SS, Sherman ME, Hildesheim A, et al. Cervical adenocarcinoma and squamous cell carcinoma incidence trends among white women and black women in the United States for 1976-2000. Cancer 2004;100:1035-1044.
118. Wright JD, Gibb RK, Geevarghese S, et al. Cervical carcinoma in the elderly: an analysis of patterns of care and outcome. Cancer 2005;103:85-91.
119. Brun JL, Stoven-Camou D, Trouette R, et al. Survival and prognosis of women with invasive cervical cancer according to age. Gynecol Oncol 2003;91:395-401.
120. Sawaya GF, Sung HY, Kearney KA, et al. Advancing age and cervical cancer screening and prognosis. J Am Geriatr Soc 2001;49:1499-1504.
121. Baalbergen A, Ewing-Graham PC, Hop WC, et al. Prognostic factors in adenocarcinoma of the uterine cervix. Gynecol Oncol 2004;92:262-267.

122. Trimble EL, Harlan LC, Clegg LX. Untreated cervical cancer in the United States. Gynecol Oncol 2005;96:271-277.
123. Ioka A, Tsukuma H, Ajiki W, Oshima A. Influence of age on cervical cancer survival in Japan. Jpn J Clin Oncol 2005;35:464-469.
124. de Rijke JM, van der Putten HW, Lutgens LC, et al. Age-specific differences in treatment and survival of patients with cervical cancer in the southeast of The Netherlands, 1986-1996. Eur J Cancer 2002;38:2041-2047.
125. Nygard JF, Skare GB, Thoresen SO. The cervical cancer screening programme in Norway, 1992-2000: changes in Pap smear coverage and incidence of cervical cancer. J Med Screen 2002;9:86-91.
126. Capelli G, De Vincenzo RI, Addamo A, et al. Which dimensions of health-related quality of life are altered in patients attending the different gynecologic oncology health care settings? Cancer 2002;95:2500-2507.
127. Nystrom L, Andersson I, Bjurstam N, et al. Long-term effects of mammography screening: updated overview of the Swedish randomised trials. Lancet 2002;359:909-919.
128. Walter LC, Lindquist K, Covinsky KE. Relationship between health status and use of screening mammography and Papanicolaoú smears among women older than 70 years of age. Ann Intern Med 2004;140:681-688.
129. Heflin MT, Oddone EZ, Pieper CF, et al. The effect of comorbid illness on receipt of cancer screening by older people. J Am Geriatr Soc 2002;50:1651-1658.
130. Walter LC, Eng C, Covinsky KE. Screening mammography for frail older women: what are the burdens? J Gen Intern Med 2001;16:779-784.
131. Young RF, Waller JB, Jr., Smitherman H. A breast cancer education and on-site screening intervention for unscreened African American women. J Cancer Educ 2002;17:231-236.
132. West DS, Greene P, Pulley L, et al. Stepped-care, community clinic interventions to promote mammography use among low-income rural African American women. Health Educ Behav 2004;31:29S-44S.
133. Valdez A, Banerjee K, Ackerson L, Fernandez M. A multimedia breast cancer education intervention for low-income Latinas. J Community Health 2002;27:33-51.
134. Hiatt RA, Pasick RJ, Stewart S, et al. Community-based cancer screening for underserved women: design and baseline findings from the Breast and Cervical Cancer Intervention Study. Prev Med 2001;33:190-203.
135. Schneider TR, Salovey P, Apanovitch AM, et al. The effects of message framing and ethnic targeting on mammography use among low-income women. Health Psychol 2001;20:256-266.
136. Simon MS, Gimotty PA, Moncrease A, et al. The effect of patient reminders on the use of screening mammography in an urban health department primary care setting. Breast Cancer Res Treat 2001;65:63-70.
137. Vacek PM, Geller BM. A prospective study of breast cancer risk using routine mammographic breast density measurements. Cancer Epidemiol Biomarkers Prev 2004;13:715-722.
138. Torres-Mejia G, De Stavola B, Allen DS, et al. Mammographic features and subsequent risk of breast cancer: a comparison of qualitative and quantitative evaluations in the Guernsey prospective studies. Cancer Epidemiol Biomarkers Prev 2005;14:1052-1059.
139. Kerlikowske K, Shepherd J, Creasman J, et al. Are breast density and bone mineral density independent risk factors for breast cancer? J Natl Cancer Inst 2005;97:368-374.
140. Maskarinec G, Pagano I, Lurie G, et al. Mammographic density and breast cancer risk: the multiethnic cohort study. Am J Epidemiol 2005;162:743-752.
141. Ursin G, Ma H, Wu AH, et al. Mammographic density and breast cancer in three ethnic groups. Cancer Epidemiol Biomarkers Prev 2003;12:332-338.

142. Roubidoux MA, Bailey JE, Wray LA, Helvie MA. Invasive cancers detected after breast cancer screening yielded a negative result: relationship of mammographic density to tumor prognostic factors. Radiology 2004;230:42-48.
143. Ziv E, Tice J, Smith-Bindman R, et al. Mammographic density and estrogen receptor status of breast cancer. Cancer Epidemiol Biomarkers Prev 2004;13:2090-2095.
144. Kavanagh AM, Cawson J, Byrnes GB, et al. Hormone replacement therapy, percent mammographic density, and sensitivity of mammography. Cancer Epidemiol Biomarkers Prev 2005;14:1060-1064.
145. Theberge I, Hebert-Croteau N, Langlois A, et al. Volume of screening mammography and performance in the Quebec population-based Breast Cancer Screening Program. CMAJ 2005;172:195-199.
146. Beam CA, Conant EF, Sickles EA. Association of volume and volume-independent factors with accuracy in screening mammogram interpretation. J Natl Cancer Inst 2003;95:282-290.
147. Barlow WE, Chi C, Carney PA, et al. Accuracy of screening mammography interpretation by characteristics of radiologists. J Natl Cancer Inst 2004;96:1840-1850.
148. Smith-Bindman R, Chu P, Miglioretti DL, et al. Physician predictors of mammographic accuracy. J Natl Cancer Inst 2005;97:358-367.
149. Pradhan AD, Manson JE, Rossouw JE, et al. Inflammatory biomarkers, hormone replacement therapy, and incident coronary heart disease: prospective analysis from the Women's Health Initiative observational study. JAMA 2002;288:980-987.
150. Lowe GD, Upton MN, Rumley A, et al. Different effects of oral and transdermal hormone replacement therapies on factor IX, APC resistance, t-PA, PAI and C-reactive protein—a cross-sectional population survey. Thromb Haemost 2001;86:550-556.
151. Yildirir A, Aybar F, Tokgozoglu L, et al. Effects of hormone replacement therapy on plasma homocysteine and C-reactive protein levels. Gynecol Obstet Invest 2002;53:54-58.
152. Vehkavaara S, Silveira A, Hakala-Ala-Pietila T, et al. Effects of oral and transdermal estrogen replacement therapy on markers of coagulation, fibrinolysis, inflammation and serum lipids and lipoproteins in postmenopausal women. Thromb Haemost 2001;85:619-625.
153. Luyer MD, Khosla S, Owen WG, Miller VM. Prospective randomized study of effects of unopposed estrogen replacement therapy on markers of coagulation and inflammation in postmenopausal women. J Clin Endocrinol Metab 2001;86:3629-3634.
154. Prelevic GM, Kwong P, Byrne DJ, et al. A cross-sectional study of the effects of hormone replacement therapy on the cardiovascular disease risk profile in healthy postmenopausal women. Fertil Steril 2002;77:945-951.
155. Ossewaarde ME, Bots ML, Bak AA, et al. Effect of hormone replacement therapy on lipids in perimenopausal and early postmenopausal women. Maturitas 2001;39:209-216.
156. Langer RD, Pradhan AD, Lewis CE, et al. Baseline associations between postmenopausal hormone therapy and inflammatory, haemostatic, and lipid biomarkers of coronary heart disease. The Women's Health Initiative Observational Study. Thromb Haemost 2005;93:1108-1116.
157. Lakoski SG, Brosnihan B, Herrington DM. Hormone therapy, C-reactive protein, and progression of atherosclerosis: data from the Estrogen Replacement on Progression of Coronary Artery Atherosclerosis (ERA) trial. Am Heart J 2005;150:907-911.
158. Barnes JF, Farish E, Rankin M, Hart DM. Effects of two continuous hormone therapy regimens on C-reactive protein and homocysteine. Menopause 2005;12:92-98.
159. Barrett-Connor E, Grady D, Sashegyi A, et al. Raloxifene and cardiovascular events in osteoporotic postmenopausal women: four-year results from the MORE (Multiple Outcomes of Raloxifene Evaluation) randomized trial. JAMA 2002;287:847-857.
160. Grady D, Ettinger B, Moscarelli E, et al. Safety and adverse effects associated with raloxifene: multiple outcomes of raloxifene evaluation. Obstet Gynecol 2004;104:837-844.

161. Nordenskjold B, Rosell J, Rutqvist LE, et al. Coronary heart disease mortality after 5 years of adjuvant tamoxifen therapy: results from a randomized trial. J Natl Cancer Inst 2005;97:1609-1610.
162. Reis SE, Costantino JP, Wickerham DL, et al. Cardiovascular effects of tamoxifen in women with and without heart disease: breast cancer prevention trial. National Surgical Adjuvant Breast and Bowel Project Breast Cancer Prevention Trial Investigators. J Natl Cancer Inst 2001;93:16-21.
163. Wenger NK, Barrett-Connor E, Collins P, et al. Baseline characteristics of participants in the Raloxifene Use for The Heart (RUTH) trial. Am J Cardiol 2002;90:1204-1210.
164. Christian RC, Harrington S, Edwards WD, et al. Estrogen status correlates with the calcium content of coronary atherosclerotic plaques in women. J Clin Endocrinol Metab 2002;87:1062-1067.
165. Akhrass F, Evans AT, Wang Y, et al. Hormone replacement therapy is associated with less coronary atherosclerosis in postmenopausal women. J Clin Endocrinol Metab 2003;88:5611-5614.
166. Rossouw JE, Anderson GL, Prentice RL, et al. Risks and benefits of estrogen plus progestin in healthy postmenopausal women: principal results from the Women's Health Initiative randomized controlled trial. JAMA 2002;288:321-333.
167. Anderson GL, Limacher M, Assaf AR, et al. Effects of conjugated equine estrogen in postmenopausal women with hysterectomy: the Women's Health Initiative randomized controlled trial. JAMA 2004;291:1701-1712.
168. Grady D, Herrington D, Bittner V, et al. Cardiovascular disease outcomes during 6.8 years of hormone therapy: Heart and Estrogen/progestin Replacement Study follow-up (HERS II). JAMA 2002;288:49-57.
169. Nilsen J, Brinton RD. Impact of progestins on estradiol potentiation of the glutamate calcium response. Neuroreport 2002;13:825-830.
170. Markham JA, Pych JC, Juraska JM. Ovarian hormone replacement to aged ovariectomized female rats benefits acquisition of the Morris water maze. Horm Behav 2002;42:284-293.
171. Gibbs RB, Nelson D, Anthony MS, Clarkson TB. Effects of long-term hormone replacement and of tibolone on choline acetyltransferase and acetylcholinesterase activities in the brains of ovariectomized, cynomologus monkeys. Neuroscience 2002;113:907-914.
172. Rapp SR, Espeland MA, Shumaker SA, et al. Effect of estrogen plus progestin on global cognitive function in postmenopausal women: the Women's Health Initiative Memory Study: a randomized controlled trial. JAMA 2003;289:2663-2672.
173. Shumaker SA, Legault C, Rapp SR, et al. Estrogen plus progestin and the incidence of dementia and mild cognitive impairment in postmenopausal women: the Women's Health Initiative Memory Study: a randomized controlled trial. JAMA 2003;289:2651-2662.
174. Yaffe K, Krueger K, Sarkar S, et al. Cognitive function in postmenopausal women treated with raloxifene. N Engl J Med 2001;344:1207-1213.
175. Grady D, Yaffe K, Kristof M, et al. Effect of postmenopausal hormone therapy on cognitive function: the Heart and Estrogen/progestin Replacement Study. Am J Med 2002;113:543-548.
176. Biglia N, Sgro L, Defabiani E, et al. The influence of hormone replacement therapy on the pathology of breast cancer. Eur J Surg Oncol 2005;31:467-472.
177. Daling JR, Malone KE, Doody DR, et al. Association of regimens of hormone replacement therapy to prognostic factors among women diagnosed with breast cancer aged 50-64 years. Cancer Epidemiol Biomarkers Prev 2003;12:1175-1181.
178. Sacchini V, Zurrida S, Andreoni G, et al. Pathologic and biological prognostic factors of breast cancers in short- and long-term hormone replacement therapy users. Ann Surg Oncol 2002;9:266-271.

179. Pappo I, Meirshon I, Karni T, et al. The characteristics of malignant breast tumors in hormone replacement therapy users versus nonusers. Ann Surg Oncol 2004;11:52-58.
180. Delgado RC, Lubian Lopez DM. Prognosis of breast cancers detected in women receiving hormone replacement therapy. Maturitas 2001;38:147-156.
181. Gertig DM, Erbas B, Fletcher A, et al. Duration of hormone replacement therapy, breast tumour size and grade in a screening programme. Breast Cancer Res Treat 2003;80:267-273.
182. Manjer J, Malina J, Berglund G, et al. Increased incidence of small and well-differentiated breast tumours in post-menopausal women following hormone-replacement therapy. Int J Cancer 2001;92:919-922.
183. Stahlberg C, Pedersen AT, Andersen ZJ, et al. Breast cancer with different prognostic characteristics developing in Danish women using hormone replacement therapy. Br J Cancer 2004;91:644-650.
184. Chen WY, Hankinson SE, Schnitt SJ, et al. Association of hormone replacement therapy to estrogen and progesterone receptor status in invasive breast carcinoma. Cancer 2004;101:1490-1500.
185. Chlebowski RT, Hendrix SL, Langer RD, et al. Influence of estrogen plus progestin on breast cancer and mammography in healthy postmenopausal women: the Women's Health Initiative Randomized Trial. JAMA 2003;289:3243-3253.
186. Chlebowski RT, Wactawski-Wende J, Ritenbaugh C, et al. Estrogen plus progestin and colorectal cancer in postmenopausal women. N Engl J Med 2004;350:991-1004.
187. Woodson K, Lanza E, Tangrea JA, et al. Hormone replacement therapy and colorectal adenoma recurrence among women in the Polyp Prevention Trial. J Natl Cancer Inst 2001;93:1799-1805.
188. McTiernan A, Martin CF, Peck JD, et al. Estrogen-plus-progestin use and mammographic density in postmenopausal women: Women's Health Initiative randomized trial. J Natl Cancer Inst 2005;97:1366-1376.
189. Harman SM, Brinton EA, Cedars M, et al. KEEPS: The Kronos Early Estrogen Prevention Study. Climacteric 2005;8:3-12.
190. Fisher B, Costantino JP, Wickerham DL, et al. Tamoxifen for the prevention of breast cancer: current status of the National Surgical Adjuvant Breast and Bowel Project P-1 study. J Natl Cancer Inst 2005;97:1652-1662.
191. King MC, Wieand S, Hale K, et al. Tamoxifen and breast cancer incidence among women with inherited mutations in BRCA1 and BRCA2: National Surgical Adjuvant Breast and Bowel Project (NSABP-P1) Breast Cancer Prevention Trial. JAMA 2001;286:2251-2256.
192. Martino S, Cauley JA, Barrett-Connor E, et al. Continuing outcomes relevant to Evista: breast cancer incidence in postmenopausal osteoporotic women in a randomized trial of raloxifene. J Natl Cancer Inst 2004;96:1751-1761.
193. Walsh JM, Cheung AM, Yang D, et al. Raloxifene and colorectal cancer. J Womens Health (Larchmt) 2005;14:299-305.
194. Campbell-Thompson M, Lynch IJ, Bhardwaj B. Expression of estrogen receptor (ER) subtypes and ERbeta isoforms in colon cancer. Cancer Res 2001;61:632-640.
195. Jassam N, Bell SM, Speirs V, Quirke P. Loss of expression of oestrogen receptor beta in colon cancer and its association with Dukes' staging. Oncol Rep 2005;14:17-21.
196. Wong NA, Malcomson RD, Jodrell DI, et al. ERbeta isoform expression in colorectal carcinoma: an in vivo and in vitro study of clinicopathological and molecular correlates. J Pathol 2005;207:53-60.
197. Slattery ML, Potter JD, Curtin K, et al. Estrogens reduce and withdrawal of estrogens increase risk of microsatellite instability-positive colon cancer. Cancer Res 2001;61:126-130.

198. Cavallini A, Notarnicola M, Giannini R, et al. Oestrogen receptor-related receptor alpha (ERRalpha) and oestrogen receptors (ERalpha and ERbeta) exhibit different gene expression in human colorectal tumour progression. Eur J Cancer 2005;41:1487-1494.
199. Slattery ML, Sweeney C, Murtaugh M, et al. Associations between ERalpha, ERbeta, and AR genotypes and colon and rectal cancer. Cancer Epidemiol Biomarkers Prev 2005;14:2936-2942.
200. Slattery ML, Ballard-Barbash R, Potter JD, et al. Sex-specific differences in colon cancer associated with p53 mutations. Nutr Cancer 2004;49:41-48.
201. Morimoto LM, Newcomb PA, White E, et al. Insulin-like growth factor polymorphisms and colorectal cancer risk. Cancer Epidemiol Biomarkers Prev 2005;14:1204-1211.
202. Holmberg L, Anderson H. HABITS (hormonal replacement therapy after breast cancer—is it safe?), a randomised comparison: trial stopped. Lancet 2004;363:453-455.
203. von Schoultz E, Rutqvist LE. Menopausal hormone therapy after breast cancer: the Stockholm randomized trial. J Natl Cancer Inst 2005;97:533-535.
204. Cascella T, Musella T, Orio F, Jr., et al. Effects of neridronate treatment in elderly women with osteoporosis. J Endocrinol Invest 2005;28:202-208.
205. Milliken LA, Going SB, Houtkooper LB, et al. Effects of exercise training on bone remodeling, insulin-like growth factors, and bone mineral density in postmenopausal women with and without hormone replacement therapy. Calcif Tissue Int 2003;72:478-484.
206. Villareal DT, Binder EF, Yarasheski KE, et al. Effects of exercise training added to ongoing hormone replacement therapy on bone mineral density in frail elderly women. J Am Geriatr Soc 2003;51:985-990.
207. Going S, Lohman T, Houtkooper L, et al. Effects of exercise on bone mineral density in calcium-replete postmenopausal women with and without hormone replacement therapy. Osteoporos Int 2003;14:637-643.
208. Prestwood KM, Kenny AM, Kleppinger A, Kulldorff M. Ultralow-dose micronized 17beta-estradiol and bone density and bone metabolism in older women: a randomized controlled trial. JAMA 2003;290:1042-1048.
209. Ettinger B, Ensrud KE, Wallace R, et al. Effects of ultralow-dose transdermal estradiol on bone mineral density: a randomized clinical trial. Obstet Gynecol 2004;104:443-451.
210. Cauley JA, Robbins J, Chen Z, et al. Effects of estrogen plus progestin on risk of fracture and bone mineral density: the Women's Health Initiative randomized trial. JAMA 2003;290:1729-1738.
211. Banks E, Beral V, Reeves G, et al. Fracture incidence in relation to the pattern of use of hormone therapy in postmenopausal women. JAMA 2004;291:2212-2220.
212. Matkovic V, Landoll JD, Badenhop-Stevens NE, et al. Nutrition influences skeletal development from childhood to adulthood: a study of hip, spine, and forearm in adolescent females. J Nutr 2004;134:701S-705S.
213. Stear SJ, Prentice A, Jones SC, Cole TJ. Effect of a calcium and exercise intervention on the bone mineral status of 16-18-y-old adolescent girls. Am J Clin Nutr 2003;77:985-992.
214. Lloyd T, Beck TJ, Lin HM, et al. Modifiable determinants of bone status in young women. Bone 2002;30:416-421.
215. Kontulainen SA, Kannus PA, Pasanen ME, et al. Does previous participation in high-impact training result in residual bone gain in growing girls? One year follow-up of a 9-month jumping intervention. Int J Sports Med 2002;23:575-581.
216. Lucas JA, Lucas PR, Vogel S, et al. Effect of sub-elite competitive running on bone density, body composition and sexual maturity of adolescent females. Osteoporos Int 2003;14:848-856.
217. Laing EM, Massoni JA, Nickols-Richardson SM, et al. A prospective study of bone mass and body composition in female adolescent gymnasts. J Pediatr 2002;141:211-216.

218. Tylavsky FA, Holliday K, Danish R, et al. Fruit and vegetable intakes are an independent predictor of bone size in early pubertal children. Am J Clin Nutr 2004;79:311-317.
219. Reid IR, Horne A, Mason B, et al. Effects of calcium supplementation on body weight and blood pressure in normal older women: a randomized controlled trial. J Clin Endocrinol Metab 2005;90:3824-3829.
220. Reid IR, Mason B, Horne A, et al. Effects of calcium supplementation on serum lipid concentrations in normal older women: a randomized controlled trial. Am J Med 2002;112:343-347.
221. Domrongkitchaiporn S, Ongphiphadhanakul B, Stitchantrakul W, et al. Risk of calcium oxalate nephrolithiasis in postmenopausal women supplemented with calcium or combined calcium and estrogen. Maturitas 2002;41:149-156.
222. Sakhaee K, Poindexter JR, Griffith CS, Pak CY. Stone forming risk of calcium citrate supplementation in healthy postmenopausal women. J Urol 2004;172:958-961.
223. Grant AM, Avenell A, Campbell MK, et al. Oral vitamin D3 and calcium for secondary prevention of low-trauma fractures in elderly people (Randomised Evaluation of Calcium Or vitamin D, RECORD): a randomised placebo-controlled trial. Lancet 2005;365:1621-1628.
224. Heaney RP, Dowell MS, Bierman J, et al. Absorbability and cost effectiveness in calcium supplementation. J Am Coll Nutr 2001;20:239-246.
225. Rozen GS, Rennert G, Dodiuk-Gad RP, et al. Calcium supplementation provides an extended window of opportunity for bone mass accretion after menarche. Am J Clin Nutr 2003;78:993-998.
226. Matkovic V, Goel PK, Badenhop-Stevens NE, et al. Calcium supplementation and bone mineral density in females from childhood to young adulthood: a randomized controlled trial. Am J Clin Nutr 2005;81:175-188.
227. Di Daniele N, Carbonelli MG, Candeloro N, et al. Effect of supplementation of calcium and vitamin D on bone mineral density and bone mineral content in peri- and post-menopause women; a double-blind, randomized, controlled trial. Pharmacol Res 2004;50:637-641.
228. Hanzlik RP, Fowler SC, Fisher DH. Relative bioavailability of calcium from calcium formate, calcium citrate, and calcium carbonate. J Pharmacol Exp Ther 2005;313:1217-1222.
229. Martini L, Wood RJ. Relative bioavailability of calcium-rich dietary sources in the elderly. Am J Clin Nutr 2002;76:1345-1350.
230. Eriksen EF, Melsen F, Sod E, et al. Effects of long-term risedronate on bone quality and bone turnover in women with postmenopausal osteoporosis. Bone 2002;31:620-625.
231. Ste-Marie LG, Sod E, Johnson T, Chines A. Five years of treatment with risedronate and its effects on bone safety in women with postmenopausal osteoporosis. Calcif Tissue Int 2004;75:469-476.
232. Ensrud KE, Barrett-Connor EL, Schwartz A, et al. Randomized trial of effect of alendronate continuation versus discontinuation in women with low BMD: results from the Fracture Intervention Trial long-term extension. J Bone Miner Res 2004;19:1259-1269.
233. Black DM, Greenspan SL, Ensrud KE, et al. The effects of parathyroid hormone and alendronate alone or in combination in postmenopausal osteoporosis. N Engl J Med 2003;349:1207-1215.
234. Bone HG, Hosking D, Devogelaer JP, et al. Ten years' experience with alendronate for osteoporosis in postmenopausal women. N Engl J Med 2004;350:1189-1199.
235. Odvina CV, Zerwekh JE, Rao DS, et al. Severely suppressed bone turnover: a potential complication of alendronate therapy. J Clin Endocrinol Metab 2005;90:1294-1301.
236. Tanko LB, Qin G, Alexandersen P, et al. Effective doses of ibandronate do not influence the 3-year progression of aortic calcification in elderly osteoporotic women. Osteoporos Int 2005;16:184-190.

237. Jamal SA, Cummings SR, Hawker GA. Isosorbide mononitrate increases bone formation and decreases bone resorption in postmenopausal women: a randomized trial. J Bone Miner Res 2004;19:1512-1517.
238. Reginster JY, Seeman E, De Vernejoul MC, et al. Strontium ranelate reduces the risk of nonvertebral fractures in postmenopausal women with osteoporosis: Treatment of Peripheral Osteoporosis (TROPOS) study. J Clin Endocrinol Metab 2005;90:2816-2822.
239. Meunier PJ, Slosman DO, Delmas PD, et al. Strontium ranelate: dose-dependent effects in established postmenopausal vertebral osteoporosis—a 2-year randomized placebo controlled trial. J Clin Endocrinol Metab 2002;87:2060-2066.
240. Meunier PJ, Roux C, Seeman E, et al. The effects of strontium ranelate on the risk of vertebral fracture in women with postmenopausal osteoporosis. N Engl J Med 2004;350:459-468.
241. McClung MR, Wasnich RD, Hosking DJ, et al. Prevention of postmenopausal bone loss: six-year results from the Early Postmenopausal Intervention Cohort Study. J Clin Endocrinol Metab 2004;89:4879-4885.
242. Quandt SA, Thompson DE, Schneider DL, et al. Effect of alendronate on vertebral fracture risk in women with bone mineral density T scores of −1.6 to −2.5 at the femoral neck: the Fracture Intervention Trial. Mayo Clin Proc 2005;80:343-349.
243. Greenspan SL, Resnick NM, Parker RA. Combination therapy with hormone replacement and alendronate for prevention of bone loss in elderly women: a randomized controlled trial. JAMA 2003;289:2525-2533.
244. Gallagher JC, Fowler SE, Detter JR, Sherman SS. Combination treatment with estrogen and calcitriol in the prevention of age-related bone loss. J Clin Endocrinol Metab 2001;86:3618-3628.
245. Deal C, Omizo M, Schwartz EN, et al. Combination teriparatide and raloxifene therapy for postmenopausal osteoporosis: results from a 6-month double-blind placebo-controlled trial. J Bone Miner Res 2005;20:1905-1911.
246. Weber AM, Abrams P, Brubaker L, et al. The standardization of terminology for researchers in female pelvic floor disorders. Int Urogynecol J Pelvic Floor Dysfunct 2001;12:178-186.
247. Ghetti C, Gregory WT, Edwards SR, et al. Pelvic organ descent and symptoms of pelvic floor disorders. Am J Obstet Gynecol 2005;193:53-57.
248. Swift SE, Tate SB, Nicholas J. Correlation of symptoms with degree of pelvic organ support in a general population of women: what is pelvic organ prolapse? Am J Obstet Gynecol 2003;189:372-377; discussion 377-379.
249. Tan JS, Lukacz ES, Menefee SA, et al. Predictive value of prolapse symptoms: a large database study. Int Urogynecol J Pelvic Floor Dysfunct 2005;16:203-209; discussion 209.
250. Nygaard I, Bradley C, Brandt D. Pelvic organ prolapse in older women: prevalence and risk factors. Obstet Gynecol 2004;104:489-497.
251. Jomaa M. Combined tension-free vaginal tape and prolapse repair under local anaesthesia in patients with symptoms of both urinary incontinence and prolapse. Gynecol Obstet Invest 2001;51:184-186.
252. Moore RD, Miklos JR. Colpocleisis and tension-free vaginal tape sling for severe uterine and vaginal prolapse and stress urinary incontinence under local anesthesia. J Am Assoc Gynecol Laparosc 2003;10:276-280.
253. Axelsen SM, Bek KM. Anterior vaginal wall repair using local anaesthesia. Eur J Obstet Gynecol Reprod Biol 2004;112:214-216.
254. Buchsbaum GM, Duecy EE. Local anesthesia with sedation for transvaginal correction of advanced genital prolapse. Am J Obstet Gynecol 2005;193:2173-2176.
255. Buchsbaum GM, Albushies DT, Schoenecker E, et al. Local anesthesia with sedation for vaginal reconstructive surgery. Int Urogynecol J Pelvic Floor Dysfunct 2006;17:211-214.

256. Dennerstein L, Dudley E, Burger H. Are changes in sexual functioning during midlife due to aging or menopause? Fertil Steril 2001;76:456-460.
257. Barber MD, Visco AG, Wyman JF, et al. Sexual function in women with urinary incontinence and pelvic organ prolapse. Obstet Gynecol 2002;99:281–289.

10

GERIATRIC UROLOGY

*Badrinath Konety, MD, MBA; George W. Drach, MD**

Urology is undergoing rapid changes with the introduction of new technology and laboratory discoveries. These changes will exert a considerable influence in the way urologic diseases are managed in the future. Not only will they dramatically shift our diagnostic and management paradigms, they will also dictate future thinking and the directions of new research. Finding answers to several key urologic questions, especially as they pertain to the geriatric patient, has never been more important, given the aging of our population and its increased longevity. The chapter on geriatric urology in *New Frontiers in Geriatrics Research*, the project publication which this supplement updates, analyzed existing knowledge regarding various important urologic conditions that particularly affect older adults and identified several key research areas and questions pertaining to each of these urologic conditions that merited further investigation. [1] In this update of that chapter we have assessed the progress made since the literature review for *New Frontiers* was completed. We have sought to determine the extent and manner in which the Key Questions in geriatric urology identified in *New Frontiers* have been addressed by ongoing research. We determined that although some questions have been directly addressed in the interim, there are several areas where results are still forthcoming or progress needs to be encouraged. We have also identified several new topics where research efforts could be directed (see the section New Horizons in Geriatric Urology, at the end of the chapter). In discussing the research results that pertain to each Key Question identified in *New Frontiers,* we also point out contradictions and further questions that have resulted from these investigations.

The three Key Questions in urology identified in *New Frontiers* are listed below. Although these questions define the general theme for analysis of all the data identified in the literature, several nuances to these questions need to be addressed in the context of the individual disease processes and our population of interest. We have attempted to clarify these nuances in this chapter.

Urol KQ1: **Research is needed to better define the pathophysiology and natural history of the most common genitourinary disorders affecting older adults. These include but are not limited to urinary incontinence, urinary tract infection, prostate diseases, urologic malignancies, sexual dysfunction, stone disease, and renal failure and transplantation.**

Urol KQ2: **Research is needed to develop and validate predictive models to identify appropriate candidates for early surgical or other more active therapies for urologic disorders versus appropriate candidates for an initial trial of more conservative treatment options.**

* Konety: Associate Professor, Departments of Urology, Epidemiology and Biostatistics, University of California at San Francisco, San Francisco, CA; Drach: Professor of Urology, Division of Urology, University of Pennsylvania, Philadelphia , PA.

Urol KQ3: **Research is needed to analyze the longitudinal outcomes of various urologic therapies, including potential risks, benefits, and costs.**

METHODS

An exhaustive and systematic literature search was performed to identify all published articles pertaining to six specific subject areas in urology. The PubMed database of the National Library of Medicine was used for all searches. The major MeSH headings used as search terms were *general urology, prostatic diseases, kidney disease, sex disorders, urinary incontinence,* and *urinary tract infections*. These MeSH headings were combined with the following MeSH terms to restrict the search to articles directly related to geriatrics: *age, geriatric assessment, aged, 80 and over, frail elderly, longevity,* and *geriatrics*. Limit specifications for the searches included age 65 years and older, English language, human, and year of publication 2000–2006. Larger search results were broken down by category of publication into clinical trial, meta-analysis, randomized controlled trial, and review articles. The numbers of articles identified by the search were general urology 44, prostatic diseases 109, kidney disease 7346, sex disorders 7940, urinary incontinence 1265, and urinary tract infections 408. An additional search of the National Library of Medicine database using search terms *65 or older, aged,* and *geriatric* among English-language articles in core clinical journals yielded 91 articles for the years 2000–2005. Additional searches to identify publications that may address the specific questions raised in *New Frontiers* were also conducted. For example, for agenda item Urol 25, the search terms included *urinary calculi, minimally invasive surgery, geriatrics,* and *elderly*. For Urol 13, the search terms were *benign prostatic hyperplasia, elderly, phytotherapy*, and *medical therapy*. Again, limits applied were publication years 2000–2005, English language, human, and age 65 years and older. These additional searches yielded well over 2500 articles. We also searched for articles on the general subject matter without the keyword *elderly* or *geriatrics* in order to capture all data on the subject. If these articles included results obtained in elderly patients even though the entire target population was not limited to those aged 65 years or older, we included them in our literature review.

All the articles identified through the various search strategies were reviewed, and those that contained data clearly relevant to the area of interest were selected by one of the authors (BRK). The article abstracts were reviewed in the context of the research agenda set forth in *New Frontiers*. Those articles that addressed the urology Key Questions and any of the proposed areas of investigation were reviewed in their entirety, and their results were summarized. Our updated understanding of the available state of evidence forms the basis for the modifications of and additions to the research agenda from *New Frontiers.*

PROGRESS IN GERIATRIC UROLOGY

URINARY INCONTINENCE

Background and Epidemiology

See *New Frontiers,* pp. 270–271.

Types of Urinary Incontinence

See *New Frontiers,* pp. 271–272.

Diagnostic Evaluation

See *New Frontiers,* pp. 272–273.

Treatment

See *New Frontiers,* pp. 273–276.

Needed Research in Urinary Incontinence

Urol 1 (Level B): **Studies are needed on the pathophysiology of nocturia, which occurs in a wide variety of conditions, including heart failure, renal failure, vascular insufficiency, sleep disorders, prostate enlargement, and polyuria of various causes.**

New Research Addressing This Question: Nocturia is one of the main complaints of most patients with benign prostatic hyperplasia (BPH). Population-based cohort studies conducted in Japanese men suggest that even in men with normal-sized prostates and no other symptoms of BPH, nocturia more than one time per night is prevalent in men aged 55 years or older and nocturia more than two times per night is prevalent in men aged 75 years or older. [2] The presence of nocturia is directly correlated with the age of the patient. It appears to be related to reduced nocturnal bladder capacity, since diurnal urine volume variation actually decreases with age. [3] Nocturnal urinary volume is also known to increase with age, and this in combination with decreased capacity could precipitate the nocturia. Of further importance, nocturia is a significant risk factor for falls among older adults. Reducing fluid intake before bedtime may be one good strategy to decrease nocturia. Other interventions to increase bladder capacity may include the administration of anticholinergics, though such medications may have central nervous system side effects that are not very desirable in this population. Some of the newer anticholinergic medications cross the blood-brain barrier to a lesser extent, mitigating some of this toxicity.

Worsening of lower urinary tract symptoms with increasing age appears to be present in both sexes. [4] Men aged 70 years or older have an International Prostate Symptom Score (IPSS) score of 7 (mild symptoms), and women have a score of 5.6 (even milder symptoms). Most of the increase in the scores in older age groups is related to increased complaints of weak stream and nocturia in men and of nocturia and urgency in women.

Modification of This Question in Light of New Research: These data further emphasize the need for studies in older persons to ascertain the pathophysiology of nocturia.

Urol 2 (Level B): **Studies are needed to establish the validity of new and existing survey instruments to assess the types and degrees of urinary incontinence in older adults.**

New Research Addressing This Question: Studies have used various survey instruments to assess the degree and impact of incontinence in older adults. Some of the tools that have been used include the Protection, Amount, Frequency, Adjustment, Body Image assessment tool, the Incontinence Impact Questionnaire, and the Urogenital Distress Inventory (UDI). [5] The Epidemiology of Prolapse and Incontinence Questionnaire attempts to identify symptoms related to overall pelvic floor dysfunction. [6] Bradley et al used a modified version of the Pelvic Floor Distress Inventory similar to the UDI to assess prevalence of incontinence in a cohort of older women participating in the Women's Health Study. They found both stress and urge urinary incontinence to be prevalent in almost 50% of the cohort with a mean age of 68 years. They identified lifestyle factors, such as daily exercise and coffee drinking, that are associated with higher likelihood of incontinence. [7]

A variety of questionnaires are available to assess the degree of urge incontinence and have been comparatively validated in a small cohort of older women with a mean age of 66 years. In comparing the Overactive Bladder Questionnaire, the Patient Perception of Bladder Condition, Urgency Questionnaire, and Primary OAB Symptom Questionnaire, Matza et al found that all were equally consistent in measuring symptom severity and better than micturition diaries. [8] Hence, these instruments could be potentially useful in evaluating elderly patients with incontinence. One must be cautious about extrapolating to an older population the accuracy of incontinence assessment questionnaires validated in a younger cohort. Prior studies suggest that as few as 4% of octogenarians who report stress urinary incontinence on a questionnaire will actually have stress incontinence demonstrable on urodynamic evaluation. [9] This further underscores the need to develop age-specific disease assessment tools for use in older persons.

One strategy employed to assess quality of life (QOL) in these patients has been to couple validated instruments (eg, the Medical Outcomes Study Short Form 36-item health survey, or SF-36) that assess QOL with indigenous short surveys that in the elderly patient assess degree of incontinence. In one such study, Ko et al determined that incontinence had significant negative impact on the global QOL as determined by the SF-36 in persons aged 65 years or older. Interestingly, the gender-based prevalence of incontinence in this population was not very different (20.9% in men, 27.5% in women). [10] The Incontinence Quality of Life (I-QOL) is an instrument specifically developed to assess the impact of incontinence on QOL. Validation studies on this instrument have included elderly patients; 46% of patients in one study of 605 respondents were in the age group 65 years or older. The impact of incontinence on QOL does not appear to vary by age. Comparison of scores obtained using I-QOL appear to correlate well with scores obtained on more generic instruments, such as the SF-36 or the SF-12, but the I-QOL is more sensitive in identifying degree of bother from the incontinence. [11] In a validation study of the I-QOL instrument conducted in 288 patients with incontinence participating in a clinical trial, 32% were aged 60 years or older. Although the data were not analyzed after age stratification, the instrument appeared to have across the board a high internal consistency and cross-sectional validity. [12] Total scores on the I-QOL instrument do appear to be higher (better) among older patients (aged 60 years or older), an effect ascribed to the adaptability of older patients to their disease. [13] This has been observed in earlier studies using more standardized instruments such as the SF-36. This finding further emphasizes the need to specifically validate such instruments in an older cohort of patients in order to determine "ceiling and floor effects." If baseline scores are already high among the older persons, there may not be much room for improvement, hence precluding identification of QOL differences by intervention. Other measures that have been used to assess outcome following incontinence surgery include the Stress, Emptying, Anatomy, Protection, and Instability score. [14]

Modification of This Question in Light of New Research: Although these results suggest that several instruments can be used adequately in an elderly population of patients, the use of targeted analysis with QOL instruments in an elderly cohort would ensure that results are valid in this population.

Urol 3 (Level B): **Systematic prospective cohort or case-control studies are needed to determine whether urodynamic and imaging techniques are associated with better outcomes in urinary incontinence in older patients.**

New Research Addressing This Question: Retrospective analysis of older patients with incontinence suggests that other than cognitive status and medications, measured bladder capacity and ability to voluntarily suppress voiding are important predictors of urge urinary incontinence.[15] These data offer additional targets for intervention in future studies. Randomized trials comparing several treatment options for incontinence in older women have used various urodynamic measures of response. However, there appears to be a disconnect between measured urodynamic response and clinical response, such as avoidance of accidents, which suggests that more comprehensive measures of bladder function beyond routine urodynamics may be required to provide a more complete picture of the disease.[16] Newer evaluation techniques, such as ambulatory urodynamics, have been incorporated into randomized clinical trials evaluating pharmacologic agents for treating urge incontinence.[17] Although the studies include older patients, none of them have specifically assessed the benefit of these investigations in a cohort of older patients. Lack of data in this regard is underscored by the fact that there is great observed variability in the frequency, type, and appropriateness of the urodynamic evaluation used by various physicians.[18] Studies analyzing the benefits of urodynamic evaluation in large cohorts of patients suggest that reliance on clinical symptoms alone will risk underdiagnosis of overactive bladder. In one study of 4500 women with overactive bladder, 1641 or 36.5% had urodynamic findings of overactive bladder. Only 27.5% of the 1641 women actually had symptoms representing bladder overactivity.[19]

Modification of This Question in Light of New Research: Urodynamic assessment may provide a more objective measure of baseline function from which relative change can be judged. It is assumed that the same normal expected baseline applies to patients of all ages. Directed determination of urodynamic parameters in an older cohort can help determine if the current approach is valid and define normal bounds for common urodynamic measurements in the older adult. This will also help better assess outcomes of therapy in this age group.

Urol 4 (Level A): **Depending on the results of studies of the impact of urodynamic and imaging techniques on outcomes (Urol 3), the effect of particular urodynamic or imaging studies on the accuracy of diagnosis and outcomes of treatment should be assessed in randomized controlled trials.**

New Research Addressing This Question: Almost all of the recent clinical trials assessing various therapeutic interventions for incontinence incorporate some objective measure of outcome assessment. Several of them use QOL and other questionnaires to assess outcome, and others use urodynamic measurements at baseline and after the intervention to assess improvement. Combinations of the two methods have also been used. There are no large studies focused on older patients (aged 65 years or older) that specifically address the validity of the various methods of outcome assessment. This is particularly true for the objective measures, such as urodynamics and radiographic evaluation. Such a comparative evaluation would allow us to define a reference standard that can be used in all studies and allow easier comparison of data across studies.

Evaluation of the benefit of routine urodynamics before initiation of therapy has been conducted in a prospective manner in women 50 to 74 years of age. Ultimate outcomes were no different in those patients who underwent pre-intervention urodynamics and in those who underwent urodynamics only following intervention. A change in diagnosis and therapy based on urodynamics was required in 26% of patients in this trial, but this did not affect final outcome. This led the authors to suggest that routine urodynamics may not be necessary, at least before initiation of first-line therapy.[20] It is unclear if these findings will apply generally to an older population, but they do provide food for thought. The accuracy of specific subjective and objective criteria to diagnose stress urinary incontinence has been evaluated in a large study of 950 women of all ages. Using urodynamic demonstration of stress incontinence as a standard, the authors were able to identify a small subset of patients who met predetermined criteria for incontinence that correlated highly with the urodynamic results.[21]

Modification of This Question in Light of New Research: Previously identified clinical diagnostic criteria have to be validated in an older cohort of patients to determine if the criteria can facilitate selection of patients who would require urodynamic evaluation.

***Urol 5 (Level A)*: Further randomized controlled trials are needed to test the efficacy and safety of both new and established anticholinergic drugs for the management of urinary incontinence in older adults.**

New Research Addressing This Question: Several of the newer agents for overactive bladder have been used safely in treating older adults. In a randomized, double blind, placebo-controlled trial, tolterodine was found to be safe and more effective than placebo in treating symptoms of overactive bladder. In this study the mean age of patients was 75 years, and a dosage of 2 mg twice a day was used.[22] Other agents, such as calcium channel blockers, have been evaluated for the treatment of urge incontinence in older patients in randomized trials and found not to be very effective.[23] Several new anticholinergic agents have demonstrated efficacy in treating detrusor overactivity. Most of them have a more benign side-effect profile than oxybutynin, which previously was the most commonly used agent. One of the main concerns with using oxybutynin is the risk of cognitive impairment in the older patient, since the drug is able to cross the blood-brain barrier. Many of the newer agents have a decreased risk of this side effect. This has been demonstrated for darifenacin in a randomized placebo-controlled trial in patients aged 65 years or older.[24] Another newer anticholinergic agent, solifenacin, has also been shown to be well tolerated in older adults. Higher plasma concentrations and areas under the curve, indicating duration of exposure, were achieved in older persons treated with solifenacin for 14 days.[25]

Modification of This Question in Light of New Research: Further specific trials targeted at the geriatric age group are required to thoroughly evaluate the effects of these agents in this population of patients.

Urol 6 (Level A): **Randomized controlled trials with large numbers of subjects will be required to determine whether acupuncture or other complementary therapies have a significant beneficial effect in treating urge or mixed urinary incontinence in older patients.**

New Research Addressing This Question: Analysis of prospective trial data indicates that behavioral therapy may be more effective than pharmacotherapy or placebo in treating older women with irritative symptoms, such as nocturia. [26] Initiating behavioral modification therapy before the occurrence of incontinence can significantly reduce the subsequent development of incontinence. This effect lasted up to a year after stopping the intervention in postmenopausal women who participated in a randomized controlled trial in which the control group received no intervention. [27] From a systematic review of four randomized trials and four before-and-after studies in the published literature, Teunissen et al reported that behavioral therapy alone or in combination with drug therapy appeared to be as effective if not better than drug therapy alone in treating incontinence. Behavioral modification appeared to consistently reduce urinary accidents in a substantial number of women aged 55 years or older, but the benefit of drug therapy was not consistent. [28] There have been no randomized controlled trials to examine the benefit of acupuncture in treating incontinence. Single-arm phase II studies in women aged 66 to 82 years suggest that such treatment can result in durable symptomatic improvement. [29] Randomized placebo-controlled trials of acupuncture for the treatment of overactive bladder have been performed with good results in younger women. [30] It remains to be seen if similar results can be achieved in older patients. Similarly, randomized trials of intravesical injection of botulinum toxin have included older patients and demonstrate promising results. However, in this study complications such as urinary retention, constipation, and dry mouth occurred in 4 patients, 3 of whom were aged 65 years or older. This suggests that complications of botulinum injection may be more common in the older patient. [31]

Modification of This Question in Light of New Research: The applicability of various conservative therapies and their relative toxicities need to be further assessed prospectively before it will be clear whether such approaches are safely applicable to older patients.

Urol 7 (Level A): **The bladder neck suspension and sling procedures have been proven effective in older women studied an average of 17 months after surgery. Prospective cohort studies with longer-term follow-up periods are needed to determine whether these procedures have sustained longevity.**

New Research Addressing This Question: Prospectively obtained objective and subjective assessment data following transvaginal urethral suspensions suggest that similar long-term outcomes (at up to 22 months) can be obtained regardless of age, even in octogenarians. [32] This substantiates prior retrospective data that suggest equivalent results following pubovaginal sling surgery in women above and below 70 years of age. [33] Needle suspension procedures using either the Raz or the Stamey technique generally do not appear to be effective in older women, as demonstrated by prior studies. [34,35] Large studies of tension-free vaginal tape for the treatment of incontinence in elderly women suggest that long-term outcomes are better for those with stress incontinence but that in women with mixed (stress plus urge) incontinence the cure rate declines to 60% at 4 years and further to 30% at 8 years. The mean age of the patients in this study was 67 years for those with mixed incontinence and 61 years for those with stress incontinence.[36] Anterior vaginal wall repair for treatment of cystocele along with a urethral sling has been reported to be successful in a majority of elderly patients at a mean follow-up of 15 months; 80% had a minimum follow-up of 6 months or more. All patients demonstrated improvement in stress urinary incontinence, but younger patients were more likely to report improvement of urge incontinence.[37] Retrospective data indicate that surgery for pelvic organ prolapse can also be safely performed in octogenarians; satisfaction was expressed by as many as 80% of patients.[38] Randomized controlled studies comparing periurethral bulking agents to the pubovaginal sling in older women demonstrate that although the morbidity of the bulking agent injection is lower, the sling is more effective in the long term.[39]

Modification of This Question in Light of New Research: This question can be dropped from the research agenda.

> *Urol 8 (Level B)*: **Prospective cohort studies are needed to explore the factors that identify which elderly patients will do better with early surgical intervention than with more conservative treatment options.**

New Research Addressing This Question: Several retrospective and prospective analyses have attempted to identify factors that will predict a favorable outcome following conservative therapy for urinary incontinence. Several anatomic parameters, such as body mass index, prior pelvic surgery, and other factors, emerge as predictors, but age is not consistently among these factors.[40]

Modification of This Question in Light of New Research: More focused prospective studies in the older age group are required to compare conservative and surgical therapy and identify the best candidates for each approach. The fact that many patients progress from conservative to surgical therapy will make these studies difficult to design and will challenge adequate accrual.

> *Urol 9 (Level A)*: **Performing randomized controlled trials to extend the studies of factors that identify appropriate candidates for early surgery for incontinence could lead to the development and validation of predictive models useful for guiding treatment decisions for various types of urinary incontinence in older patients (see also the Key Questions, at the beginning of the chapter).**

New Research Addressing This Question: Prior studies have identified several factors that can predict the success of various interventions, such as pelvic floor exercises for the treatment of incontinence. Severity of symptoms at baseline, urodynamic criteria such as leak-point pressure, and pharmacologic history can all determine the likelihood of response to pelvic floor exercises.[41] Other predictors that are particularly relevant to stress urinary incontinence being treated with behavioral therapy include literacy level and prior surgery. Interestingly, the baseline urodynamic parameters, race, age, medical history, and obstetric history do not seem to consistently predict outcomes of behavioral therapy.[42] The diagnosis of urge incontinence may be facilitated by utilizing a model that includes both symptoms and demographic data, such as age and gender.[43] The presence of urgency and urge incontinence at baseline bodes ill for older men (60 to 89 years) in particular, as they have a higher relative risk of 10-year mortality even after controlling for comorbidity and lifestyle factors.[44] The increased risk of mortality can probably be attributed to secondary events such as falls and injuries that could stem from the voiding problems. This emphasizes the need to identify and treat urge incontinence in older patients to limit the risk of secondary adverse events that can occur as a result of the urgency and urge incontinence. This can be facilitated by the use of predictive models in this population.

Modification of This Question in Light of New Research: Future studies could focus on practice patterns and barriers to implementation of existing models or diagnostic criteria to treat voiding dysfunction and predict outcomes in the geriatric age group.

URINARY TRACT INFECTIONS

See *New Frontiers,* pp. 278–280.

Urol 10 (Level B): **Additional research is needed to clarify the operational definitions of urinary tract infection and of asymptomatic bacteriuria.**

New Research Addressing This Question: Previous studies indicate that 24% of noninstitutionalized older adults, who constitute about 95% of the geriatric age group, will develop a urinary tract infection (UTI) during a 2-year observation period.[45] Most research, however, is focused on the 5% who are institutionalized. Approximately 50% of women and 30% of men in the institutionalized geriatric population have asymptomatic bacteriuria that does not typically require treatment, though several antibiotic-based therapeutic intervention studies nevertheless include such patients. Though pyuria often accompanies a positive urine culture in this setting, less than 10% of febrile institutionalized elderly persons without an indwelling catheter and with asymptomatic bacteriuria will benefit from a treatment of their presumed UTI.[46] Diagnosis of UTI in this population relies on symptoms, signs, and clinical judgment, rendering it hard to interpret the efficacy of many therapies. Misinterpretation of nonspecific signs and symptoms may lead to the false diagnosis of a UTI in many of these individuals with asymptomatic bacteriuria.[47]

Modification of This Question in Light of New Research: Additional work is needed to clarify the criteria for defining a UTI in older patients. Provider education is also necessary in order to prevent overtreatment and emergence of resistant strains of bacteria.

Urol 11 (Level B): **The natural history and potential risks of urinary tract infection or asymptomatic bacteriuria and forms of preventive therapy warrant further study (see the Key Questions, at the beginning of the chapter).**

New Research Addressing This Question: Several studies have attempted to evaluate various preventive nonantibiotic therapies to manage UTI and bacteriuria. Dessole et al randomized postmenopausal women to placebo versus estriol vaginal suppositories and determined that women in the treatment group had significantly lower rates of significant bacteriuria (14% versus 45%, $P < .001$). The average age of participants was 58 years (treated) and 56 years (control). Improvements were also observed in colposcopic examinations and urethral pressure profiles.[48] The use of oral nitrofurantoin macrocrystals appears to be much more effective in preventing UTI than the use of vaginal estriol pessaries. In a randomized comparison of the two treatment approaches, Raz et al discovered that UTI rates as well as the rates of bacteriuria were significantly lower in those treated with nitrofurantoin; 90% of patients in the estriol group and 84% of patients in the nitrofurantoin group were 60 years of age. [49] The prevention of UTI following surgery does not appear to be facilitated by the use of a suprapubic tube rather than a urethral catheter, and often patients may need to be recatheterized per urethra after developing a complication following removal of the suprapubic catheter. This limits the use of this approach. [50] Data from the Heart and Estrogen/Progestin Replacement Study (HERS) suggests that oral hormone replacement does not impact the risk of UTI in postmenopausal women. Higher UTI frequencies were observed in women in the hormone therapy arm than in those receiving placebo, though the difference was not statistically significant. [51] Hence, it does appear that urinary antiseptic therapy with mild agents such as nitrofurantoin may be as effective as, if not better than, topical or systemic hormonal therapy for prevention of UTI.

Modification of This Question in Light of New Research: Future research should focus on the prophylactic role of agents such as cranberry juice and changes in local hygiene in preventing UTI through prospective trials in the geriatric age group. A combined approach adding antibacterials to prevention may yield better results.

Urol 12 (Level A): **Research on new antibiotic agents for the treatment of urinary tract infection should include randomized controlled trials specifically designed to assess the safety and efficacy of these drugs in geriatric patient populations.**

New Research Addressing This Question: Antibiotic use is very prevalent among older adults residing in nursing homes. This contributes to increased risk of resistance, costs, side effects, and drug interactions. The prevalence of antibiotic use is estimated to be between 8% and 17%. [52–56] Trials to test algorithm-based approaches to govern the use of antibiotics in geriatric residents of long-term-care facilities are under way, and once completed, they will enable the establishment of standard protocols to manage this common problem in this population. [56] Vogel et al randomized 183 women aged 65 years or older to receive either a short (3-day) course of ciprofloxacin or a 7-day course of ciprofloxacin. These researchers discovered that bacterial eradication rates were no different between the groups, at 98% and 93%, respectively. [57] Treatment-related side effects were much lower in those receiving the shorter course of antibiotics. This suggests that in older women with uncomplicated UTI, a 3-day course of oral ciprofloxacin is adequate and less toxic. In a randomized comparison, oral ciprofloxacin was found to be more effective in eradicating both the clinical symptoms of UTI and bacteriuria when compared with trimethoprim/sulfamethoxazole in women aged 65 years or older. [58] Fewer adverse effects were also observed in women receiving ciprofloxacin. These findings contradict those from previous studies which suggest that short-term antibiotic therapy is inadequate for the older adult, with 75% of patients having positive urine cultures at 6 months post-treatment when a 3-day course is used. [59] A systematic review of 13 trials evaluating different durations of antibiotic therapy for uncomplicated symptomatic UTI in elderly women indicated that single-dose therapy is less effective than a short (3- to 7-day) course of therapy but is better accepted by patients. There appears to be no significant difference in efficacy between a short (above) or long (7- to 14-day) course of therapy. [60] Hence, it appears that for uncomplicated UTI in older women, a short 3-day course of oral ciprofloxacin may be the optimal treatment.

Funguria is relatively prevalent among older persons since many of them are residents of long-term-care facilities and have indwelling catheters. The presence of other comorbid illness, such as diabetes mellitus, can also contribute to the development of funguria. [61] *Candida albicans* is most commonly involved (52% of cases), and *C. glabrata* is the second most common (16%). Removal of the catheter can result in resolution of the funguria in many cases, and up to 75% of cases resolve with no treatment. Amphotericin bladder irrigation can eradicate funguria in 54% of cases, whereas oral fluconazole is effective in 45% of cases. In a randomized study, patients with an average age of 70 years took oral fluconazole or placebo for the treatment of asymptomatic or minimally symptomatic candidal UTI. A 14-day course of oral fluconazole eradicated the UTI in 50% of patients, but eradication occurred in 29% of the placebo group. [62] Still, most patients with asymptomatic funguria may require no treatment other than removal of the catheter. Those needing treatment can be managed with oral fluconazole, and amphotericin B bladder irrigation is reserved for the recalcitrant cases.

Modification of This Question in Light of New Research: This question can be dropped from the research agenda.

PROSTATE DISEASES

Benign Prostatic Hyperplasia

See *New Frontiers,* pp. 280–282.

Prostate Cancer

See *New Frontiers,* pp. 282–284.

Needed Research in Prostate Disease

Urol 13 (Level A): **Randomized controlled trials in elderly men are needed to compare phytotherapies with placebo or with established medical therapies for benign prostatic hyperplasia.**

New Research Addressing This Question: Although there are very few well-conducted randomized trials of phytotherapy versus medical therapy for BPH, the available evidence is controversial. Gross et al determined that conversion from phytotherapy to α-blockers such as tamsulosin is well tolerated and more effective in providing symptom relief. [63] An international study randomizing patients to saw palmetto or tamsulosin revealed equivalent improvements with both therapies up to 1 year of follow-up. [64] Comparison of α-blockers and other natural agents such as eviprostat also do not demonstrate any objective or subjective benefit of using the herbal agents. [65] A meta-analysis of 11 randomized trials and 2 single-arm studies published before 2000 suggested that saw palmetto may yield symptomatic as well as uroflow improvements significantly greater than placebo alone. [66] However, at least one recent randomized prospective study comparing saw palmetto with placebo revealed that there were no significant differences in symptomatic improvement or urinary flow rates between the treatment and placebo groups. [67] Systematic analysis of the randomized studies using *Pygeum africanum*, another common phytotherapy for BPH, also revealed that this agent may result in slight improvement in symptoms of BPH. [68] However, none of the studies have compared the agent with standard medical therapy for BPH, and most studies are small, with short follow-up. Hence, it is hard to make definitive conclusions regarding its efficacy. Botanically derived 5-α-reductase inhibitors have also been compared with placebo and pharmacologic 5-α-reductase inhibitors, demonstrating equivalent effects in terms of symptom improvement. Agents such as β-sitosterols and Cernilton (rye grass pollen extract) also appear to be effective in providing symptomatic relief in men with BPH while being well tolerated. However, the available randomized studies are poorly conducted, and long-term data are lacking. [69,70]

Modification of This Question in Light of New Research: Future studies should focus on the benefits of phytotherapy in older men with BPH and their specific toxicities in this population, given older men's higher likelihood of having limited mobility and cognitive impairment as well as other comorbidities. The effect and extent of interaction of various phytotherapeutic agents with conventional medications is also essential to discern, given that many older men are taking multiple medications.

> *Urol 14 (Level A)*: **Randomized trials in elderly men are needed to compare minimally invasive surgical therapies for benign prostatic hyperplasia with the gold-standard procedure, transurethral resection of the prostate.**

New Research Addressing This Question: Several minimally invasive alternatives to transurethral resection of the prostate (TURP) have emerged. TURP was long considered the gold-standard surgical therapy for BPH. In the two randomized comparisons of TURP with transurethral needle ablation of the prostate (TUNA), both symptomatic improvement and urine flow rates were found to be better among patients undergoing TURP, but the differences were not substantial. Improvements achieved following TUNA appeared to last 5 years, though the number of patients followed up to that time point was low in at least one of the studies. Both these studies enrolled men with a mean age over 65 years. [71,72] A meta-analysis of 13 published studies of TUNA concluded that TUNA is a reasonable alternative to TURP or medical therapy for men with severely symptomatic BPH, and that perhaps it is more cost-effective. The analysis also suggested that it might be a good choice for men who do not want medical therapy or TURP or who are poor surgical candidates. [73] In a similar manner, a systematic review of six randomized clinical studies involving 540 men compared TURP with microwave therapy in men with symptomatic BPH. Results suggested that transurethral microwave therapy (TUMT) is a reasonable short-term alternative with acceptable side effects, but improvements in both symptom score and uroflow rate were substantially better with TURP. However, almost all of these studies had inadequate reporting of methods and varied widely in enrollment criteria. Side effects were fewer in the microwave therapy group. [74] The attractiveness of both the minimally invasive methods is that they can be performed as an outpatient procedure in the office. Men who fail either of these therapies can usually be salvaged with TURP. Randomized comparisons of gold-standard surgical therapy for BPH, ie, TURP, with newer methods of transurethral resection, such as laser vaporization and holmium laser enucleation (HOLEP), have been performed. In men with larger prostates (> 40 g), the three approaches appear to be equally effective in terms of objective and subjective symptom relief at 6 months and 1 year.[75] Both HOLEP and laser vaporization tend to have lower perioperative morbidity and blood loss. Other studies confirm the similarity in outcomes. HOLEP appears to result in more irritative voiding symptoms but has shorter hospital stay and catheterization time. Duration of surgery may be longer with a HOLEP.[76] The average age of men in these trials was 65 years. Overall, minimally invasive therapies may be particularly attractive for older men with multiple comorbidities since they can be performed as an outpatient procedure under local anesthesia, and complications are minimal.

Modification of This Question in Light of New Research: This question can be dropped from the research agenda.

> *Urol 15 (Level A)*: **Randomized controlled trials are needed to compare outcomes of early transurethral resection of the prostate with outcomes of initial medical therapy followed by subsequent transurethral resection of the prostate when clinically necessary.**

New Research Addressing This Question: There are no studies comparing initial TURP with medical therapy followed by TURP. It would probably be very difficult to pursue such studies at this time, given data indicating that medical therapy is effective in many men with BPH. Data do suggest that patients initially treated with α-blockers are more likely to progress to TURP than those treated with 5-α-reductase inhibitors.[77] Retrospective analysis of the effect of medical therapy on surgical treatment of BPH suggests that men are on average 5 years older with larger glands when undergoing surgery for BPH. The advent of medical therapy has decreased the use of TURP by 17% over the past decade, but open surgery for BPH is more often required now than it was 10 years ago (19% versus 29%).[78]

Modification of This Question in Light of New Research: It is increasingly important to define strict criteria for monitoring the efficacy of medical therapy and to establish guidelines for switching to surgical alternatives, particularly in older men where some deliberation may be required before embarking on surgical interventions. A large proportion of these men are already old when starting medical therapy, and by the time surgical therapy becomes necessary, their comorbidities and general functional status may also have changed, thereby restricting therapeutic alternatives.

> *Urol 16 (Level B)*: **Prospective cohort studies and decision-analysis models are needed to identify the characteristics that predispose an older patient with benign prostatic hyperplasia to benefit from early transurethral resection of the prostate (see the Key Questions, at the beginning of the chapter).**

New Research Addressing This Question: Cost-effectiveness models suggest that cost equivalence with medical therapy may be reached by some of the minimally invasive therapies, such as TUNA, within 3 to 5 years. Naslund et al determined that TUNA is cost-equivalent to medical management combined with α-blockers and 5-α-reductase inhibitors after about 2.5 years of therapy.[79] Cost comparisons of TUMT with TURP suggest that total costs during a 3-year follow-up period are lower for TUMT than for TURP, though the risk of retreatment is higher with TUMT. The main explanation for the difference is the outpatient delivery of TUMT, which significantly reduces costs over those with inpatient TURP.[80] Cost-utility analysis using Markov models suggests that risk-averse patients are likely to choose medical management and that non–risk-averse patients will choose TUMT. Neither type of patient will choose TURP.[81]

Modification of This Question in Light of New Research: These data are probably applicable to men in the geriatric age group, but additional functional and cognitive concerns have to be taken into consideration while evaluating these cost-utility data. It would be reasonable to assume that to a large extent the available cost-utility data will hold true, albeit with some modifications, in older men. Hence, this question can be dropped from the research agenda.

Urol 17 (Level B): **Because screening for prostate cancer is so widespread, it may be very difficult to design a randomized controlled trial comparing prostate-specific antigen screening with rectal examination alone, using risks, benefits, and costs as outcome measures. Therefore, the decision as to when to stop routine screening for prostate cancer in elderly men may depend on prospective cohort studies.**

New Research Addressing This Question: PSA levels clearly increase with increasing noncancerous prostate volume. Since prostate volume increases with age, there is an indirect link between PSA and age.[82] Hence, it is hard to interpret elevated PSA values in older men. There are currently no data to indicate a survival benefit to screening for prostate cancer. Ongoing studies in Europe—European Randomized Study of Screening for Prostate Cancer (ERSPC)]—and the United States—Prostate, Lung, Colorectal and Ovarian Screening Trial (PLCO)—are expected to provide data that clarifies this issue in the next few years. However, the proportion of older men is limited in both of these studies. Currently there appears to be an age-related decline in routine PSA testing and screening for prostate cancer, with lower rates being observed in the older age group. However, the rate of persistent PSA testing is small but not insignificant. Observational cross-sectional studies indicate a 3% to 5% rate of PSA testing in men aged 75 years or older.[83,84] The rate of PSA-based screening and the use of different types of therapy also vary by region, with rates of screening in men aged 75 years or older being much higher in Florida.[85]

Modification of This Question in Light of New Research: Further cohort studies are needed establish and ratify an age to stop screening for prostate cancer (as is done for cervical cancer) and develop a uniform and systematic approach to evaluation and treatment of prostate cancer in older men.

Urol 18 (Level A): **Because there is so much uncertainty regarding the best treatment plan for localized or locally metastatic prostate cancer, it is justified and indeed necessary to design randomized clinical trials in large populations of elderly men, with subgroup analyses, to examine the effects of clinical characteristics on treatment decisions.**

New Research Addressing This Question: A well-controlled clinical study with 10-year follow-up suggests a long-term benefit with regard to disease progression and survival in men who undergo radical prostatectomy for prostate cancer in comparison with watchful waiting.[86,87] All the patients enrolled in this study were men aged 75 years or younger with a mean age of 64 years (± 5.1) in each of the two groups. The survival and delayed progression benefits were not restricted by age. The majority of these men had clinically detectable cancers, and very few were identified by routine screening. This raises concerns regarding the applicability of these data in the current context of screening-detected prostate cancer, which is the more likely scenario at the present time. However, the results cannot be generalized to men aged 75 years or older.

Modification of This Question in Light of New Research: Randomized clinical trials of therapeutic alternatives are very hard to conduct in prostate cancer. This will be especially true for older men, in whom risk-stratified therapy is being utilized increasingly, with watchful waiting being the main recourse in those with low-risk disease. Furthermore, the clinical criteria (PSA, Gleason grade, disease stage) that are currently used to risk stratify younger patients are equally applicable to older patients. Hence, this question can be dropped from the research agenda.

OTHER GENITOURINARY MALIGNANCIES

See *New Frontiers,* pp. 285–286.

Urol 19 (Level A): **Randomized clinical trials are needed to determine the overall safety and long-term efficacy of less invasive therapy for bladder and renal malignancies in older adults, comparing these with the standard procedures (radical cystectomy and radical nephrectomy).**

New Research Addressing This Question: Several observational uncontrolled cohort studies report that radical cystectomy and radical nephrectomy can be performed in elderly patients with outcomes comparable to those observed in younger patients. There does appear to be an increase in complication and mortality rates following radical cystectomy in older adults, but in well-selected individuals these differences are not significant.[88,89] In larger population-based studies, age does appear to be an independent predictor of negative outcomes following radical cystectomy.[90] Although several studies have suggested that a bladder-sparing approach to treat muscle-invasive bladder cancer is as effective as cystectomy, these studies have not been randomized, nor have they specifically enrolled older patients. The same is true for the evaluation of minimally invasive therapies, such as cryoablation and radiofrequency ablation, for kidney tumors. All of these are now recognized as viable therapeutic alternatives in older patients. Surveillance of small renal masses is also considered acceptable in patients with small exophytic masses (< 3 cm) that are easily accessible percutaneously and do not involve the collecting system.

Modification of This Question in Light of New Research: Future studies should concentrate on the evaluation of bladder-sparing therapy for the treatment of bladder cancer and minimally invasive therapy for the management of renal masses in older patients. The prospective evaluation of surveillance with delayed treatment as a management option in biopsy-proven renal cancer, particularly in older individuals, is also important.

Urol 20 (Level A): **Predictive outcomes models to identify who would most benefit from the various forms of therapy for bladder and renal malignancies need to be developed and validated (see the Key Questions, at the beginning of the chapter).**

New Research Addressing This Question: There are predictive algorithms that can help identify patients who are more likely to respond to surgical and nonsurgical therapy for renal cancer.[91,92] Because age is not used as a predictive variable in these models, they have not been specifically validated in cohorts of different age groups. Similar predictive nomograms to predict outcomes from therapy for bladder cancer are under development, but none are currently available.

Modification of This Question in Light of New Research: Further research in this area is required to develop and validate predictive algorithms for cancer-specific outcomes for bladder and kidney cancers in older patients.

SEXUAL DYSFUNCTION

Male Sexual Dysfunction

See *New Frontiers,* pp. 286–287.

Female Sexual Dysfunction

See *New Frontiers,* p. 287.

Influence of Comorbid Disease

See *New Frontiers,* pp. 287–288.

Treatment of Sexual Dysfunction

See *New Frontiers,* p. 288.

Needed Research in Sexual Dysfunction

Urol 21 (Level B): **Most of the studies that examine the relationship between sexual dysfunction and comorbid conditions are small retrospective reviews or case series, and they typically do not focus on elderly subjects. Larger, well-designed prospective cohort studies will be necessary to confirm these associations in older adult populations (see the Key Questions, at the beginning of the chapter).**

New Research Addressing This Question: Several population-based studies suggest that erectile dysfunction (ED) is very prevalent in older men.[93,94] More recent data estimates that 77% of men aged 75 years or older may have some form of ED.[93] Secondary analysis of data from the Prostate Cancer Prevention Trial indicates that at least 47% of men aged 55 years or older report some form of erectile dysfunction.[94] In this study, the development of new-onset ED was reported by 65% of men at 7 years of follow-up and was a significant predictor of cardiovascular disease. The presence of ED has also been linked to a 75% higher risk of peripheral vascular disease.[95] In the study by Blumentals et al, which was a retrospective analysis of over 12,000 men with and without ED, the odds of developing peripheral vascular disease and its association with ED was found to increase with increasing age.[95] In men with diabetes mellitus, the presence of ED may even be the most effective predictor of asymptomatic coronary artery disease.[96] The presence of chronic stable liver disease does not appear to increase the risk of ED.[97] The presence of

ED as documented on self-reported questionnaires such as the International Index of Erectile Function is prevalent in 71% of men with diabetes and 67% of men with hypertension.[98] Even the presence of mere dyslipidemia and depression can increase the prevalence of ED.[99,100] Lower urinary tract dysfunction has been linked to the presence of ED in men of various ages.[101,102] It is reasonable to assume that this would be true for older men, though specific data are not available.

Modification of This Question in Light of New Research: There are now excellent epidemiologic data linking ED to various comorbidities. Although these data do not focus on populations of elderly men, it would be reasonable to assume that the results would hold true across age groups. This question can be dropped from the research agenda.

Urol 22 (Level B): **Time series (before-and-after) studies may be sufficient to assess the effect of sildenafil on sexual function of women aged 65 to 74, 75 to 84, and 86 years and older.**

New Research Addressing This Question: Sildenafil citrate has been found to be effective in treating female sexual arousal disorder, a form of female sexual dysfunction. In one prospective randomized trial, postmenopausal women up to age 71 years were enrolled, but the data were not analyzed by age strata and hence do not allow us to assess the efficacy of this approach specifically in older women.[103] These positive results have not been consistent.[104,105]

Modification of This Question in Light of New Research: More detailed studies focused on elderly postmenopausal women are necessary in order to determine if therapy with a phosphodiesterase 5 (PDE 5) inhibitor such as sildenafil would be of benefit in women who complain of sexual dysfunction.

Urol 23 (Level B): **Time series (before-and-after) studies may be sufficient to assess the effect of sildenafil on sexual function of men aged 65 to 74, 75 to 84, and 86 years and older.**

New Research Addressing This Question: PDE 5 inhibitors appear to work equally well in older men (aged 60 years or older), but the rate of improvement may be faster in younger men.[106] The proportion of men 65 years or older who report improvement of ED with sildenafil therapy is similar to that for men who are a decade younger but considerably lower than that for men in their 20s.[107] An analysis of combined data from five large, randomized, placebo-controlled studies of sildenafil indicates that this agent is equally safe and efficacious in men aged 65 years or older and in younger men.[108] Tadalafil, another long-acting PDE 5 inhibitor, has been evaluated in men aged 65 years or older and found to be safe and efficacious.[109]

Modification of This Question in Light of New Research: This question can be dropped from the research agenda.

Urol 24 (Level B): **Prospective clinical series are needed to examine the use of intracavernosal injections, vacuum erection devices, and penile prostheses by men who are nonresponsive to sildenafil or are ineligible to use it.**

New Research Addressing This Question: In assessing preferences for the treatment of ED, researchers find that older men seem to prefer injection therapy over oral medications.

Dropout rates following oral therapy are as high as 78%, whereas those for injection therapy and vacuum erection devices are much lower, at 48% and 29%, respectively.[110] This has to be borne in mind when counseling older men regarding therapy for ED. In older men considering intracorporeal injections, the combination of prostaglandin E_1 (PGE_1), phentolamine, and papaverine appears to be more effective than PGE_1 alone.[111] Intracorporeal injection with PGE_1 such as alprostadil can improve erectile function in men who have failed PDE 5 inhibitors such as sildenafil.[112] This study included men up to 80 years of age, but it is not clear if equivalent response rates were obtained in men of all ages. However, intracorporeal injection therapy appears to work better than intraurethral PGE pellets.[113] This suggests that intracorporeal injections are a better first-line salvage therapy in men who fail oral agents such as PDE 5 inhibitors. It would be reasonable to assume that this would hold true for both older and younger men until further verification is available.

Sequential therapy is a very attractive concept for managing ED, given the variety of treatment options and the graded invasiveness of the actual therapeutic alternatives. It ranges from oral agents to surgical intervention. At least one prospective study of sequential treatment consisting of oral agents, followed by vacuum erection device, followed by intracorporeal injections, and ending with implantation of penile prosthesis suggests that short-term complete symptomatic improvement is achievable in 91% of patients. Forty-five percent of the men in this study were over the age of 60 and had diabetes mellitus. The results, however, were not analyzed by age strata, again making it difficult to estimate the benefit of such a program in elderly men.[114]

Modification of This Question in Light of New Research: Even though many of the studies described were not restricted to older men, it would be reasonable to assume that the results would hold true in older men. However, there are unique concerns regarding the applicability of various types of therapy in older men who may have some degree of cognitive impairment, dexterity issues, or partner issues. The feasibility of using these second-line therapies for ED and the barriers to adherence need to be investigated in order to determine the best second-line alternatives for older men.

STONE DISEASE

See *New Frontiers,* pp. 289–290.

***Urol 25 (Level B)*: Cohort studies are needed to evaluate the safety and clinical efficacy of minimally invasive surgical techniques in older adults with stone disease.**

New Research Addressing This Question: Studies suggest a peak in incidence of urinary calculi between the ages of 40 and 60 years. More recent studies suggest a later peak in incidence at 60 to 70 years, with stone rates declining dramatically thereafter.[115–117] The composition of the stones also tends to vary by age. Calcium oxalate stones predominate during the years of peak stone incidence, but uric acid stones are more frequent in the older age group.[118] Other stones such as cystine may be found more often with increasing age. Age-related changes in stone composition follow similar patterns in men and women. The incidence of struvite stones appears to be high at the extremes of age.[118] These findings have been corroborated by other studies in the geriatric population.[119] Higher excretion of urinary calcium may also be prevalent in older adults, contributing to stone formation, though stone recurrence rates are no higher than for younger adults.[119] Interestingly, increased oral calcium intake does not appear to increase the risk of stone formation in postmenopausal women. The presence of hypertension and low magnesium intake do contribute to a higher stone risk in postmenopausal women.[120]

These data have significant implications for stone management and prevention in the older adult. One potential explanation for the higher incidence of uric acid stones is the greater prevalence of metabolic syndrome with insulin resistance and acidic urine pH in older adults, with almost 40% of people aged 60 years or older demonstrating these features.[121,122] Better control of metabolic syndrome in the older adult, along with control of infection and decreasing placement of indwelling catheters, may help decrease stone formation. Recurrent bladder stone formation has been linked to catheter encrustation by biofilm formed by organisms such as *Proteus mirabilis*, which tends to occur quite rapidly after replacement of long-term indwelling catheters.[123] Decreased use of catheters or their frequent replacement with prompt attention to symptoms suggestive of bladder stones may help mitigate this problem. Estrogen replacement may decrease urinary calcium excretion and calcium oxalate saturation.[124] Studies suggest that the lower stone rates observed in women in general may be due to lower urinary excretion of calcium, oxalate, and dissociated uric acid or to higher levels of citrate. Estrogen replacement in postmenopausal women restores the urinary milieu to premenopausal levels, thereby decreasing stone risk.[124]

Modification of This Question in Light of New Research: In terms of specific therapeutic approaches to the management of stone disease, there were no reports identified through our literature search that examined these issues in geriatric patients or any analysis that described the results in an age-stratified manner with sample sizes large enough to make the results generally applicable. Studies addressing these issues in the geriatric population are recommended.

Renal Transplantation

The Older Adult as Donor

See *New Frontiers,* pp 290–291.

The Older Adult as Recipient

See *New Frontiers,* pp. 291–292.

Needed Research in Renal Transplantation

Urol 26 (Level B): **The role of renal transplantation in older adults has grown recently, with the expansion of both donor and recipient age limits and other clinical criteria. Research is needed to clarify the unique needs of geriatric transplant patients, particularly with regard to immunosuppression and clinical outcomes. The effect of age of the kidney donor, age of the recipient, methods and degrees of immunosuppression, and the presence of concomitant disease need to be evaluated in prospective cohort studies.**

New Research Addressing This Question: With increasing requirement for donor kidneys, there is a strong push in the transplant community to expand the donor pool by utilizing cadaveric kidneys from older donors. Large-scale database analysis does suggest that kidneys from older donors have lower graft survival and greater delay in normalization of renal function post-transplant. [125] A prolonged cold ischemia time may be one of the factors responsible for the less satisfactory function observed in these donor kidneys. However, it should be pointed out that in the context of kidney donors, all individuals aged 55 to 60 years are typically included in the older age group. In some large European series, about 14% of all donors are classified as older (60 years or older). [126] The proportion of recipients in the United States who were older (aged 64 years or older) was approximately 9% in 2000. [127] Older donor age is an independent predictor of delayed graft function, chronic allograft nephropathy, and creatinine level at 1 year. There is some indication that cardiovascular morbidity and subsequent mortality are also increased in recipients of kidneys from older donors. [126] Several centers are advocating the concept of "old for old," with kidneys from older donors being placed in older recipients. The Eurotransplant Senior Programme that was launched in January 1999 in order to increase the acquisition of kidneys from older (65 years or older) donors and transplant them into older (65 years or older) recipients. This program outlines strict criteria for the acceptance of older kidneys for transplantation. Several innovative approaches are being tested under this program. [128] The use of dual kidney transplantation if the donor glomerular filtration rate (GFR) is below 50 to 70 mL/min is increasing in popularity; several small cohort studies demonstrate graft survival and function equivalent to that of single kidney transplants with high GFR into elderly recipients. [129] Some cohort studies even suggest that the best dialysis-free outcomes and lowest rejection rates are present in older recipients and donor grafts from older patients, respectively. [130,131] If the Eurotransplant Senior Program criteria are followed and the donors and recipients are well matched, early evidence suggests that outcome in terms of graft survival may be identical to that achieved in transplants that were matched for human leukocyte antigens (HLA). [128] Graft survival rates of 86% have been observed in the participants of the program (age matched but not necessarily HLA matched), in comparison with 79% in control groups (HLA matched and age matched). [132] Three-year graft survival was 64% for "old for old" transplants versus 67% for HLA-matched transplants into older recipients. These rates were further enhanced to 80% or better if initial graft function was good. It is interesting to note that the presence of comorbidities in the recipients or interventions to correct these (eg, coronary artery bypass grafting for coronary artery disease) does not seem to affect outcomes.

There is also evidence to suggest that using less atherogenic and less nephrotoxic immunosuppressive regimens can yield graft survival rates comparable to those achieved in younger patients who are transplanted with kidneys from younger donors. [133] The recognition of the importance of initial graft function as a predictor of subsequent graft survival, particularly in elderly recipients of kidneys from older donors, has led to the investigation of various strategies to delay the use of strong immunosuppressive agents, such as tacrolimus and cyclosporine. [134] Decreasing or delaying the use of calcineurin inhibitors appears to enhance the survival of old-for-old transplants. These strategies largely appear to be successful. [135,136] The less vigorous baseline immune response status of older patients may also be beneficial in this regard, with decreased risk of acute rejection (as low as 6% in some series) along with the need to use less exogenous immunosuppression. [127]

Despite the encouraging results from kidney transplantation using older donors and recipients, there are several concerns. The concerns lie more on the merit of pursuing transplants in older recipients rather than the use of kidneys from older donors per se. Recipient age continues to be an independent predictor of graft survival; however, the absolute effect of age on 5-year graft survival, though statistically significant, is small at 2.1%.[137] The larger concern may be the fact that older recipients are more prone to develop chronic allograft nephropathy, which still limits enthusiasm for pursuing transplantation in older recipients.

Modification of This Question in Light of New Research: Most of these data are based on cohort studies, and even though truly randomized prospective trials may be difficult to accrue patients to, further investigation is clearly needed to establish criteria and standards to guide transplantation in the elderly age group.

NEW HORIZONS IN GERIATRIC UROLOGY

ANDROPAUSE

Studies suggest that serum total testosterone levels as well as free testosterone levels decline with age in most men aged 40 to 69 years. There are corresponding increases observed in sex hormone–binding globulin levels. It is estimated that the prevalence of true symptomatic androgen deficiency is 6% to 12%.[138] That would mean a total of 2.4 million men with androgen deficiency, or 480,000 new cases per year. Treatment of such androgen deficiency usually relies on androgen supplementation that carries some concern regarding the risk for either promoting or initiating the growth of unsuspected prostate cancer in these men. Supplementation with dihydrotestosterone gel appears to be acceptable, as it can increase muscle strength and does not appear to affect prostate volume or prostate-specific antigen levels.[139] This is an area of great clinical interest that needs additional research.

Urol 27 (Level A): **The benefit of androgen supplementation in the aging male needs to be determined. The appropriate agents that can be used for androgen supplementation, dose, duration of therapy, and necessary monitoring for concomitant diseases such as benign prostatic hyperplasia and prostate cancer need to be better examined in randomized clinical trials.**

Urol 28 (Level B): **Observational studies will be required to determine the impact of androgen supplementation on the risk of subsequent development of prostate cancer or symptomatic benign prostatic hyperplasia.**

Urol 29 (Levels B, A): **Observational case-control cohort studies will be required to assess the risk and prevalence of osteoporosis in aging men with low sex steroid hormone levels. This could lead to further randomized trials of agents to treat such osteoporosis if it is present.**

ASSESSMENT OF LIFE EXPECTANCY

A reasonably accurate assessment of remaining life expectancy on an individual patient basis is required before initiating therapy for many men or women with various urologic conditions and particularly for issues such as prostate cancer screening. Prostate cancer treatment decisions also often hinge on the likelihood of 10-year life expectancy. Current studies suggest that clinicians can underestimate life expectancy an average of 33% of the time and overestimate it 3.9% of the time. [140] This indicates that certain therapeutic and preventive interventions may be denied to elderly patients on the basis of incorrect estimates of life expectancy. In another study conducted in Canada, physicians were asked to review 18 different patient scenarios and predict life expectancy. Eighty-two percent of the responses correctly estimated life expectancy as being greater than or less than 10 years. However, 67% of responses were accurate within 3 years of actual and only 31% were within 1 year of actual lifespan, evaluated on the basis of Markov modeling. [141] The average error in predicted life expectancy ranged between 2.4 and 5.2 years. Hence, it could be very useful for most medical decision making but particularly for urology to develop tools to assist in more accurate estimation of remaining life expectancy.

> ***Urol 30 (Level B)*: Observational cohort studies to test the accuracy of tools to measure life expectancy in several real-life situations would be useful for more informed therapeutic and other management decisions in treating the older adult.**

REFERENCES

1. Solomon DH, LoCicero J, 3rd, Rosenthal RA (eds): New Frontiers in Geriatrics Research: An Agenda for Surgical and Related Medical Specialties. New York: American Geriatrics Society, 2004 (online at http://www.frycomm.com/ags/rasp).
2. Ukimura O, Kojima M, Inui E, et al. A statistical study of the American Urological Association symptom index for benign prostatic hyperplasia in participants of mass screening program for prostatic diseases using transrectal sonography. J Urol 1996;156:1673-1678.
3. Kawauchi A, Tanaka Y, Soh J, et al. Causes of nocturnal urinary frequency and reasons for its increase with age in healthy older men. J Urol 2000;163:81-84.
4. van Haarst EP, Heldeweg EA, Newling DW, Schlatmann TJ. A cross-sectional study of the international prostate symptom scores related to age and gender in Dutch adults reporting no voiding complaints. Eur Urol 2005;47:334-339.
5. Teunissen D, van Weel C, Lagro-Janssen T. Urinary incontinence in older people living in the community: examining help-seeking behaviour. Br J Gen Pract 2005;55:776-782.
6. Lukacz ES, Lawrence JM, Buckwalter JG, et al. Epidemiology of prolapse and incontinence questionnaire: validation of a new epidemiologic survey. Int Urogynecol J Pelvic Floor Dysfunct 2005;16:272-284.
7. Bradley CS, Kennedy CM, Nygaard IE. Pelvic floor symptoms and lifestyle factors in older women. J Womens Health (Larchmt) 2005;14:128-136.
8. Matza LS, Thompson CL, Krasnow J, et al. Test-retest reliability of four questionnaires for patients with overactive bladder: the Overactive Bladder Questionnaire (OAB-q), Patient Perception of Bladder Condition (PPBC), Urgency Questionnaire (UQ), and the Primary OAB Symptom Questionnaire (POSQ). Neurourol Urodyn 2005;24:215-225.
9. Kirschner-Hermanns R, Scherr PA, Branch LG, et al. Accuracy of survey questions for geriatric urinary incontinence. J Urol 1998;159:1903-1908.

10. Ko Y, Lin SJ, Salmon JW, Bron MS. The impact of urinary incontinence on quality of life of the elderly. Am J Manag Care 2005;11:S103-S111.
11. Finkelstein MM, Skelly J, Kaczorowski J, Swanson G. Incontinence Quality of Life Instrument in a survey of primary care physicians. J Fam Pract 2002;51:952.
12. Patrick DL, Martin ML, Bushnell DM, et al. Quality of life of women with urinary incontinence: further development of the Incontinence Quality of Life Instrument (I-QOL). Urology 1999;53:71-76.
13. Hunskaar S, Vinsnes A. The quality of life in women with urinary incontinence as measured by the Sickness Impact Profile. J Am Geriatr Soc 1991;39:378-382.
14. Raz S. SEAPI QMM incontinence classification system. Neurourol Urodyn 1992;11:187-199.
15. Rosenberg LJ, Griffiths DJ, Resnick NM. Factors that distinguish continent from incontinent older adults with detrusor overactivity. J Urol 2005;174:1868-1872.
16. Goode PS, Burgio KL, Locher JL, et al. Urodynamic changes associated with behavioral and drug treatment of urge incontinence in older women. J Am Geriatr Soc 2002;50:808-816.
17. Chapple CR, Abrams P. Comparison of darifenacin and oxybutynin in patients with overactive bladder: assessment of ambulatory urodynamics and impact on salivary flow. Eur Urol 2005;48:102-109.
18. Duggan PM, Wilson PD, Norton P, et al. Utilization of preoperative urodynamic investigations by gynecologists who frequently operate for female urinary incontinence. Int Urogynecol J Pelvic Floor Dysfunct 2003;14:282-287; discussion 286-287.
19. Digesu GA, Khullar V, Cardozo L, Salvatore S. Overactive bladder symptoms: do we need urodynamics? Neurourol Urodyn 2003;22:105-108.
20. Holtedahl K, Verelst M, Schiefloe A, Hunskaar S. Usefulness of urodynamic examination in female urinary incontinence—lessons from a population-based, randomized, controlled study of conservative treatment. Scand J Urol Nephrol 2000;34:169-174.
21. Weidner AC, Myers ER, Visco AG, et al. Which women with stress incontinence require urodynamic evaluation? Am J Obstet Gynecol 2001;184:20-27.
22. Malone-Lee JG, Walsh JB, Maugourd MF. Tolterodine: a safe and effective treatment for older patients with overactive bladder. J Am Geriatr Soc 2001;49:700-705.
23. Naglie G, Radomski SB, Brymer C, et al. A randomized, double-blind, placebo controlled crossover trial of nimodipine in older persons with detrusor instability and urge incontinence. J Urol 2002;167:586-590.
24. Lipton RB, Kolodner K, Wesnes K. Assessment of cognitive function of the elderly population: effects of darifenacin. J Urol 2005;173:493-498.
25. Krauwinkel WJ, Smulders RA, Mulder H, et al. Effect of age on the pharmacokinetics of solifenacin in men and women. Int J Clin Pharmacol Ther 2005;43:227-238.
26. Johnson TM, 2nd, Burgio KL, Redden DT, et al. Effects of behavioral and drug therapy on nocturia in older incontinent women. J Am Geriatr Soc 2005;53:846-850.
27. Diokno AC, Sampselle CM, Herzog AR, et al. Prevention of urinary incontinence by behavioral modification program: a randomized, controlled trial among older women in the community. J Urol 2004;171:1165-1171.
28. Teunissen TA, de Jonge A, van Weel C, Lagro-Janssen AL. Treating urinary incontinence in the elderly—conservative therapies that work: a systematic review. J Fam Pract 2004;53:25-30, 32.
29. Bergstrom K, Carlsson CP, Lindholm C, Widengren R. Improvement of urge- and mixed-type incontinence after acupuncture treatment among elderly women—a pilot study. J Auton Nerv Syst 2000;79:173-180.
30. Emmons SL, Otto L. Acupuncture for overactive bladder: a randomized controlled trial. Obstet Gynecol 2005;106:138-143.

31. Ghei M, Maraj BH, Miller R, et al. Effects of botulinum toxin B on refractory detrusor overactivity: a randomized, double-blind, placebo controlled, crossover trial. J Urol 2005;174:1873-1877; discussion 1877.
32. Carey JM, Leach GE. Transvaginal surgery in the octogenarian using cadaveric fascia for pelvic prolapse and stress incontinence: minimal one-year results compared to younger patients. Urology 2004;63:665-670.
33. Carr LK, Walsh PJ, Abraham VE, Webster GD. Favorable outcome of pubovaginal slings for geriatric women with stress incontinence. J Urol 1997;157:125-128.
34. Peattie AB, Stanton SL. The Stamey operation for correction of genuine stress incontinence in the elderly woman. Br J Obstet Gynaecol 1989;96:983-986.
35. Nitti VW, Bregg KJ, Sussman EM, Raz S. The Raz bladder neck suspension in patients 65 years old and older. J Urol 1993;149:802-807.
36. Holmgren C, Nilsson S, Lanner L, Hellberg D. Long-term results with tension-free vaginal tape on mixed and stress urinary incontinence. Obstet Gynecol 2005;106:38-43.
37. Bukkapatnam R, Shah S, Raz S, Rodriguez L. Anterior vaginal wall surgery in elderly patients: outcomes and assessment. Urology 2005;65:1104-1108.
38. Schweitzer KJ, Vierhout ME, Milani AL. Surgery for pelvic organ prolapse in women of 80 years of age and older. Acta Obstet Gynecol Scand 2005;84:286-289.
39. Maher CF, O'Reilly BA, Dwyer PL, et al. Pubovaginal sling versus transurethral Macroplastique for stress urinary incontinence and intrinsic sphincter deficiency: a prospective randomised controlled trial. BJOG 2005;112:797-801.
40. Truijen G, Wyndaele JJ, Weyler J. Conservative treatment of stress urinary incontinence in women: who will benefit? Int Urogynecol J Pelvic Floor Dysfunct 2001;12:386-390.
41. Cammu H, Van Nylen M, Blockeel C, et al. Who will benefit from pelvic floor muscle training for stress urinary incontinence? Am J Obstet Gynecol 2004;191:1152-1157.
42. Burgio KL, Goode PS, Locher JL, et al. Predictors of outcome in the behavioral treatment of urinary incontinence in women. Obstet Gynecol 2003;102:940-947.
43. Gray M, McClain R, Peruggia M, et al. A model for predicting motor urge urinary incontinence. Nurs Res 2001;50:116-122.
44. Nuotio M, Tammela TL, Luukkaala T, Jylha M. Urgency and urge incontinence in an older population: ten-year changes and their association with mortality. Aging Clin Exp Res 2002;14:412-419.
45. Ruben FL, Dearwater SR, Norden CW, et al. Clinical infections in the noninstitutionalized geriatric age group: methods utilized and incidence of infections. The Pittsburgh Good Health Study. Am J Epidemiol 1995;141:145-157.
46. Nicolle LE. Urinary infections in the elderly: symptomatic of asymptomatic? Int J Antimicrob Agents 1999;11:265-268.
47. Walker S, McGeer A, Simor AE, et al. Why are antibiotics prescribed for asymptomatic bacteriuria in institutionalized elderly people? A qualitative study of physicians' and nurses' perceptions. CMAJ 2000;163:273-277.
48. Dessole S, Rubattu G, Ambrosini G, et al. Efficacy of low-dose intravaginal estriol on urogenital aging in postmenopausal women. Menopause 2004;11:49-56.
49. Raz R, Colodner R, Rohana Y, et al. Effectiveness of estriol-containing vaginal pessaries and nitrofurantoin macrocrystal therapy in the prevention of recurrent urinary tract infection in postmenopausal women. Clin Infect Dis 2003;36:1362-1368.
50. Baan AH, Vermeulen H, van der Meulen J, et al. The effect of suprapubic catheterization versus transurethral catheterization after abdominal surgery on urinary tract infection: a randomized controlled trial. Dig Surg 2003;20:290-295.
51. Brown JS, Vittinghoff E, Kanaya AM, et al. Urinary tract infections in postmenopausal women: effect of hormone therapy and risk factors. Obstet Gynecol 2001;98:1045-1052.

52. Setia U, Serventi I, Lorenz P. Nosocomial infections among patients in a long-term care facility: spectrum, prevalence, and risk factors. Am J Infect Control 1985;13:57-62.
53. Franson TR, Duthie EH, Jr., Cooper JE, et al. Prevalence survey of infections and their predisposing factors at a hospital-based nursing home care unit. J Am Geriatr Soc 1986;34:95-100.
54. Warren JW, Palumbo FB, Fitterman L, Speedie SM. Incidence and characteristics of antibiotic use in aged nursing home patients. J Am Geriatr Soc 1991;39:963-972.
55. Zimmer JG, Bentley DW, Valenti WM, Watson NM. Systemic antibiotic use in nursing homes: a quality assessment. J Am Geriatr Soc 1986;34:703-710.
56. Loeb M, Brazil K, Lohfeld L, et al. Optimizing antibiotics in residents of nursing homes: protocol of a randomized trial. BMC Health Serv Res 2002;2:17.
57. Vogel T, Verreault R, Gourdeau M, et al. Optimal duration of antibiotic therapy for uncomplicated urinary tract infection in older women: a double-blind randomized controlled trial. CMAJ 2004;170:469-473.
58. Gomolin IH, Siami PF, Reuning-Scherer J, et al. Efficacy and safety of ciprofloxacin oral suspension versus trimethoprim-sulfamethoxazole oral suspension for treatment of older women with acute urinary tract infection. J Am Geriatr Soc 2001;49:1606-1613.
59. Tzias V, Dontas AS, Petrikkos G, et al. Three-day antibiotic therapy in bacteriuria of old age. J Antimicrob Chemother 1990;26:705-711.
60. Lutters M, Vogt N. Antibiotic duration for treating uncomplicated, symptomatic lower urinary tract infections in elderly women. Cochrane Database Syst Rev 2002:CD001535.
61. Kauffman CA, Vazquez JA, Sobel JD, et al. Prospective multicenter surveillance study of funguria in hospitalized patients. The National Institute for Allergy and Infectious Diseases (NIAID) Mycoses Study Group. Clin Infect Dis 2000;30:14-18.
62. Sobel JD, Kauffman CA, McKinsey D, et al. Candiduria: a randomized, double-blind study of treatment with fluconazole and placebo. The National Institute of Allergy and Infectious Diseases (NIAID) Mycoses Study Group. Clin Infect Dis 2000;30:19-24.
63. Gross AJ, Busse M, Leonard J, Schumacher H. Switch from phytotherapy to tamsulosin in patients with lower urinary tract symptoms suggestive of benign prostatic hyperplasia (LUTS/BPH). Prostate Cancer Prostatic Dis 2005;8:210-214.
64. Debruyne F, Koch G, Boyle P, et al. Comparison of a phytotherapeutic agent (Permixon) with an alpha-blocker (Tamsulosin) in the treatment of benign prostatic hyperplasia: a 1-year randomized international study. Eur Urol 2002;41:497-506; discussion 506-497.
65. Yamanishi T, Yasuda K, Kamai T, et al. Single-blind, randomized controlled study of the clinical and urodynamic effects of an alpha-blocker (naftopidil) and phytotherapy (eviprostat) in the treatment of benign prostatic hyperplasia. Int J Urol 2004;11:501-509.
66. Boyle P, Robertson C, Lowe F, Roehrborn C. Meta-analysis of clinical trials of permixon in the treatment of symptomatic benign prostatic hyperplasia. Urology 2000;55:533-539.
67. Bent S, Kane C, Shinohara K, et al. Saw palmetto for benign prostatic hyperplasia. N Engl J Med 2006;354:557-566.
68. Wilt T, Ishani A, Mac Donald R, et al. Pygeum africanum for benign prostatic hyperplasia. Cochrane Database Syst Rev 2002:CD001044.
69. Wilt T, Ishani A, MacDonald R, et al. Beta-sitosterols for benign prostatic hyperplasia. Cochrane Database Syst Rev 2000:CD001043.
70. Wilt T, Mac Donald R, Ishani A, et al. Cernilton for benign prostatic hyperplasia. Cochrane Database Syst Rev 2000:CD001042.
71. Hill B, Belville W, Bruskewitz R, et al. Transurethral needle ablation versus transurethral resection of the prostate for the treatment of symptomatic benign prostatic hyperplasia: 5-year results of a prospective, randomized, multicenter clinical trial. J Urol 2004;171:2336-2340.

72. Chandrasekar P, Virdi JS, Kapasi F. Transurethral needle ablation of the prostate (TUNA)—a prospective randomized study, long-term results [abstract]. J Urol 2003;169:463. Abstract 1754.
73. Boyle P, Robertson C, Vaughan ED, Fitzpatrick JM. A meta-analysis of trials of transurethral needle ablation for treating symptomatic benign prostatic hyperplasia. BJU Int 2004;94:83-88.
74. Hoffman RM, MacDonald R, Monga M, Wilt TJ. Transurethral microwave thermotherapy vs transurethral resection for treating benign prostatic hyperplasia: a systematic review. BJU Int 2004;94:1031-1036.
75. Gupta N, Sivaramakrishna, Kumar R, et al. Comparison of standard transurethral resection, transurethral vapour resection and holmium laser enucleation of the prostate for managing benign prostatic hyperplasia of >40 g. BJU Int 2006;97:85-89.
76. Montorsi F, Naspro R, Salonia A, et al. Holmium laser enucleation versus transurethral resection of the prostate: results from a 2-center, prospective, randomized trial in patients with obstructive benign prostatic hyperplasia. J Urol 2004;172:1926-1929.
77. Souverein PC, Erkens JA, de la Rosette JJ, et al. Drug treatment of benign prostatic hyperplasia and hospital admission for BPH-related surgery. Eur Urol 2003;43:528-534.
78. Vela-Navarrete R, Gonzalez-Enguita C, Garcia-Cardoso JV, et al. The impact of medical therapy on surgery for benign prostatic hyperplasia: a study comparing changes in a decade (1992-2002). BJU Int 2005;96:1045-1048.
79. Naslund MJ, Carlson AM, Williams MJ. A cost comparison of medical management and transurethral needle ablation for treatment of benign prostatic hyperplasia during a 5-year period. J Urol 2005;173:2090-2093; discussion 2093.
80. De La Rosette JJ, Floratos DL, Severens JL, et al. Transurethral resection vs microwave thermotherapy of the prostate: a cost-consequences analysis. BJU Int 2003;92:713-718.
81. Manyak MJ, Ackerman SJ, Blute ML, et al. Cost effectiveness of treatment for benign prostatic hyperplasia: an economic model for comparison of medical, minimally invasive, and surgical therapy. J Endourol 2002;16:51-56.
82. Bo M, Ventura M, Marinello R, et al. Relationship between prostatic specific antigen (PSA) and volume of the prostate in the benign prostatic hyperplasia in the elderly. Crit Rev Oncol Hematol 2003;47:207-211.
83. McNaughton Collins M, Stafford RS, Barry MJ. Age-specific patterns of prostate-specific antigen testing among primary care physician visits. J Fam Pract 2000;49:169-172.
84. Dyche DJ, Ness J, West M, et al. Prevalence of prostate specific antigen testing for prostate cancer in elderly men. J Urol 2006;175:2078-2082.
85. McNaughton Collins M, Barry MJ, Zietman A, et al. United States radiation oncologists' and urologists' opinions about screening and treatment of prostate cancer vary by region. Urology 2002;60:628-633.
86. Holmberg L, Bill-Axelson A, Helgesen F, et al. A randomized trial comparing radical prostatectomy with watchful waiting in early prostate cancer. N Engl J Med 2002;347:781-789.
87. Bill-Axelson A, Holmberg L, Ruutu M, et al. Radical prostatectomy versus watchful waiting in early prostate cancer. N Engl J Med 2005;352:1977-1984.
88. Soulie M, Straub M, Game X, et al. A multicenter study of the morbidity of radical cystectomy in select elderly patients with bladder cancer. J Urol 2002;167:1325-1328.
89. Chang SS, Alberts G, Cookson MS, Smith JA, Jr. Radical cystectomy is safe in elderly patients at high risk. J Urol 2001;166:938-941.
90. Konety BR, Dhawan V, Allareddy V, Joslyn SA. Impact of hospital and surgeon volume on in-hospital mortality from radical cystectomy: data from the health care utilization project. J Urol 2005;173:1695-1700.

91. Kattan MW, Reuter V, Motzer RJ, et al. A postoperative prognostic nomogram for renal cell carcinoma. J Urol 2001;166:63-67.
92. Motzer RJ, Bacik J, Schwartz LH, et al. Prognostic factors for survival in previously treated patients with metastatic renal cell carcinoma. J Clin Oncol 2004;22:454-463.
93. Saigal CS, Wessells H, Pace J, et al. Predictors and prevalence of erectile dysfunction in a racially diverse population. Arch Intern Med 2006;166:207-212.
94. Thompson IM, Tangen CM, Goodman PJ, et al. Erectile dysfunction and subsequent cardiovascular disease. JAMA 2005;294:2996-3002.
95. Blumentals WA, Gomez-Caminero A, Joo S, Vannappagari V. Is erectile dysfunction predictive of peripheral vascular disease? Aging Male 2003;6:217-221.
96. Gazzaruso C, Giordanetti S, De Amici E, et al. Relationship between erectile dysfunction and silent myocardial ischemia in apparently uncomplicated type 2 diabetic patients. Circulation 2004;110:22-26.
97. Simsek I, Aslan G, Akarsu M, et al. Assessment of sexual functions in patients with chronic liver disease. Int J Impot Res 2005;17:343-345.
98. Giuliano FA, Leriche A, Jaudinot EO, de Gendre AS. Prevalence of erectile dysfunction among 7689 patients with diabetes or hypertension, or both. Urology 2004;64:1196-1201.
99. Rosen RC, Fisher WA, Eardley I, et al. The multinational Men's Attitudes to Life Events and Sexuality (MALES) study: I: prevalence of erectile dysfunction and related health concerns in the general population. Curr Med Res Opin 2004;20:607-617.
100. Shiri R, Koskimaki J, Hakkinen J, et al. Effects of age, comorbidity and lifestyle factors on erectile function: Tampere Ageing Male Urological Study (TAMUS). Eur Urol 2004;45:628-633.
101. Barqawi A, O'Donnell C, Kumar R, et al. Correlation between LUTS (AUA-SS) and erectile dysfunction (SHIM) in an age-matched racially diverse male population: data from the Prostate Cancer Awareness Week (PCAW). Int J Impot Res 2005;17:370-374.
102. Elliott SP, Gulati M, Pasta DJ, et al. Obstructive lower urinary tract symptoms correlate with erectile dysfunction. Urology 2004;63:1148-1152.
103. Berman JR, Berman LA, Toler SM, et al. Safety and efficacy of sildenafil citrate for the treatment of female sexual arousal disorder: a double-blind, placebo controlled study. J Urol 2003;170:2333-2338.
104. Basson R, McInnes R, Smith MD, et al. Efficacy and safety of sildenafil citrate in women with sexual dysfunction associated with female sexual arousal disorder. J Womens Health Gend Based Med 2002;11:367-377.
105. Basson R, Brotto LA. Sexual psychophysiology and effects of sildenafil citrate in oestrogenised women with acquired genital arousal disorder and impaired orgasm: a randomised controlled trial. BJOG 2003;110:1014-1024.
106. Fujisawa M, Sawada K. Clinical efficacy and safety of sildenafil in elderly patients with erectile dysfunction. Arch Androl 2004;50:255-260.
107. Rendell MS, Rajfer J, Wicker PA, Smith MD. Sildenafil for treatment of erectile dysfunction in men with diabetes: a randomized controlled trial. Sildenafil Diabetes Study Group. JAMA 1999;281:421-426.
108. Wagner G, Montorsi F, Auerbach S, Collins M. Sildenafil citrate (VIAGRA) improves erectile function in elderly patients with erectile dysfunction: a subgroup analysis. J Gerontol A Biol Sci Med Sci 2001;56:M113-M119.
109. Brock GB, McMahon CG, Chen KK, et al. Efficacy and safety of tadalafil for the treatment of erectile dysfunction: results of integrated analyses. J Urol 2002;168:1332-1336.
110. Finelli A, Hirshberg ED, Radomski SB. The treatment choice of elderly patients with erectile dysfunction. Geriatr Nephrol Urol 1998;8:15-19.

111. Richter S, Vardi Y, Ringel A, et al. Intracavernous injections: still the gold standard for treatment of erectile dysfunction in elderly men. Int J Impot Res 2001;13:172-175.
112. Shabsigh R, Padma-Nathan H, Gittleman M, et al. Intracavernous alprostadil alfadex (EDEX/VIRIDAL) is effective and safe in patients with erectile dysfunction after failing sildenafil (Viagra). Urology 2000;55:477-480.
113. Shabsigh R, Padma-Nathan H, Gittleman M, et al. Intracavernous alprostadil alfadex is more efficacious, better tolerated, and preferred over intraurethral alprostadil plus optional actis: a comparative, randomized, crossover, multicenter study. Urology 2000;55:109-113.
114. Israilov S, Shmuely J, Niv E, et al. Evaluation of a progressive treatment program for erectile dysfunction in patients with diabetes mellitus. Int J Impot Res 2005;17:431-436.
115. Robertson WG, Peacock M, Heyburn PJ. Clinical and metabolic aspects of urinary stone disease in Leeds. Scand J Urol Nephrol Suppl 1980;53:199-206.
116. Koide T, Itatani H, Yoshioka T, et al. Clinical manifestations of calcium oxalate monohydrate and dihydrate urolithiasis. J Urol 1982;127:1067-1069.
117. Daudon M, Donsimoni R, Hennequin C, et al. Sex- and age-related composition of 10 617 calculi analyzed by infrared spectroscopy. Urol Res 1995;23:319-326.
118. Daudon M, Dore JC, Jungers P, Lacour B. Changes in stone composition according to age and gender of patients: a multivariate epidemiological approach. Urol Res 2004;32:241-247.
119. Usui Y, Matsuzaki S, Matsushita K, Shima M. Urolithiasis in geriatric patients. Tokai J Exp Clin Med 2003;28:81-87.
120. Hall WD, Pettinger M, Oberman A, et al. Risk factors for kidney stones in older women in the southern United States. Am J M ed Sci 2001;322:12-18.
121. Abate N, Chandalia M, Cabo-Chan AV, Jr., et al. The metabolic syndrome and uric acid nephrolithiasis: novel features of renal manifestation of insulin resistance. Kidney Int 2004;65:386-392.
122. Ford ES, Giles WH, Dietz WH. Prevalence of the metabolic syndrome among US adults: findings from the third National Health and Nutrition Examination Survey. JAMA 2002;287:356-359.
123. Sabbuba NA, Stickler DJ, Mahenthiralingam E, et al. Genotyping demonstrates that the strains of *Proteus mirabilis* from bladder stones and catheter encrustations of patients undergoing long-term bladder catheterization are identical. J Urol 2004;171:1925-1928.
124. Heller HJ, Sakhaee K, Moe OW, Pak CY. Etiological role of estrogen status in renal stone formation. J Urol 2002;168:1923-1927.
125. Woo YM, Gill JS, Johnson N, et al. The advanced age deceased kidney donor: current outcomes and future opportunities. Kidney Int 2005;67:2407-2414.
126. Oppenheimer F, Aljama P, Asensio Peinado C, et al. The impact of donor age on the results of renal transplantation. Nephrol Dial Transplant 2004;19 Suppl 3:iii11-15.
127. Friedman AL, Goker O, Kalish MA, et al. Renal transplant recipients over aged 60 have diminished immune activity and a low risk of rejection. Int Urol Nephrol 2004;36:451-456.
128. Cohen B, Smits JM, Haase B, et al. Expanding the donor pool to increase renal transplantation. Nephrol Dial Transplant 2005;20:34-41.
129. Boggi U, Barsotti M, Collini A, et al. Kidney transplantation from donors aged 65 years or more as single or dual grafts. Transplant Proc 2005;37:577-580.
130. Moreso F, Ortega F, Mendiluce A. Recipient age as a determinant factor of patient and graft survival. Nephrol Dial Transplant 2004;19 Suppl 3:iii16-20.
131. Oniscu GC, Brown H, Forsythe JL. How old is old for transplantation? Am J Transplant 2004;4:2067-2074.
132. Smits JM, Persijn GG, van Houwelingen HC, et al. Evaluation of the Eurotransplant Senior Program: the results of the first year. Am J Transplant 2002;2:664-670.

133. Arbogast H, Huckelheim H, Schneeberger H, et al. A calcineurin antagonist-free induction/maintenance strategy for immunosuppression in elderly recipients of renal allografts from elderly cadaver donors: long-term results from a prospective single centre trial. Clin Transplant 2005;19:309-315.
134. Gentil MA, Osuna A, Capdevila L, et al. Safety and efficacy of delayed introduction of low-dose tacrolimus in elderly recipients of cadaveric renal transplants from donors over 55 years of age. Transplant Proc 2003;35:1706-1708.
135. Bosmuller C, Ollinger R, Mark W, et al. Excellent results with calcineurin inhibitor-free initial immunosuppression in old recipients of old kidneys. Transplant Proc 2005;37:881-883.
136. Segoloni GP, Messina M, Squiccimarro G, et al. Preferential allocation of marginal kidney allografts to elderly recipients combined with modified immunosuppression gives good results. Transplantation 2005;80:953-958.
137. Gjertson DW. A multi-factor analysis of kidney graft outcomes at one and five years post-transplantation: 1996 UNOS update. Clin Transpl 1996:343-360.
138. Araujo AB, O'Donnell AB, Brambilla DJ, et al. Prevalence and incidence of androgen deficiency in middle-aged and older men: estimates from the Massachusetts Male Aging Study. J Clin Endocrinol Metab 2004;89:5920-5926.
139. Ly LP, Jimenez M, Zhuang TN, et al. A double-blind, placebo-controlled, randomized clinical trial of transdermal dihydrotestosterone gel on muscular strength, mobility, and quality of life in older men with partial androgen deficiency. J Clin Endocrinol Metab 2001;86:4078-4088.
140. Wilson JR, Clarke MG, Ewings P, et al. The assessment of patient life-expectancy: how accurate are urologists and oncologists? BJU Int 2005;95:794-798.
141. Krahn MD, Bremner KE, Asaria J, et al. The ten-year rule revisited: accuracy of clinicians' estimates of life expectancy in patients with localized prostate cancer. Urology 2002;60:258-263.

11

GERIATRIC ORTHOPEDICS

*Susan Day, MD; Robert Karpman, MD**

Research on orthopedic management of elderly patients is of critical importance, given the high risk for musculoskeletal disorders among older adults. For a summary of the incidence and prevalence of musculoskeletal disorders among adults aged 65 and older, see the opening section of the chapter on geriatric orthopedics in *New Frontiers in Geriatrics Research* (p. 303).[1] This chapter updates that review of research in geriatric orthopedics, noting for each topic the new research that has been described in the literature. Research in geriatric orthopedics conducted since the publication of *New Frontiers* suggests no new research topics for the research agenda in this area and no new Key Questions for this specialty.

With regard to the Key Questions posed in *New Frontiers* (see below), there is still much to be learned regarding the influence of aging on fracture healing. Augmentation of fracture healing in aged bone requires further investigation. Techniques of internal fixation have received some study. Locking plates, plates that have screw holes that are threaded which allow screws to lock into the plate, have been shown to be useful in treating fractures when bone quality is poor. They have been shown to be helpful in achieving fracture union with minimal complications in proximal humeral,[2] humeral diaphyseal,[3] and distal radius factures.[4] Randomized clinical trials are needed to compare this method of treatment in other osteoporotic fractures.

***Ortho KQ1*: How can implant fixation in osteoporotic bone be improved?**

***Ortho KQ2*: How can fracture healing in the aged person be enhanced?**

***Ortho KQ3*: How can the outcomes after fracture be optimized in elderly patients?**

METHODS

A search was conducted on the National Library of Medicine's PubMed database for the years 2000 to 2005; limits applied to the search were age greater than 65 and articles in English. The key words used were *osteoporosis, total hip arthroplasty, total knee arthroplasty, total shoulder arthroplasty, vertebroplasty, spinal stenosis, distal radius fractures, osteoarthritis, foot and ankle, fracture healing.*

* Day: Clinical Instructor, Michigan State University, Grand Rapids Orthopaedics Residency Program, Grand Rapids, MI; Karpman: Vice-President of Medical Affairs, Caritas Holy Family Hospital, Methuen, MA.

PROGRESS IN GERIATRIC ORTHOPEDICS

NORMAL MUSCULOSKELETAL AGING AND THE AGING ATHLETE

See *New Frontiers,* p. 304.

Ortho 1 (Level B): **Observational studies are needed to define the normal range of motion of the extremities in older people without musculoskeletal disease. Such studies should also examine the range of motion necessary for activities of daily living and instrumental activities of daily living.**

Ortho 2 (Level D): **Observational studies of older athletes are needed to define the incidence and nature of sports-related injuries in older athletes and to examine the utility of arthroscopy in the treatment of knee and shoulder injuries.**

New Research Addressing These Questions: No reports of new research on these questions were identified.

Modification of These Questions in Light of New Research: These items should remain unchanged on the research agenda for geriatric orthopedics.

FACTORS THAT INFLUENCE POSTOPERATIVE OUTCOME

See *New Frontiers,* p. 305.

Ortho 3 (Level B): **Observational and case-control studies are needed to determine the elements of preoperative evaluation and treatment that are associated with reduction in mortality in older orthopedic surgery patients.**

Ortho 4 (Level B): **Case-control studies are needed to compare the incidence of malnutrition among older hip fracture patients to that in the general population of older adults. Databases examining risk factors for hip fracture should be expanded (when possible) to include detailed nutritional measures.**

Ortho 5 (Levels B, A): **Observational studies using multivariate regression analysis are needed to identify which nutritional deficiencies (eg, calcium, protein) appear to be predictive of bad outcomes following hip surgery in older patients. Randomized controlled trials based on these findings are then needed to determine the type and duration of nutritional supplementation that would most effectively improve surgical outcome and fracture healing.**

New Research Addressing These Questions: No reports of new research on these questions were identified.

Modification of These Questions in Light of New Research: These items should remain unchanged on the research agenda for geriatric orthopedics.

DEGENERATIVE JOINT DISEASE

See *New Frontiers,* pp. 306–307.

Ortho 6 (Level B): **Basic studies are needed to determine the mechanism of action of hylan and hyaluronate injections in providing long-term pain relief from knee arthritis. Additional clinical studies are needed to examine the long-term effect on cartilage in older persons during repeated courses of treatment.**

Ortho 7 (Level A): **A randomized clinical trial is needed to examine if hylan and hyaluronate injections delay or reduce the likelihood of total knee arthroplasty in elderly patients.**

Ortho 8 (Level B): **Existing databases should be examined (or expanded) in an effort to determine the independent contribution that hip or knee osteoarthritis holds as a risk factor for falls by older people.**

Ortho 9 (Level B): **Databases examining the effects of joint replacement surgery should assess baseline and postoperative rates of falling to determine the effects of replacement on falls risk in older persons.**

Ortho 10 (Level B): **Further laboratory and clinical studies of COX-2 inhibitors should examine the effects of these agents in older persons on fracture healing, tissue healing (eg, after rotator cuff injury), and on bony ingrowth (into joint replacements).**

Ortho 11 (Level B): **Case-control studies should examine the surgical and functional outcome in older patients for various methods of fixation and various surgical approaches in total hip replacement. Such studies should examine the outcomes for cementless components in osteoporotic bone.**

Ortho 12 (Levels B, A): **Observational studies are needed to define the outcome of revision hip surgery in elderly patients. Careful reporting of factors associated with outcome would help define future level A studies to further define the optimal approach to this problem.**

Ortho 13 (Level D): **Basic laboratory studies are needed to define the influence of age on the cellular response to wear debris.**

Ortho 14 (Level B): **Observational studies are needed to define the type of hip procedure (cemented or uncemented) that is associated with the lower incidence of periprosthetic fractures in elderly patients. Additional observational studies are needed to generate information on the outcomes of various treatments for periprosthetic fractures in preparation for hypothesis-testing studies.**

Ortho 15 (Level B): **Observational studies are needed to define the**

subpopulation of older patients who might respond to arthroscopy or meniscectomy.

Ortho 16 (Level B): **Observational studies are needed to identify older patients at risk for less than optimal outcome after total knee arthroplasty, for example, those with peripheral vascular disease or neuropathy.**

Ortho 17 (Level B): **Additional observational studies focused on patients aged 85 years and over who undergo total knee arthroplasty are needed to identify risk factors for postoperative morbidity and to begin to define interventional strategies to reduce that risk.**

Ortho 18 (Level D): **Case-control studies are needed to determine whether metal-backed or all-polyethylene tibial components should be used in arthroplasty for elderly patients and whether there are indications for each.**

Ortho 19 (Level B): **Observational studies of older patients undergoing treatment for comminuted distal femur fractures are needed to examine the possible utility of total knee arthroplasty as a reconstructive procedure in this setting.**

Ortho 20 (Level B): **Observational studies are needed to further define those benefits of total knee arthroplasty (eg, increased range of motion, increased strength, decreased pain) which serve to improve gait and balance. Ultimately, such studies may begin to determine whether or not total knee arthroplasty helps to reduce the risk of hip fracture.**

Ortho 21 (Level B): **Case-control or focused cohort studies are needed to compare functional outcomes in older people with shoulder disease who do not undergo surgery with those who undergo rotator cuff surgery, hemiarthroplasty, or total shoulder replacement. Key outcomes for comparison include improved function and decreased pain. Such studies should address how the desired outcomes may change with age, from those aged 65 to 75 years to those aged 90 years and over.**

Ortho 22 (Level A): **Randomized controlled clinical trials are needed of the various preventive regimens (alone or in combination) to identify the safest and most effective treatment strategy for preventing thromboembolism after joint replacement surgery in older patients. Such studies should also address how long deep-vein thrombosis prophylaxis should continue in elderly patients who have had recent total joint replacements or hip fracture.**

Ortho 23 (Level B): **Further retrospective studies are needed to examine risk factors beyond age and poor bone quality for periprosthetic fractures. Case-control studies could possibly suggest protective factors, such as the nature of the implant (cemented or uncemented) and the use of antiresorptive therapies.**

Ortho 24 (Level A): **Randomized controlled trials are needed to determine with certainty whether specific prostheses or antiresorptive therapies would be effective at minimizing the risk of periprosthetic fracture.**

Ortho 25 (Level B): **Observational studies and subgroup analyses are needed to determine if features of periprosthetic infections are different in elderly patients and to examine differences in outcome for elderly patients when specific established or emerging approaches are used.**

New Research in Surgical Treatment of Degenerative Joint Disease: See *New Frontiers,* p. 307.

Arthroplasty of either the hip or knee performed in elderly patients 89 years of age and older was found to have a perioperative complication rate of 14% in a review of 101 arthroplasties performed in this age group. [5] Significantly improved function and decreased pain has been demonstrated following total hip arthroplasty [5,6] and total knee arthroplasty [5] in the very elderly patient.

New Research in Degenerative Disease of the Hip: See *New Frontiers,* pp. 307–308.

In patients aged 75 years and older, cementless fixation has been found to be successful. Tapered, cementless femoral components have been found, in one study, to have 100% survivability at 5 years in patients aged 75 years and older. [7] These tapered, cementless stems have also been found to be successful in treating periprosthetic fractures. [8] In a study evaluating the use of a modular, proximally porous-coated femoral stem and a cementless acetabular component in 135 patients, no revisions for loosening were needed at 5 years. [9] Still another study found 100% survivability of the acetabular and femoral component 78 months postoperatively in patients older than 80 years. [10] Hemiarthroplasty performed for femoral neck fracture can also be successfully treated with a cementless stem. A retrospective review of over 250 patients with cementless bipolar hemiarthroplasties found that all but two had stable stems with bony ingrowth and a low revision rate at 3.5 years. [11]

A retrospective review of 60 patients treated with a total hip arthroplasty for a femoral neck fracture found that they did not have greater perioperative morbidity than 30 patients who had total hip arthroplasty for osteoarthritis. [12] Likewise, a separate study of 51 patients with subcapital hip fractures treated by total hip replacement found function on follow-up that was comparable to that of osteoarthritic patients treated by total hip replacement. [13]

Patients evaluated following total hip arthroplasty have been found to have improved balance during gait and sit-to-stand activities. Control of trunk velocity, however, was not improved by total hip replacement. [14]

New Research in Degenerative Disease of the Knee: See *New Frontiers,* pp. 308–309.

A review of 110 total knee arthroplasties in 90 patients aged 80 years and older found that after 10 years, even though 96% had complete pain relief and 91% had an excellent knee score, only 14% had an excellent function score. [15]

Cementless fixation has also been evaluated with respect to total knee arthroplasty. One prospective study evaluating a hydroxyapatite-coated, cementless total knee replacement found that at 5 years, patients aged 75 years and older had results equivalent to those of younger patients.[16]

In a review of 6 patients, constrained total knee arthroplasty was reported to be a successful method for treating periarticular distal femur and proximal tibia fractures.[17]

New Research in Degenerative Disease of the Shoulder: See *New Frontiers,* pp. 309–310.

A meta-analysis found that after 2 years of follow-up, total shoulder arthroplasty performed better than hemiarthroplasty for osteoarthritis of the shoulder.[18] Arthroscopic acromioplasty for chronic rotator cuff tears has been shown to be helpful when conservative measures have failed.[19]

New Research in Complications of Joint Replacement Surgery: See *New Frontiers,* pp. 310–312. No reports of new research on this topic were found.

Modification of Questions on Degenerative Joint Disease in Light of New Research: The recent research on various aspects of the surgical treatment of degenerative joint disease in the elderly patient summarized herein indicates no need for changes or deletions in the research agenda for this important topic.

DEGENERATIVE SPINE DISEASE

See *New Frontiers,* pp. 315–316.

> ***Ortho 26 (Level B)*: Observational studies are needed to examine the impact of aging on bone fusion or fracture healing and to begin examining strategies to augment the bone healing response after fusion or fracture. Candidate strategies include growth factors.**

> ***Ortho 27 (Level B)*: Case-control or focused cohort studies are needed to refine understanding of which patients benefit (in terms of symptom control and function) most from spinal decompression versus conservative management. Important covariates include duration of symptoms and degree of neurologic deficits and perhaps the degree of osteoporosis. Such studies should attempt to clarify when elderly patients should be referred for spinal decompression in order to experience maximum benefit.**

New Research Addressing These Questions: No reports of new research on these questions were identified.

Modification of These Questions in Light of New Research: These items should remain unchanged on the research agenda for geriatric orthopedics.

DEGENERATIVE DISEASE OF THE FOOT AND ANKLE

See *New Frontiers,* pp. 316–317.

> ***Ortho 28 (Level B)*: Observational studies examining how foot and ankle deformity influence gait and balance in the older person are**

needed. Those deformities that are associated with significant gait problems should be the focus of research on surgical and nonsurgical approaches to these conditions. Appropriate outcome measures (eg, healing, gait improvement) from specific techniques of foot and ankle reconstruction need to be defined. In addition, more study is needed to identify characteristics of footwear that maximize balance.

***Ortho 29 (Level C)*: Controlled trials are needed to identify safe and effective treatment for fungal disease of the foot.**

New Research Addressing These Questions: No reports of new research on these questions were identified.

Modification of These Questions in Light of New Research: These items should remain unchanged on the research agenda for geriatric orthopedics.

BONE INSUFFICIENCY AND FALLS

See *New Frontiers,* pp. 317–318.

***Ortho 30 (Level A)*: Adequately powered randomized clinical trials are needed to determine if falls-prevention strategies for older persons will translate into fracture reduction for treated patients.**

***Ortho 31 (Level A)*: Cohort studies or randomized controlled trials are needed to compare the functional recovery of patients whose fractures occur close to a joint and who are treated with either total joint replacement or standard care.**

***Ortho 32 (Level B)*: Methodologic studies are needed to describe outcomes with various approaches to fixation in osteopenic bone.**

New Research Addressing These Questions: No reports of new research on these questions were identified.

Modification of These Questions in Light of New Research: These items should remain unchanged on the research agenda for geriatric orthopedics.

FRACTURES OF THE HIP

See *New Frontiers,* pp. 318–321.

***Ortho 33 (Level B)*: Observational studies are needed to examine the effect of shortening of the fractured limb on gait and balance.**

***Ortho 34 (Level B)*: Observational studies are needed to learn whether modalities such as electrical stimulation or ultrasound can speed the fracture healing response in the older patient and therefore decrease fracture collapse or hardware failure.**

***Ortho 35 (Level B)*: Methodologic studies are needed to identify elderly patients with hip fracture who are at high risk for operative intervention and postoperative complications and to devise clinical pathways for their care. Database analyses of the pre-hospital,**

in-hospital, and rehabilitation periods of elderly orthopedic patients should be performed to identify clinical management strategies that result in decreased morbidity and improved functional recovery.

Ortho 36 (Level A): **Controlled trials are needed to compare outcomes using cement and noncemented hardware for hemiarthroplasty. Additional controlled trials are needed to compare techniques for repair of intertrochanteric hip fractures.**

Ortho 37 (Level B): **Current clinical databases should be expanded to include long-term and functional outcomes of older orthopedic surgical patients recovering from hip fracture.**

New Research Addressing These Questions: Treatment of femoral neck fractures remains varied. A survey of 442 orthopedic surgeons found that, in general, surgeons preferred internal fixation for younger patients and arthroplasty for older patients. However, there was disagreement about the treatment of patients 60 to 80 years old with a displaced fracture, and there was disagreement on the optimal implants for internal fixation or arthroplasty.[20]

Total hip arthroplasty was shown to have better outcomes with less need for revision surgery than open reduction internal fixation in a randomized controlled trial performed at 4 years postoperatively.[21] A prospective cohort study found that those who had total hip arthroplasty had a better functional outcome than those who had internal fixation or hemiarthroplasty.[22]

Modification of These Questions in Light of New Research: The recent research summarized here on the treatment of hip fracture in older patients indicates no need for changes or deletions in the research agenda for this topic.

FRACTURES OF THE WRIST

See *New Frontiers,* pp. 322–323.

Ortho 38 (Level B): **Observational studies are needed to compare operative with nonoperative management to suggest which method is better with regard to outcome (time to union and function) following wrist fracture in the older patient.**

Ortho 39 (Level D): **Descriptive studies are needed to determine the range of motion and strength of the wrist necessary for good activities of daily living function in older persons.**

Ortho 40 (Level D): **Case series describing outcomes with various fixation methods are needed to suggest the best fixation method for wrist fractures in older patients.**

Ortho 41 (Level C): **Controlled trials of various graft materials are needed to determine the best graft material to supplement wrist fracture internal fixation in older patients.**

New Research Addressing These Questions: Volar plating of displaced distal radius fractures was shown, in one follow-up study, to have a higher incidence of fracture collapse but lower rate of hardware complications than dorsal plating.[23]

Modification of These Questions in Light of New Research: The research agenda regarding the treatment of wrist fractures in older patients should remain unchanged, and further research is still needed.

FRACTURES OF THE SPINE

See *New Frontiers,* pp. 323–324.

> *Ortho 42 (Level A)*: **Randomized controlled trials are needed to compare vertebroplasty with current usual care (no treatment) in older patients. The studies should compare indications (acute and or chronic pain) for vertebroplasty, complications, benefits, and long-term effects of each approach, and they should also examine the effects on adjacent vertebrae (eg, fracture, deformity) following vertebroplasty.**

New Research Addressing These Questions: Vertebroplasty for vertebral compression fractures has been shown to be helpful in reducing pain. A prospective study of 167 patients who received 207 vertebroplasty treatments to stabilize vertebral compression fractures found a significant improvement in pain, reduction in the need for analgesics, and increased mobility.[24] A nonrandomized trial comparing percutaneous vertebroplasty with conservative therapy found a 53% reduction in pain and a 29% improvement in physical function 24 hours after the procedure. Within 24 hours, 24% of treated individuals were able to cease pain medication.[25] A study looking at long-term outcome following vertebroplasty found a slightly increased risk of vertebral fracture adjacent to the cemented vertebra.[26]

Modification of These Questions in Light of New Research: The recent research described here regarding the treatment of spinal fractures in older patients indicates no need for changes or deletions in the research agenda for this topic.

FRACTURES OF THE PROXIMAL HUMERUS

See *New Frontiers,* pp. 324–325.

> *Ortho 43 (Level B)*: **Observational studies are needed to more clearly define what constitutes a good outcome following a proximal humerus fracture in the older patient.**

> *Ortho 44 (Level A)*: **Controlled studies are needed to compare operative with nonoperative repair of proximal humerus fractures in older patients.**

***Ortho 45 (Level A)*: Controlled studies are needed to compare various operative repairs for proximal humerus fractures in older patients.**

New Research Addressing These Questions: No reports of new research on these questions were identified.

Modification of These Questions in Light of New Research: These items should remain unchanged on the research agenda for geriatric orthopedics.

REFERENCES

1. Day S. Geriatric orthopedics. In Solomon DH, LoCicero J, 3rd, Rosenthal RA (eds): New Frontiers in Geriatrics Research: An Agenda for Surgical and Related Medical Specialties. New York: American Geriatrics Society, 2004, pp. 303-338 (online at http://www.frycomm.com/ags/rasp).
2. Bjorkenheim JM, Pajarinen J, Savolainen V. Internal fixation of proximal humeral fractures with a locking compression plate: a retrospective evaluation of 72 patients followed for a minimum of 1 year. Acta Orthop Scand 2004;75:741-745.
3. Ring D, Kloen P, Kadzielski J, et al. Locking compression plates for osteoporotic nonunions of the diaphyseal humerus. Clin Orthop Relat Res 2004:50-54.
4. Arora R, Lutz M, Fritz D, et al. Palmar locking plate for treatment of unstable dorsal dislocated distal radius fractures. Arch Orthop Trauma Surg 2005;125:399-404.
5. Pagnano MW, McLamb LA, Trousdale RT. Primary and revision total hip arthroplasty for patients 90 years of age and older. Mayo Clin Proc 2003;78:285-288.
6. Berend ME, Thong AE, Faris GW, et al. Total joint arthroplasty in the extremely elderly: hip and knee arthroplasty after entering the 89th year of life. J Arthroplasty 2003;18:817-821.
7. Berend KR, Lombardi AV, Mallory TH, et al. Cementless double-tapered total hip arthroplasty in patients 75 years of age and older. J Arthroplasty 2004;19:288-295.
8. Mulay S, Hassan T, Birtwistle S, Power R. Management of types B2 and B3 femoral periprosthetic fractures by a tapered, fluted, and distally fixed stem. J Arthroplasty 2005;20:751-756.
9. Sporer SM, Obar RJ, Bernini PM. Primary total hip arthroplasty using a modular proximally coated prosthesis in patients older than 70: two to eight year results. J Arthroplasty 2004;19:197-203.
10. Pieringer H, Labek G, Auersperg V, Bohler N. Cementless total hip arthroplasty in patients older than 80 years of age. J Bone Joint Surg Br 2003;85:641-645.
11. Bezwada HP, Shah AR, Harding SH, et al. Cementless bipolar hemiarthroplasty for displaced femoral neck fractures in the elderly. J Arthroplasty 2004;19:73-77.
12. Abboud JA, Patel RV, Booth RE, Jr., Nazarian DG. Outcomes of total hip arthroplasty are similar for patients with displaced femoral neck fractures and osteoarthritis. Clin Orthop Relat Res 2004:151-154.
13. Mishra V, Thomas G, Sibly TF. Results of displaced subcapital fractures treated by primary total hip replacement. Injury 2004;35:157-160.
14. Majewski M, Bischoff-Ferrari HA, Gruneberg C, et al. Improvements in balance after total hip replacement. J Bone Joint Surg Br 2005;87:1337-1343.
15. Joshi AB, Markovic L, Gill G. Knee arthroplasty in octogenarians: results at 10 years. J Arthroplasty 2003;18:295-298.
16. Dixon P, Parish EN, Chan B, et al. Hydroxyapatite-coated, cementless total knee replacement in patients aged 75 years and over. J Bone Joint Surg Br 2004;86:200-204.

17. Nau T, Pflegerl E, Erhart J, Vecsei V. Primary total knee arthroplasty for periarticular fractures. J Arthroplasty 2003;18:968-971.
18. Bryant D, Litchfield R, Sandow M, et al. A comparison of pain, strength, range of motion, and functional outcomes after hemiarthroplasty and total shoulder arthroplasty in patients with osteoarthritis of the shoulder: a systematic review and meta-analysis. J Bone Joint Surg Am 2005;87:1947-1956.
19. De Baere T, Dubuc JE, Joris D, Delloye C. Results of arthroscopic acromioplasty for chronic rotator cuff lesion. Acta Orthop Belg 2004;70:520-524.
20. Bhandari M, Devereaux PJ, Tornetta P, 3rd, et al. Operative management of displaced femoral neck fractures in elderly patients: an international survey. J Bone Joint Surg Am 2005;87:2122-2130.
21. Blomfeldt R, Tornkvist H, Ponzer S, et al. Comparison of internal fixation with total hip replacement for displaced femoral neck fractures: randomized, controlled trial performed at four years. J Bone Joint Surg Am 2005;87:1680-1688.
22. Haentjens P, Autier P, Barette M, Boonen S. Predictors of functional outcome following intracapsular hip fracture in elderly women.: a one-year prospective cohort study. Injury 2005;36:842-850.
23. Rozental TD, Blazar PE. Functional outcome and complications after volar plating for dorsally displaced, unstable fractures of the distal radius. J Hand Surg [Am] 2006;31:359-365.
24. Do HM, Kim BS, Marcellus ML, et al. Prospective analysis of clinical outcomes after percutaneous vertebroplasty for painful osteoporotic vertebral body fractures. AJNR Am J Neuroradiol 2005;26:1623-1628.
25. Diamond TH, Champion B, Clark WA. Management of acute osteoporotic vertebral fractures: a nonrandomized trial comparing percutaneous vertebroplasty with conservative therapy. Am J Med 2003;114:257-265.
26. Legroux-Gerot I, Lormeau C, Boutry N, et al. Long-term follow-up of vertebral osteoporotic fractures treated by percutaneous vertebroplasty. Clin Rheumatol 2004;23:310-317.

12

GERIATRIC REHABILITATION

*Laura W. Lee, MD, MBA; Hilary C. Siebens, MD**

Rehabilitation focuses on enhancing function and minimizing disability by means of various therapeutic interventions. Goals include optimizing quality of life and functional independence. Geriatric rehabilitation addresses not only impairments stemming from acute events, such as stroke or hip fracture, but also the deleterious effects of chronic diseases and gradually progressive disability. A better scientific understanding of rehabilitation care and efficacy is warranted, not only for improving the care of patients but also in forming optimal health care policy. For example, a critical current debate concerns which patients benefit from inpatient rehabilitation facility (IRF) care and which benefit more from skilled nursing facility (SNF) care. Evidence to help answer this question is limited. Another issue concerns the assessments and treatments that need to be done, and paid for, during the progressive disability trajectory experienced by many older adults. These issues point to the need for better definitions of rehabilitation treatments, improved measurement of treatment efficacy, and optimal timing and settings for treatments.

We are recommending no changes in the Key Questions for geriatric rehabilitation that were posed in *New Frontiers in Geriatric Research.* [1,2] However, as we note in the section Progress in the Key Research Questions in Geriatric Rehabilitation, major studies evaluating ways to prevent or reduce functional decline in older persons suggest fruitful avenues for further research addressing one of these important issues.

This chapter also summarizes recent progress in research addressing the 29 agenda items for geriatric rehabilitation from *New Frontiers,* that is, reports published between 2000 and 2005. Given the growth of research in this field, only selected contributions could be included for review. Brief summary statements have been made about each report cited, and readers are encouraged to look at articles of interest as a check on the conclusions we have drawn from them.

In the final section of the chapter, New Horizons in Geriatric Rehabilitation, we recommend new areas for research not covered in *New Frontiers,* discussing recent relevant reports and adding six new items to the rehabilitation research agenda.

METHODS

A literature search was conducted on the National Library of Medicine's PubMed database covering articles published in journals from January 2000 to June 2005. This search combined MeSH headings denoting advanced age (aged, geriatric, or 65 or older) with the terms *rehabilitation, rehabilitation nursing,* or *physical medicine and rehabilitation.* Also, references cited in these articles and pertinent rehabilitation texts were reviewed. Articles were chosen for inclusion herein on the basis of two criteria: the strength of their methodology and the relevance of the topic to improving the clinical care and knowledge base of geriatric rehabilitation.

*Lee: Assistant Professor, Department of Physical Medicine and Rehabilitation, University of Virginia Health Systems, Charlottesville, VA; Siebens: Clinical Professor of Physical Medicine and Rehabilitation, University of Virginia, Charlottesville, VA.

PROGRESS IN KEY RESEARCH QUESTIONS IN GERIATRIC REHABILITATION

See *New Frontiers,* pp. 359–361.

***Rehab KQ1*: What is the process in elderly persons underlying the development of disability and the factors influencing the disablement process?**

New Research Addressing This Key Question: Several major studies have evaluated approaches to decrease mortality, hospitalization, and functional decline in older patients. A British study tested geriatric assessments—of all older patients in a practice or of a group targeted on the basis of symptoms and problems—and two management strategies in 106 general practices in the United Kingdom including 33,326 patients aged 75 or older (mean age 81.4 years). In one comprehensive study testing geriatric assessment through brief questionnaires followed by more detailed assessments (either of all patients or of a targeted group), no significant differences were found to have been achieved in mortality, hospitalization, or nursing home admission. There were only very small benefits in mobility and morale, which were probably not clinically significant, but there was a small, likely clinically meaningful improvement in social interaction. [3] However, a meta-analysis of 18 trials involving 13,447 community-dwelling persons aged 65 years and older was able to demonstrate prevention of functional decline. This occurred, however, only in younger people, in those with a lower mortality risk, and in those who received a multidimensional geriatric assessment in the home and in-home follow-up visits. Interventions included primary prevention (eg, immunizations and exercise recommendations), secondary prevention (eg, detection of untreated problems), and tertiary prevention (eg, improvement of medication use). These results indicate that targeting interventions earlier, before advanced age or increased risk of mortality, can prevent functional decline. [4] More work is needed to research cost-effective strategies to implement these approaches.

Modification of This Key Question in Light of New Research: We recommend keeping Rehab KQ1 unchanged. The studies cited add new insights into this very important issue, and further research along these lines would be valuable.

***Rehab KQ2*: What are the costs and benefits of targeting treatment at differing aspects of the disablement process in elderly persons?**

New Research Addressing This Key Question: We are not able to comment, on the basis of our literature review, on this important and complex issue. Now that much is known about the development of disability, perhaps more extensive work on the costs and benefits of interventions will be feasible.

Modification of This Key Question in Light of New Research: We recommend keeping Rehab KQ2 unchanged.

***Rehab KQ3*: What are the relative merits of diverse rehabilitative treatments targeted at similar aspects of the disablement process in elderly patients?**

New Research Addressing This Key Question: As with Rehab KQ2, we cannot comment yet on the relative merits of different treatments for similar disabling factors.

Modification of This Key Question in Light of New Research: We recommend keeping Rehab KQ3 unchanged.

PROGRESS IN THE THEORETICAL UNDERPINNINGS FOR GERIATRIC REHABILITATION

See *New Frontiers,* pp. 339–343. For discussion of three new items for the research agenda, see the theoretical underpinnings subsection in New Horizons in Geriatric Rehabilitation at the end of the chapter.

Rehabilitation for older adults has received substantial attention in the past 5 years as the cadre of researchers focusing on the older population has grown. In addition, a major policy change by Medicare in 2002 whereby inpatient rehabilitation facilities came under the prospective payment system forced the rehabilitation community to focus more on the study of cost-effective interventions for disability. The treatment of acute-onset moderate or severe disability is challenged with changing reimbursement policies. Fortunately, the field has some standard outcome measures that are being used to help evaluate the cost-effectiveness of care. However, measuring the costs of not rehabilitating patients appropriately is not as easy as measuring the costs of not treating acute illnesses. Moreover, many older adults experience gradually progressive disability, making it hard to identify optimal timing and types of rehabilitation.

Interventions used in geriatric rehabilitation include exercise, adaptive techniques and equipment, assistive technology, physical modalities, orthotic and prosthetic devices, and psychologic and social interventions. A detailed review of only the two most commonly used interventions, exercise and assistive technology, is provided herein. Key rehabilitation personnel who assess patients and use these interventions include rehabilitation nurses, physical therapists (PTs), occupational therapists (OTs), speech language pathologists, rehabilitation psychologists, therapeutic recreation therapists, as well as others, such as social workers, case managers, pharmacists, and dietitians.

Exercise programs are used to increase joint flexibility, muscular strength, and aerobic endurance, but exercises may be used for more specific purposes, such as preserving bone density through weight bearing, reducing joint pain through strengthening of the surrounding muscles, and increasing coordination after a stroke. Different types of exercises have varying levels of data supporting their efficacy for specific conditions.

Adaptive techniques involve modifying a task so that it can be performed despite physical limitations. Adaptive techniques often are combined with assistive technology. Their combined use enables the person to interact more favorably with the environment. Rehabilitation specialists often make recommendations about which devices will be most helpful in improving function and facilitating independence.

Physical modalities use physical processes to treat impairments. For example, ultrasound providing deep heat, transcutaneous electrical nerve stimulation, whirlpool, massage, and applications of heat or cold are modalities that are used routinely during therapies. Research data on the efficacy of many physical modalities is limited.

Orthotic devices are externally applied and act to support the musculoskeletal system. Examples are inserts or specially adapted shoes for arthritic problems of the feet, splinting and padding for overuse syndromes such as carpal tunnel syndrome, and bracing to support an unstable or weak joint, such as an ankle-foot orthosis used after a stroke. Prosthetics are devices that act to substitute or replace a missing body part. Examples include below-knee leg prosthesis or below-elbow prosthesis.

Psychologic assessments and interventions assist patients' coping and adaptation. Social interventions assist family members in dealing with losses and adapting to the new needs of the family member who now has a disability.

***Rehab 1 (Level B)*: The first step required, in support of all other recommended research efforts, is to develop uniform terminology, so that multisite research consortia can be formed to allow faster progress, as was done in the field of cancer research over the past 50 years.**

New Research Addressing This Question: An increasing number of papers have discussed rehabilitation research in relation to the International Classification of Functioning, Disability and Health (ICF).[5] What has been groundbreaking in this classification is that patients' functioning is now seen as being associated with, and not merely as a consequence of, a health condition. Functioning and health are also considered not only in association with an underlying health condition, but also in association with personal and environmental factors. All aspects of patient experience, including body function and structures as well as personal and environmental factors, are covered. This bio-psycho-social view is not new to a number of medical fields, such as rehabilitation and prevention. What is new is that we now have a globally agreed-on, etiologically neutral framework and a classification both on the individual and population levels.[6]

To date, much of the work in using the ICF has been to identify core sets of components that are to be measured across and within certain general diagnostic categories like chronic conditions and musculoskeletal disorders.[7,8] These approaches should lead to new research insights, since theoretical models have been the basis of this practical classification system of relevant patient and environmental variables.

Disability, like any human condition, is an extremely complex, multifaceted phenomenon, and standard terminology depends, to some extent, on underlying assumptions and models. See the discussion of the Health Environmental Integration model under Rehab 10.

One taxonomy of rehabilitation interventions has been developed by DeJong et al.[9] The authors used an experience-driven, bottom-up, inductive approach led by front-line opinion and scientific evidence to develop a taxonomy of physical therapy, occupational therapy, speech therapy, nursing, and social work or case management interventions during inpatient rehabilitation. These were then used to collect data about the process of care as part of a major study on the "black box" of rehabilitation in stroke (see Rehab 11).[10] This work contributes significantly to the ongoing development of uniform terminology.

Modification of This Question in Light of New Research: We recommend keeping this question on the research agenda without modification, as findings of such research are still needed.

***Rehab 2 (Levels B, A)*: Hypothesis-testing research is needed to determine the costs and benefits of treatment that is targeted generically at the disability versus treatment that addresses the underlying diseases and impairments.**

New Research Addressing This Question: Our literature review yielded no papers that studied a specific disabling condition and compared disability-level treatments with treatments of the underlying disease and impairment.

Modification of This Question in Light of New Research: This is an important issue. For example, situations occur in which clinicians want to help a patient with trouble walking because of an arthritic, deformed, mildly painful spine. An assistive device, like a rollator, could well get the patient walking more easily and safely and at very low cost. However, should more diagnostic work and more specific treatment target the chronic back condition, believed to be osteoarthritis? We recommend keeping this question on the research agenda without modification, as findings of such research are still needed.

Rehab 3 (Level B): **If it is important to individualize treatment on the basis of underlying cause (see Rehab 2), then additional research will be needed to identify the most efficient diagnostic methods to distinguish among causes of disability, with an eye to identifying characteristics that may affect treatment planning and outcomes. For example, a sudden acute event may need condition-specific treatment, whereas a slow decline in function may be amenable to treatment at the level of disability.**

New Research Addressing This Question: Our literature review did not identify any studies addressing the efficiency of diagnosing the cause of disability.

Modification of This Question in Light of New Research: We recommend keeping this question on the research agenda without modification, as findings of such research are still needed.

Rehab 4 (Level B): **Mechanistic studies are needed on the physiologic processes underlying geriatric disability and on the potential effect of the biology of aging on response to rehabilitation, particularly for sarcopenia and recovery from acute illness.**

New Research Addressing This Question: One study, though not a physiologic study, clearly showed that the overall process of hospitalization caused permanent decline in activities of daily living (ADL) function in 10% of disabled women at 6 months after hospitalization and beyond. [11] This was after controlling for other factors, such as the illnesses themselves and the effects of aging per se, known to be associated with hospital-related functional decline. Another study contributes to earlier research documenting functional decline in relation to hospitalizations for conditions not known to cause sudden disability. [12] These reports contribute to the growing literature on predictors of the functional decline after hospitalizations. [13]

Modification of This Question in Light of New Research: We recommend keeping this question on the research agenda without modification, as findings of such research are still needed. Additional work will be needed to determine what aspects of hospitalization have these detrimental effects and to identify cost-effective interventions.

Rehab 5 (Levels B, A): **Hypothesis-generating research followed by hypothesis-testing research is needed to better define the point in the disablement process when treatment is optimally instituted and**

whether or not optimal timing differs according to the disablement process (catastrophic versus progressive) or the underlying condition.

New Research Addressing This Question: Bean et al have shown that residents in SNFs, like community-dwelling persons, who develop impairments in the range of motion and strength of any limb experience a concurrent step-wise loss in ADLs. [14]

In older adults living in the community, disability can have a waxing-waning course. [15] Understanding this is necessary in the design of research strategies and in targeting clinical interventions. Ongoing epidemiologic studies are clarifying the natural history of, and risk factors for, progressive and catastrophic disability. In elegant work from the Women's Health and Aging Study, measures of lower- and upper-extremity function, excepting grip strength, significantly predicted the onset of progressive ADL disability. However, only walking speed was found to be significantly associated with the onset of catastrophic ADL disability. Overall, progressive disability was easier to predict than catastrophic disability. [16]

In a 4-year longitudinal study, the disabling consequences of depression were described. Rapid declines in function occurred if depressive symptoms remained persistently elevated. [17] These results demonstrate the importance of further research to help clinicians better distinguish temporary and more permanent depression and use appropriate interventions in each case.

Modification of This Question in Light of New Research: We recommend keeping this question on the research agenda without modification, as findings of such research are still needed.

***Rehab 6 (Level B)*: A longitudinal, nationally representative cohort study is needed to define the disabling impact of different diseases and conditions at the societal level, stratified by age group and major categories of interest to geriatrics (eg, nursing home residents versus community dwellers). This information will allow better prioritization of research endeavors in geriatric rehabilitation.**

New Research Addressing This Question: Trends in disability in older adults have been systematically reviewed and show the encouraging news that disability rates are declining about 2% per year. [18,19] The US Census Bureau report *65+ in the United States: 2005* also confirms that older adults today differ markedly from prior generations. [20] The percentage of people aged 65 years and older who report "a substantial limitation in a major life activity" fell from 26.2% in 1982 to 19.7% in 1999. Poverty levels have decreased from 35% of people aged 65 and older living in poverty in 1959 to 10% in 2003. Very worrisome, however, are the effects of the increase in divorce rates among older Americans, as well as increasing obesity and the lack of decreased poverty across all population groups. Reasons for the drop in disability rates are not fully clear, though increased educational levels may play an important role. The increase in high school graduates among older adults is substantial—from 17% in 1950 to 71.5% in 2003.

The number of older adults will continue to increase; estimates are that 20% of Americans will be aged 65 years or older by 2030. Unfortunately, a substantial number of adults will nonetheless experience disability, requiring focused secondary and tertiary prevention efforts as well as appropriate rehabilitative care.

Large administrative databases, despite their limitations, and other large data sources, like the Medicare Current Beneficiary Survey, may be promising sources for rehabilitation outcomes research and for understanding the social impact of specific clinical conditions.[21] For example, 20% of the entire Medicare population has at least one health-related activity limitation. Medicare enrollees' health care costs increase as the number of activity limitations increases through greater frequency of all health care utilization events (eg, hospitalizations, outpatient visits) rather than an increase in the intensity or cost of those events.[22] A valid method has been developed for using ICD–9 codes to identify secondary conditions in Medicare patients.[23] This increases the ability to use Medicare administrative data to evaluate health care issues in a large population (as well as aspects of health care delivery).

Modification of This Question in Light of New Research: We recommend keeping this question on the research agenda without modification, as findings of such research are still needed.

***Rehab 7 (Level B)*: Observational and cohort studies are needed to identify the key social and environmental risk factors for current disability or progression into disability for the older patient, and the influence of these factors on rehabilitation outcomes.**

New Research Addressing This Question: Social relationships are intimately involved with multiple aspects of rehabilitation and living with disability. Under certain conditions, lack of social supports contributes to significant morbidity when certain illnesses occur. As described below, social supports have impact on outcomes from hip fractures and other conditions.

Progress is occurring in relation to the study of environments and their mitigating or exacerbating contributions to disablement. One barrier has been the difficulty of establishing appropriate measures of patients' environments. Promising new instruments are in development. These environmental taxonomies include physical, attitudinal, and policy factors. Different environmental levels include the micro (personal), meso (community, services), and macro (societal, systems) levels described in 1977 by Bronfenbrenner.[24,25] One new measure focuses on patient self-report of personal environments.[26] Eight physical environmental components affect older adults as they move around in their communities, and these components can contribute to varying levels of mobility disability.[27]

Preliminary studies are evaluating the adaptations that would be needed to different types of housing depending on the disability a person has and how that disability will change over time. For example, Lansley et al conclude that home environments can facilitate independence through appropriately selected adaptations and assistive technology.[28]

Modification of This Question in Light of New Research: We recommend keeping this question on the research agenda while separating the question into two parts, one focusing on social relationships and one on the physical environment.

***Rehab 8 (Level B)*: Cross-sectional studies and longitudinal cohort studies of the relations between caregiving and outcomes are needed.**

New Research Addressing This Question: Special considerations can arise in goal setting for any rehabilitation patient who requires significant family involvement—either because of cognitive impairment or significant needs for physical help, or both. In these situations, family goals are important perspectives to consider. In one assessment of an outpatient geriatric setting, low agreement was found in treatment goals between physicians and the family caregivers.[29] It is important to assess whether a similar discordance occurs in rehabilitation settings that take care of frail older patients.

Research on caregivers for patients with chronic, progressive cognitive impairment, like dementia, is substantial, and its review is beyond the scope of this chapter. However, documented outcomes for family caregivers of stroke patients have shown mental distress similar to that experienced by the caregivers of Alzheimer's disease patients when caregiver burdens are similar.[30] Some level of family conflict was reported by 66% of caregivers of stroke survivors 3 to 9 months following the stroke. In 32% of families, general family functioning was measured as ineffective. The caregiver's mental health was poorer when stroke survivors had significant motor and memory or behavior problems.[31] Newer stroke therapies, as well as chronic disabilities, all put burdens of care on families. Increased understanding of these burdens as well as interventions to alleviate some of the problems are required.

A better understanding of caregivers' experiences is needed, since they involve so much more than simple support of ADLs and instrumental ADLs. Navigating the health care systems and providing emotional support are among the many demanding tasks assumed by caregivers.[32] Research is needed on these dimensions so that rehabilitation programs can identify interventions that help offset the demands of caregiving. In a survey of caregiving in the United States, about 75% of caregivers were for individuals aged 50 years and over, and contrary to expectations, 40% of caregivers were men.[33]

Modification of This Question in Light of New Research: We recommend keeping this question on the research agenda without modification, as findings of such research are still needed.

***Rehab 9 (Level B)*: Adequate investigation of such factors as coping strategies, attitudes, and the cost versus the benefits of assistive technology and improved access will require both qualitative and quantitative research, and considerable work is needed to develop methods for combining the results of both these research traditions.**

New Research Addressing This Question: A classic study, described in *When Walking Fails* by Lisa Iezzoni, MD, represents rigorous research that synthesizes the qualitative and quantitative approaches needed to cover the multiple dimensions of mobility problems faced by adults with chronic conditions. Iezzoni describes situations involving both younger and older adults; many themes apply to both groups. Through her work she inspires individuals to lead full lives despite mobility problems.[34] Specific research needs regarding health care delivery and access to appropriate services become clear on reading this superb report.

Functional health as people age can be better when self-perceptions are better.[35] Negative self-perceptions can interfere with healthy behaviors, such as the initiation of exercise.[36] Research in both these areas—improving self-perceptions and behavioral change for exercise—is needed and will likely require qualitative and quantitative approaches.

Psychologic conditions are common comorbidities during rehabilitation. As part of a study on psychiatric disorders and psychosocial burden in rehabilitation patients, 205 of 910 patients with musculoskeletal conditions who were receiving inpatient rehabilitation were interviewed. Prevalence rates for psychologic problems were 31.1% for these patients during the first 4 weeks of the survey. The most prevalent conditions were anxiety, affective disorders, and substance-related problems. [37] Research will need to clarify which psychologic interventions during rehabilitation might help achieve better outcomes.

Modification of This Question in Light of New Research: We recommend that this question be kept without change on the research agenda. Qualitative research is needed to generate hypotheses on the nature of older patients' experiences during rehabilitation, including their perceptions of access to services (see also the research described under Rehab 22). Such work needs to explore treatment approaches that relieve suffering when possible, including evaluations and interventions for patients' coping styles and self-management abilities.

Rehab 10 (Levels B, A): Research is needed to articulate a clear theory or model of rehabilitation treatment that can then be tested.

New Research Addressing This Question: We are unaware of any new theory or model of rehabilitation treatment per se. However, one next-generation health model may serve as the basis for a model of rehabilitation treatment. In the Health Environmental Integration model, the health of any person depends on the health of the environment along with other factors. [38] Figure 12.1 depicts the four interlocking spheres of health environmental integration—the body, the mind, the physical environment, and the social environment. Stineman refers to this model as an eco-biopsychosocial model. It was built within the framework of the World Health Organization medical and disablement models and adds concepts from other biomedical, biopsychosocial, and disablement models, from organic unity theory, and from the concept of health-related quality of life. This synthesis includes models mentioned in *New Frontiers* and provides an understandable framework from which to study patients with disabilities and the care they receive in rehabilitation. [1,38]

One empiric, practical model to guide rehabilitation planning and teamwork is the Siebens Domain Management Model. This model organizes patients' health-related problems into four domains: medical and surgical issues; mental status, emotions, and coping

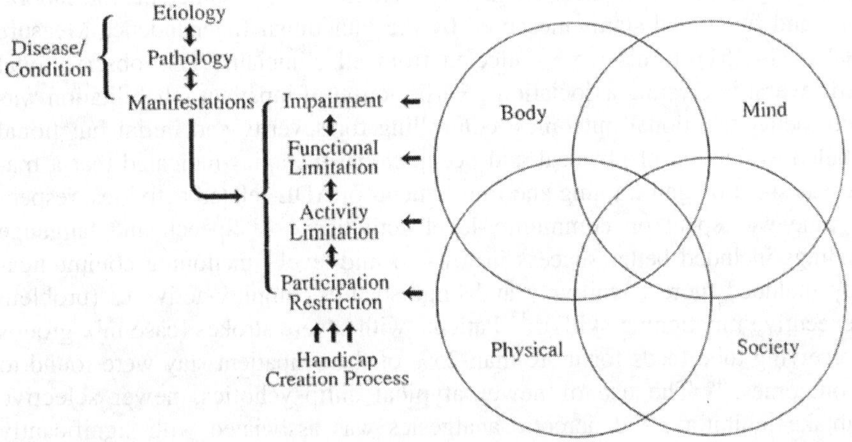

Figure 12.1—Spheres of health environmental integration. (Source: Stineman MG. A model of health environmental integration. Top Stroke Rehabil 2001;8:34–45. Reprinted with permission.)

issues; physical function issues; and living environment issues.[39,40] Errors in the management of patients with disability can occur from the lack of critical information in any one of these four domains.[41]

Modification of This Question in Light of New Research: We recommend keeping this question on the research agenda without modification, as findings of such research are still needed.

***Rehab 11 (Level B)*: Research is needed to delineate the components of the rehabilitation "black box" (eg, the dosage of rehabilitation).**

New Research Addressing This Question: Several studies focusing on stroke have started to examine in detail the "black box" of rehabilitation. For example, Bode et al analyze the type of therapy received. In general, they found that OTs spent more time in impairment-related activities, and PTs and speech language pathologists spent more time on function-related activities. More detail about the actual time spent for patients included 74% in OT, PT, and speech therapy, 10.6% in education (nursing), 7.2% in social work activities, 5% in therapeutic recreation, 2.2% in psychologic services, and 0.5% in chaplaincy activities. Overall, these amounts of therapy time were similar in the IRF and SNF units. However, this study was performed before the implementation of the prospective payment system. The level of impairment did not appear to contribute to the amount of therapy received.[42]

A major study has identified many of the components of IRF care processes, the "black box," and has related these to patient outcomes. In the Post-Stroke Rehabilitation Outcomes Project, seven IRFs participated, including one in New Zealand, and 1291 patients were studied. The study method, Practice-Based Evidence–Clinical Practice Improvement (PBE-CPI) developed by Susan Horn, has been used in numerous other studies, but this was the first time it was applied to a rehabilitation setting.[43] Detailed process factors were collected from chart review, and additional point-of-care forms were completed by clinicians about treatments. Patient factors were collected through detailed chart review by use of the Comprehensive Severity Index and standard abstraction of information deemed relevant by the study clinicians. Outcomes included length of stay, some specific laboratory indicators, and functional status measured by the Functional Independence Measure (FIM). A total of 141,511 forms were collected from all clinicians. This observational study revealed several interesting associations. Earlier onset of inpatient rehabilitation was associated with better functional outcomes, controlling for severity and initial functional status.[44] Detailed evaluation of physical and occupational therapies indicated that a majority of time was spent on gait training and impairment- or ADL-related activities, respectively. Little time was spent on community-level activities.[45,46] Speech and language pathology findings included better success in low- to mid-level functioning communicators if therapy included more cognitively and linguistically complex activities (problem solving and executive functioning skills).[47] Patients with severe strokes (case mix groups 108 to 114) receiving tube feeds for more than 25% of their inpatient stay were found to have better outcomes.[48] The use of newer atypical antipsychotics, newer selective serotonin-reuptake inhibitors, and narcotic analgesics was associated with significantly greater increase in motor FIM scores.[49] Overall, early onset of rehabilitation and early gait training (within the first 3 hours of therapy) as well as increased time spent on more complex activities were definitely associated with better functional outcomes, controlling for multiple other variables.[50] All these reports contribute to our understanding of practice variation among sites. The findings challenge traditional rehabilitation thinking, that is, that therapies must focus on simpler activities before advancement to more complex ones can occur.

Modification of This Question in Light of New Research: We recommend keeping this question on the agenda. Continued research is needed to define the therapeutic components of rehabilitation programs. The promising research methodology of PBE-CPI should be evaluated further. Additionally, work to standardize the components of rehabilitation therapies that are determined to be good or best practices should be conducted to allow for future clinical trials.

PROGRESS IN THE COMPONENTS OF REHABILITATION

See *New Frontiers,* pp. 345–353. For discussion of two new items for the research agenda, see the components of rehabilitation subsection in New Horizons in Geriatric Rehabilitation at the end of the chapter.

In the chapter on the research agenda in geriatric rehabilitation in *New Frontiers*, the components of rehabilitation were divided into structure (setting, providers), process of care (interventions), and outcomes. This was based on Donabedian's model for studying quality of care.[51] The following questions refer to studies in these areas. Five years ago little was discussed about outcomes; however, more work on outcomes has occurred since then, research that is discussed at the end of this chapter (see the section New Horizons in Geriatric Rehabilitation).

Rehab 12 (Levels B, A): **Hypothesis-generating research followed by hypothesis-testing research is needed to identify the critical factors responsible for the more optimal outcomes seen in some settings.**

New Research Addressing This Question: The new research approach using Clinical Practice Improvement has led to insights in the rehabilitation process and will be helpful in studying different sites of care. This approach uses a practice-based evidence research method that collects detailed patient-based information, detailed clinical care delivery (process) information, and outcomes measures on large patient populations.[10,52] Analyses of these observational data identify associations among patient characteristics, treatment interventions, and specific outcomes. Findings can be tested in rigorous trials and used to improve care processes directly. Given the complexities and variations among patients requiring rehabilitation, the Clinical Practice Improvement approach is a promising research method.

Rehabilitation care spans multiple settings and offers varying intensity of treatment: from rehabilitation units in acute care hospitals or freestanding rehabilitation hospitals to subacute rehabilitation units in nursing homes to rehabilitation services offered by nursing homes or home health services to outpatient rehabilitation services. Medicare policy changes for acute inpatient rehabilitation facilities, SNFs, and home health services have led to changes in care delivery. These changes and the multiplicity of sites highlight the need for research to identify optimal care settings for different types of rehabilitation patients.

Acute inpatient rehabilitation offers approximately 3 hours of therapy per day, while SNFs offer an average of 1 hour per day. There have been few controlled studies comparing the efficacy of treatments of differing intensity for specific types of disabilities. Research on this topic has been difficult because IRFs report their outcomes using the FIM at admission and discharge, whereas SNFs report their outcomes using the Minimum Data Set assessed in a different time frame. Prospective randomized controlled trials on intensity of treatment are difficult because the patient populations that tend to go to IRFs and SNFs may not be similar.

One systematic Cochrane review covered the large topic of rehabilitation setting, "care home versus hospital and own home environments for rehabilitation of older people." No conclusions could be drawn as to optimal location for rehabilitation. Comparability between intervention and control groups was weak. [53] However, studies are being done on characteristics and outcomes of specific care settings.

Several descriptive studies of different rehabilitation care providers have been published between 2000 and 2005. Chen et al reported on subacute rehabilitation occurring in 1996 and 1997. Their results show that this type of care, offered in units in acute hospitals, rehabilitation hospitals, and SNFs, provided slightly different amounts of minutes of therapy per day and that functional gains occurred in the three diagnostic groups evaluated—stroke, orthopedic, and debility. Greater gains were weakly associated with more minutes of therapy and longer lengths of stay. This research documents outcomes under former cost-based reimbursement. [54]

Comparing the results of these earlier SNF units, often referred to as subacute units with daily reimbursements approaching IRF levels, with the results of current skilled nursing units would be interesting. One study in 2002 of patients admitted to SNFs did show a relationship between therapy intensity and rehabilitation outcomes. [55] One evaluation of hip fracture patient rehabilitation between March 2002 and June 2003 compared IRF outcomes with SNF outcomes, controlling for cognitive status, social supports, and other variables. Prefracture FIM scores were similar (85.0 ± 10.5 and 85.2 ± 8.0) for IRF (n = 42) and SNF (n = 32) patients, respectively. IRF lengths of stay were shorter (12.8 days versus 36.2 days), and IRF patients were more likely to reach 95% of their pre-fracture motor FIM score by 12 weeks. [56]

Leach et al have raised the possibility that the outcomes of rehabilitation for older orthopedic patients may be better for some patients in managed care than in fee-for-service systems. Lengths of stay can be shorter in managed care. Very few patients, however, were included in this analysis (N = 34). [57] A more recent study directly compared IRF and SNF outcomes for total joint replacement surgery. The study design was a retrospective chart review on 87 pairs of patients who were matched for age, gender, type of surgery, and FIM score at admission. Mean lengths of stay were shorter in the IRFs (10.3 ± 3.3 days versus 20 ± 10.8 days, $P < .005$), and a larger number of IRF patients were discharged to home (89.5% versus 79.1%, $P = .029$). The mean locomotion score and distance walked were greater as well for the IRF patients. [58] More studies will help clarify the respective strengths of SNF and IRF rehabilitation for joint replacements. One ongoing study that will include 2400 patients is using practice-based evidence and the Clinical Practice Improvement method. Results are expected in 2007. [59]

One special population requiring a unique rehabilitation approach is older patients with resolving acute medical or surgical conditions, multiple comorbidities, and severe deconditioning. The term *slow stream rehabilitation* has been applied to programs caring for these patients, usually for several months. These patients can get discharged to their desired discharge locations, often to home. Predictors of successful discharge included higher initial level of functioning, good vision, and having sufficient help at home.[60] More research on these types of patients will be necessary to determine which ones will benefit from a long period of inpatient care and progressive rehabilitation and which patients are reaching end-stage disability for which purely compensatory management is appropriate.

Modification of This Question in Light of New Research: We recommend keeping this question on the research agenda without modification, as findings of such research are still needed.

> *Rehab 13 (Levels B, A)*: **Hypothesis-generating research followed by hypothesis-testing research is needed to examine the effect of changes in Medicare reimbursement changes on access to rehabilitation and the quality of rehabilitative care.**

New Research Addressing This Question: One study examined nursing home rehabilitation services before and after the establishment of the prospective payment system in the state of Ohio. Rehabilitation services did decrease. The types of patients admitted to SNFs changed and included more patients with chronic medical and surgical conditions. The study found that patients less likely to receive any therapies before the prospective payment system was installed tended to get some therapies after it was in effect.[61]

Modification of This Question in Light of New Research: We recommend keeping this question on the research agenda without modification, as findings of such research are still needed.

> *Rehab 14 (Level A)*: **Randomized trials are needed to investigate the trade-offs of using less costly paraprofessionals to provide rehabilitation treatment, of using streamlined teams, and of using diverse strategies for team coordination and communication.**

New Research Addressing This Question: Rehabilitation providers during inpatient care work as a multidisciplinary team. Team functioning and contribution to care are being evaluated both within and beyond the field of rehabilitation medicine. In one study of stroke rehabilitation, three of ten measures of team functioning were found to be significantly associated with patient functional improvement—task orientation, order and organization, and utility of quality information. Patient length of stay was found to be associated with a single measure of team effectiveness.[62] With measures now available to assess team functioning, ongoing research will be able to assess team functioning and evaluate interventions to improve team effectiveness.

Modification of This Question in Light of New Research: We recommend keeping this question on the research agenda without modification, as findings of such research are still needed.

> *Rehab 15 (Levels B, A)*: **Observational studies followed by randomized trials are needed to identify which conditions are best treated with a team approach (eg, disability resulting from multiple medical prob-**

lems or a condition like stroke that causes multiple physical impairments) versus which conditions are treated equally well by a single provider (eg, disability due to a single condition causing a limited physical impairment like osteoarthritis of the knee).

New Research Addressing This Question: Our literature review found no studies evaluating this issue directly.

Modification of This Question in Light of New Research: We recommend keeping this question on the research agenda without modification, as findings of such research are still needed.

***Rehab 16 (Level A)*: Randomized controlled trials are needed to examine whether specific kinds of resistive exercise, modes of exercise delivery, and combinations of treatments (eg, psychosocial intervention plus exercise intervention) might enhance functional outcomes for older persons, and which functional outcomes are affected to the greatest extent.**

New Research Addressing This Question: A large number of studies of exercise have been reported since publication of *New Frontiers.* Description of these studies below is organized as follows: first, the benefits of exercise, and then according to the types of exercise studied—resistance, aerobic, balance, flexibility, and functionally based exercise.

There is substantial evidence that regular physical activity has a number of health benefits, especially for community-dwelling older adults with or without chronic conditions.[63] Physiologic changes associated with aging are similar to those seen with physical inactivity and can, in many instances, be ameliorated with exercise. At the physiologic level, exercise can improve aerobic capacity, increase maximal cardiac output, and reduce resting blood pressure. Exercise can also translate into improving functional performance, self-efficacy, and disability. Nevertheless, it should be noted that increasing physical activity and exercise do not always result in similar levels of increased function, as the relationship between degree of exercise and physical function may depend on baseline levels of function; those more deconditioned are able to benefit more from exercise than those already at high levels of function.

Strength training has been a focus of considerable research in geriatrics and is considered the most established means of enhancing and maintaining function in older adults.[64–73] This is due, in part, to the strong evidence that muscle mass and strength declines with age. Work has been done to characterize the underlying physiology behind the change in muscle mass, but the cause of age-related decline in muscle mass, *sarcopenia*, remains unclear. Much of the interest in resistive exercises has been generated because they have been shown to improve a number of physiologic parameters important to older persons, including insulin sensitivity, bone mineral density, aerobic capacity, and muscle strength.[74–78] Guidelines that correlate intensity of exercise and a particular level of function will be useful for further research. Musculoskeletal injuries can occur, as was shown in one study of high-intensity, home-based quadriceps resistance exercise in 243 frail older adults.[79]

Studies indicate that muscle power may correlate better than strength with mobility and function and thus may be a more sensitive indicator of a person's mobility and function.[80] Muscle power, which is the product of force times velocity, is different from muscle strength, which is measured by the force exerted by the muscle. Muscle power seems to decline more than strength with advanced age, but power seems to be responsive to exercises that include velocity training.[81–83]

Aerobic capacity is decreased in older adults, but this age-associated impairment can be reversed through aerobic exercise. For example, Keysor and Jette report that 70% of studies of aerobic conditioning in older adults showed improvements in aerobic capacity, but the effect of aerobic exercise on body composition is less consistent.[84] Studies of aerobic exercise for specific conditions commonly seen in older adults have demonstrated beneficial effects. For example, a meta-analysis showed that aerobic exercise significantly reduces systolic and diastolic blood pressure in normotensive and hypertensive older adults.[85] Aerobic and weight-bearing exercise as a method of rehabilitation for coronary heart disease and increasing insulin sensitivity are additional examples.[86–88] Haykowsky et al reported that aerobic exercise training improves relative peak Vo_2 as much as strength training in older women, although aerobic exercise did not seem as effective as strength training for increasing muscle strength.[89] With regard to long-term outcomes, a small study found that benefits of 14 weeks of aerobic endurance training included improvements in Vo_2 max and body composition, but gains were reversed after 1 year.[90] It may be that, to optimally improve function, aerobic exercise should be combined with other forms of training. One study noted that an exercise program consisting of endurance, strength, balance, and flexibility training performed at a senior center had greater gains on performance tests than home-based training, although motivation and compliance as well as group support also may have influenced results.[91]

Balance exercises address multiple deficits, including muscular weakness, vestibular dysfunction, and neurologic abnormality. These exercises are increasingly important, given the clear association of poor balance, fear of falling, and actual falls.[92] Balance exercises appear to be most effective when performed as part of a comprehensive approach. For instance, Tai Chi has been demonstrated as efficacious in lessening the incidence of injurious falls, but the exact mechanism is unclear. Balance training in specific conditions, like idiopathic Parkinson's disease, can improve balance but is even more effective when combined with strength training.[93] For community-dwelling seniors, a minimally supervised home-based exercise program improved dynamic balance 33.8% ± 14.4% in exercisers versus 11.5% ± 23.7% in control persons. No differences occurred in strength, gait speed, or cardiovascular endurance. The authors, citing other studies as well, point out that meaningful improvements in functional performance, as measured by the Physical Performance Test, can occur through improvement in balance in the absence of increased motor strength.[94]

Another randomized controlled outpatient exercise study for community-dwelling seniors involved exercises classes three times a week for 6 months and home exercise, then classes just once a week during months 7 to 12 and home exercise, and then only home exercises during months 13 to 18. Although balance was improved at 12 months, this difference was lost by 18 months when participants were doing only the home exercise program.[91] This shows how easily gains from exercise can be lost. Further research will eventually help clarify the ideal, minimal amount of exercise necessary to maintain adequate balance as the body ages.

Isolated studies of flexibility in older adults remain limited. One creative line of research has evaluated hip flexibility in relation to gait. Gait studies in older adults, in those who do and do not fall, are defining the contributions of static and dynamic hip range of motion in changing walking patterns as people age. Standing hip characteristics are similar in younger and older adults, but hip extension is decreased in older adults. The decrease in peak hip extension appears to be a mostly dynamic phenomenon. Subtle hip flexion contractures may contribute to the decrease.[95,96]

The limitations of just increasing range of motion in frail older people were demonstrated in one randomized controlled trial of exercise. Older volunteers, mean age 83 years, were randomized into an outpatient exercise program or a control home program that included only range-of-motion exercise. All the participants were identified as frail by scoring over 17 and under 33 on the Physical Performance Test. Range of motion improved in major joint groups in the control group, but there were no other benefits in overall function, balance, or walking.[97]

Recent data suggests that specific task-based training may lead to better function more effectively than specific exercises per se. The benefits of exercise are known to decline once the exercise is stopped. One randomized controlled trial therefore focused on training healthy older women by the use of exercises in movement patterns from daily activities. These included moving with a vertical component, moving with a horizontal component, carrying an object, and changing between lying, sitting, and standing positions. This program was compared with a resistance-exercise training group and with a control group that continued their usual daily activities. By the end of a 12-week training period, those who were functionally trained maintained better daily activity performance than did those in the control group. This gain persisted at 6 months after the training program ended as well.[98] The benefits from task training, in comparison with resistance training, depends on the type of patient and the goals. For example, task training on reaching for stroke survivors yielded better movements in more impaired persons, whereas those at a higher level benefited more from resistive exercise training.[99] The importance of task training, focusing on gait, in stroke rehabilitation has been highlighted by Horn et al and evaluated in relation to balance self-efficacy.[50,100] These types of research are beginning to sort out the complex relationships between functionally based task training and more specific exercise training.

A parallel to this concept of functionally based exercise for people with physical disabilities has been observed in able-bodied persons. Physiologic benefits can occur from changes in lifestyle physical activity.[101,102] A person does not necessarily have to participate in a structured, vigorous exercise program in order to become more fit. Thus, activity that is functionally based—be it during a rehabilitation program or part of regular physical activity—is beneficial.

Modification of This Question in Light of New Research: We recommend dividing this question into two sections—general exercise interventions involving the whole person and specific exercise interventions involving specific body systems (eg, muscle, tendons). It should remain on the research agenda.

***Rehab 17 (Level A)*: Randomized trials are needed on the health, functional, and quality-of-life benefits of aerobic exercise in older persons who are already disabled. The study population should be homogeneous with regard to amount and type of disability, and methodologic consideration should be given to how to deal with**

underlying medical conditions in the population and the differences they might produce in response to exercise. The outcome measures should be clearly specified; they might include physiologic parameters such as blood pressure, body composition, oxygen-carrying capacity, measures of physical function such as 6-minute walk distance, self-reported difficulty with activities of daily living, and measures of health-related quality of life like the Medical Outcomes Study 36-item Short Form 36 (SF 36).

New Research Addressing This Question: Exercise training was found to be effective in older adults with cognitive impairment and dementia in one meta-analytic review. [103] We found no reports of randomized controlled trials.

Modification of This Question in Light of New Research: We recommend keeping this question on the research agenda without modification, as findings of such research are still needed.

***Rehab 18 (Levels B, A)*: Hypothesis-generating research (eg, databases, cohort studies, case series) followed by hypothesis-testing research is needed to examine the benefits of differing types of exercise for specific conditions.**

New Research Addressing This Question: Musculoskeletal rehabilitation studies need to compare exercise with other treatments, such as manual therapy or manipulation. For example, one small randomized controlled trial compared manipulation therapy with exercise therapy for painful osteoarthritis of the hip. After 5 weeks of therapy, twice a week, pain reduction was found to be greater with manual therapy than with exercise therapy (odds ratio 1.92, 95% confidence interval 1.30 to 2.60). This difference remained at 17 and 29 weeks later. However, in both treatment groups, equal numbers of patients went on to receive total joint replacement surgery. [104] More work will be needed to sort out optimal treatments. The goal of manual therapy is to loosen a tight joint capsule and surrounding tissues around an arthritic joint. This is the proposed mechanism for decreasing pain. Perhaps a combination of manual and exercise therapy would yield better results.

More work on specific types of strengthening exercises will help determine cost-effective approaches. For example, in one study of knee osteoarthritis, concentric strengthening was compared with concentric-eccentric isokinetic training. Both were found to reduce pain and increase function. Stair climbing and descending, however, improved more in the concentric-eccentric group. [105]

Resistance training can benefit patients with neurologic diseases. In adults with Parkinson's disease, resistance training was found to increase muscle strength as much as in control persons of similar age. Speed of gait improved despite the Parkinson's disease and not in the control persons. [106] In long-term stroke survivors, high-intensity resistance training was found to improve function. [107]

Modification of This Question in Light of New Research: We recommend keeping this question on the research agenda without modification, as findings of such research are still needed.

***Rehab 19 (Levels B, A)*: Observational and cohort studies are greatly needed to identify effect size for key outcomes, which devices are**

promising enough to merit later comparative clinical trials, and what long-term follow-up shows among older people using assistive devices. These should be followed by randomized trials of the most promising devices.

New Research Addressing This Question: Salient characteristics of assistive technology (AT) highlighted in *New Frontiers* included a significant increase in the use of these technologies—an increase far greater than increases in the US population—but little research on actual use by older persons. Cross-sectional data from six national surveys of community-dwelling adults aged 65 and older show estimates of use of any device to be 14% to 18%.[108] In one retrospective longitudinal study 74% of 85-year-olds were using assistive devices, and this increased to 92% by the age of 90.[109] The most commonly used devices were for bathing and mobility. According to a 2001 survey, 6.2% of Medicare beneficiaries obtained mobility assistive technology. Average prices ranged from $52 for canes to $6,208 for power wheelchairs.[110]

AT is often not used once prescribed or is ill fitting. For example, one survey of 42 nursing home residents using wheelchairs identified 93 instances of inadequate equipment. Yet 86% of users were mostly satisfied with their wheelchairs.[111] The process of wheelchair provision may contribute to shortcomings. When wheelchairs are provided through a multifactorial approach involving experienced therapists, a prescription based on medical conditions and function, and additional therapy for training, new wheelchair owners were found to use their wheelchairs more often.[112] More formalized community-based wheelchair skills training that includes caregivers does improve users' skills.[113] For older persons for whom manual wheelchair use becomes difficult, power-assisted wheelchairs may be an excellent option to improve wheelchair mobility.[114] In a study of another common assistive device—a long-handled bath sponge—86% of patients used the device, and a variety of reasons accounted for the lack of use by the remaining 14%.[115]

The concept of usability defined by the International Organization for Standardization includes effectiveness, efficiency, satisfaction, and context of use. This construct can be applied to all assistive products, even clothing. For example, one study of orthopedic shoe use at 3 months in 93 older adults with degenerative arthritis in their feet added measures of efficiency (how easy shoes were to put on) and satisfaction (whether shoes were considered attractive) to usual measures of effectiveness (increase in stance duration, decrease in skin abnormalities). The fit of the logistic regression model predicting show use had an R^2 value of 34.9% when only effectiveness variables were used. Adding the efficiency variable and then the satisfaction variable increased the R^2 to 43.3% and 56.3%, respectively.[116] This type of research approach may improve both the successful development and use of new assistive products.

Rollators, a frame with four large tires, are especially effective, yet they are probably underused in the United States as assistive devices to compensate for balance problems. In Sweden 4% of the total population uses them, and in Denmark, 6.4% of people aged 56 to 84 years use them.[117] In one study, 89 users reported frequent device use and general satisfaction. Some users, however, reported having problems in handling the rollator, concerns with its weight, and difficulty in transporting it on a bus or folding it for car use.[118]

Some studies suggest that besides improving functional independence, AT can reduce the amount of human help a person requires. One randomized controlled trial showed this to be the case for frail elderly persons, many of whom had been discharged the prior year from an inpatient rehabilitation program. Home environmental modifications were combined with AT devices after a home assessment by an occupational therapist.[119] Another study analyzed data from the National Long Term Care Survey in 1994 and found persons with disability who used AT used fewer hours of personal assistance. Since this was a cross-sectional study, this association of greater AT use and fewer hours of assistance may not be causal.[120] Another research model, using data from the 1994–1995 National Health Interview Survey Disability Supplement, suggested that AT does reduce informal care hours for persons who are unmarried, better educated, or have better cognitive abilities. However, these same persons used more formal care hours. Therefore, the authors caution against concluding that AT might be a means of offsetting care costs for older disabled persons.[121]

For community-dwelling older adults, occupational therapy is an effective way to help patients obtain effective assistive devices. A systematic review demonstrated clear benefit when occupational therapy, as part of a home hazards assessment of functional ability, not only suggested the use of particular assistive devices but also subsequently helped train the person in behavioral changes to use the devices effectively.[122]

Modification of This Question in Light of New Research: We recommend keeping this question on the research agenda, as findings of such research are still needed. Overall, research in assistive device outcomes will require more development of outcome measures. Concepts to be covered include usability, quality of life, social role performance,[123] effectiveness, social significance, and subjective well-being.[124]

PROGRESS IN REHABILITATION FOR SPECIFIC CONDITIONS

See *New Frontiers,* pp. 353–359. For discussion of one new item for the research agenda, see the subsection on rehabilitation for specific conditions in New Horizons in Geriatric Rehabilitation at the end of the chapter

In this section of the rehabilitation chapter in *New Frontiers*, the discussion covered themes in several common disabling conditions: arthritic and related musculoskeletal problems, stroke, cardiac disease, hip fracture, amputation, deconditioning, sarcopenia and frailty, falls, and pain. Pertinent new research on these topics is described under the next ten agenda items.

***Rehab 20 (Level B)*: Epidemiologic and observational studies of older patients with specific disabling conditions are needed in order to identify risk factors and to select key outcomes for measurement in future clinical trials.**

New Research Addressing This Question: According to the Nagi model, one of the earliest models of disability, the disabling process starts with a particular pathophysiology that leads to an impairment, then to a functional limitation, and finally to a disability.[125] A societal limitation could then be present as well. This simpler, linear model of disability contrasts with a rehabilitation research model that uses a "transdomain" approach that evaluates simultaneously the impairment, functional limitation, and disability.[126] This research approach then clarifies contributing factors to disabilities and possible therapeutic approaches. For example, the relatively "simple" act of sit-to-stand performance depends on impairments in the person, chair-related factors, and compensatory strategies if impairments or chair factors are contributing to a functional disability. As chair seat height is lowered, the more functionally impaired person is less able to perform the task despite an increasing use of compensatory strategies. [127] This research has helped dissect the components of disability, showing that environmental factors as well as person's physiology contribute to functional limitations and disability. Rehabilitation clinicians have always known, from gross observation, that chair height plays a critical role in a patient's independence in transferring out of a chair. This research dissects this phenomenon more completely in a way that will help in the design of more effective rehabilitation strategies.

As disability becomes more widespread and affects a greater number of different populations, more emphasis in studies of disability is being placed on the prevention of disability. Such studies borrow from the traditional public health model and its focus on populations (Figure 12.2). [128,129] The three categories of disability prevention are primary (preventing the disease or pathophysiology), secondary (reducing disability risk factors, effectively treating early or asymptomatic disease, delaying progression of aging-related conditions such as diabetes mellitus, osteoarthritis), and tertiary (limiting progression of already present disability, or preventing additional impairments). [130] After appropriate diagnostic and prevention treatment strategies have been discovered, the health care delivery system needs to be designed to provide appropriate, cost-effective services.

The research on geriatric rehabilitation-related disability prevention and treatment interventions is growing rapidly, especially given the increasing recognition of the multiple

Pathology Impairment Functional Limitation Disability

Primary Prevention

Secondary Prevention

Tertiary Prevention

Figure 12.2—The disablement process (Verbrugge and Jette) is depicted in the top line. The public health prevention model below it correlates prevention with points in the disablement process. (Sources: Verbrugge LM, Jette AM. The disablement process. Soc Sci Med 1994;38:1–14. Figure from Magaziner J. Epidemiology of musculoskeletal conditions. Bethesda, MD: Interagency Committee on Disability Research, 2006. Reprinted with permission.)

factors contributing to disablement (eg, in the ICF). For older adults, "enabling" environments include a growing number of assisted-living facilities.[131] These vary in structure and services; they offer options for older adults who, for various reasons, need to change home environments.

A special complexity in understanding disability prevention and rehabilitation needs in older adults is the result of the interactions of frailty and multiple comorbidities. Recent detailed epidemiologic research has shown both the independence of frailty, comorbidities, and disability among seniors and their varying overlapping presence in some individuals.[132] (See Figure 12.3.) As the understanding of the underlying pathophysiology increases, targeting prevention strategies and interventions will be possible.

One new comorbidity index, the Geriatric Index of Comorbidity, combines the number of diseases and their severity.[133] This particular measure was found to have greater concurrent validity with disability and to be a better predictor of mortality than other measures in common use.

Modification of This Question in Light of New Research: We recommend keeping this question on the research agenda without modification, as findings of such research are still needed.

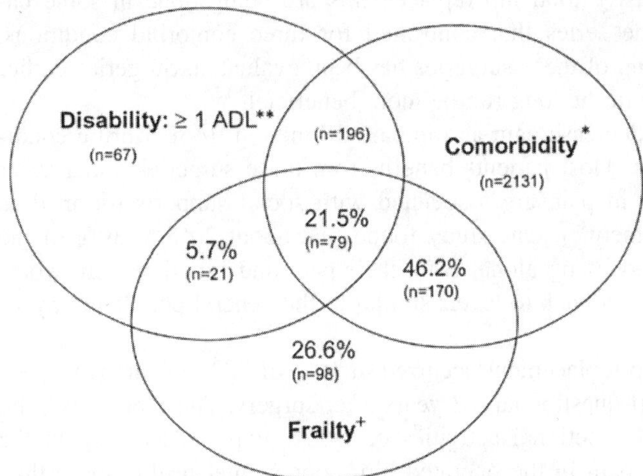

Figure 12.3—Venn diagram displaying the extent of overlap of frailty with activities of daily living disability and comorbidity (≥ 2 diseases). Total represented: 2762 subjects who had comorbidity, disability, or frailty (or two or all three). The number in each group is indicated in parentheses.

+ = Frail: overall N = 368 frail subjects (both cohorts).

* = Cormorbidity: overall N = 2576 with two or more out of the following nine diseases: myocardial infarction, angina, congestive heart failure, claudication, arthritis, cancer, diabetes, hypertension, chronic obstructive pulmonary disease. Of these, 249 were also frail.

** = Disabled: overall N = 363 with a disability in activities of daily living. Of these, 100 were frail.

(Source: Fried LP, Tangen CM, Walston J, et al. Frailty in older adults: evidence for a phenotype. J Gerontol A Biol Sci Med Sci 2001;56(3):M146–M156. Copyright © The Gerontological Society of America. Reproduced with permission of the publisher.)

Rehab 21 (Levels B, A): **Observational and cohort studies are needed to define the efficacy and safety of specific types of exercise, assistive devices, and orthotics for arthritic and musculoskeletal conditions. These studies could lead later to controlled trials comparing the most promising interventions.**

New Research Addressing This Question: Estimates are that the prevalence of osteoarthritis will increase by 50% by 2020.[134] Because osteoarthritis affects multiple joints, research challenges include identifying which specific joints are being studied, as back, knees, hip, feet, and hands can all be affected. And although sometimes emphasis has been on mechanical effects as contributory, there may well be metabolic components. For example, in obese patients with osteoarthritis of the knee, there is also an increased incidence of osteoarthritis in non-weight-bearing joints. Exercise is now accepted as a core component of any rehabilitation regimen because of its benefits, such as delaying the onset of ADL disability.[135] The American Geriatrics Society has published a guideline reviewing the consensus on exercise in osteoarthritis.[136]

Total joint replacements to treat advanced disease will likely be performed more frequently in our aging population. Some studies have looked at specific components of this type of surgery. Minimally invasive total hip replacements are being done in some patients, generally younger. In one series that controlled for three comorbid conditions, recovery was very fast.[137] Timing of these surgeries has been evaluated. Surgeries earlier in the course of the disease may in the long run be more beneficial.[138]

Currently, joint replacements decrease pain and impaired function from arthritic conditions in both the knees and hips. Most patients benefit from these surgeries, but greater gains in function and decreases in pain are associated with social supports (defined as being married or living with someone). One study found that about 20% to 30% of the patients were both unmarried and living alone. Both their pain and function were worse initially at 1 month after surgery but back to levels similar to the general population by 12 months.[139]

Poorer outcomes after total hip replacement occurred in 10% of 922 patients who were re-evaluated through a self-report questionnaire 3 years after surgery. These patients, who had moderate difficulty with all functional activities or worse, experienced pain in the back or lower extremity, severe pain in the operated hip, poor mental health, more than one common geriatric problem, and obesity, and all also had less than college education.[140]

One randomized controlled trial compared a structured exercise program both before and after total hip replacement surgery with usual care in Australia. The exercise group received two supervised clinic sessions a week and were to repeat the activities at home two times a week for a total of 8 weeks before surgery. These structured exercises were continued for 12 weeks after surgery. The control group received only the instruction from hospital therapists. Both groups were comparable in basic demographics, neither group had surgical complications, and the same surgeons operated on the patients in both the intervention and control groups. At 24 weeks after surgery, both stride length and speed of gait were greater in the exercise group.[141]

A Canadian study evaluated clinic-based total knee replacement rehabilitation, comparing it with a home program that was taught to patients during the 5- to 7-day hospitalization. No differences were found between the two groups.[142]

Pain management from total knee replacement during inpatient rehabilitation was found to be improved in a randomized trial using oxycodone twice a day. Patients were able to walk further and had lengths of stay 2.3 days shorter, on average.[143] In total knee replacements, the use of continuous passive motion machines and slider boards has not been associated with better range of motion at discharge, 3, or 6 months.[144]

The effects of dehydration can be marked in older orthopedic rehabilitation patients. Length of stay was significantly longer for patients with azotemia (BUN/creatine $\geq$ 20) and orthostatic hypotension (13.6 $\pm$ 2.7 days versus 7.2 $\pm$ 2.8 days) than for patients without these conditions. Discharge function was similar in the two groups.[145] These huge differences in length of stay indicate a real need to evaluate this problem and possible early interventions in more detail.

Little work has been done focusing on patients' subjective experience before, during, and after joint replacement. One such study used grounded theory in interviewing 9 patients with varied total knee replacement experiences. Patients' experiences were summarized as "enduring," "thinking twice," and "keeping faith."[146] Better understanding of these experiences may lead directly to changes in the prehabilitation, hospitalization, and postoperative phases of the patients' joint replacements.

Modification of This Question in Light of New Research: We recommend keeping this question on the research agenda without modification, as findings of such research are still needed.

Rehab 22 (Levels B, A): **Observational and cohort studies are needed in the rehabilitation of musculoskeletal conditions to obtain preliminary data on the effects of the location of the physical therapy, the level of expertise of therapists needed, and how much is accomplished by education of elderly patients. This could lead eventually to controlled trials assessing these variables.**

New Research Addressing This Question: Our literature review found no reports addressing this issue.

Modification of This Question in Light of New Research: We recommend keeping this question on the research agenda without modification, as findings of such research are still needed.

Rehab 23 (Levels B, A): **Hypothesis-generating research followed by hypothesis-testing research is needed to identify the key components facilitating better outcomes that are seen in some settings and to identify ways to optimize treatment and outcomes among elderly patients unable to tolerate therapy in a stroke unit or rehabilitation hospital.**

New Research Addressing This Question: A major study has identified many of the components of inpatient IRF care processes for stroke patients and has related these to patient outcomes.[43] (See the discussion under Rehab 11.) Multiple aspects of more effective treatment components were identified.

The usage patterns of anticoagulant, antihypertensive, nonsteroidal anti-inflammatory, and antiplatelet agents in the Post-Stroke Rehabilitation Outcome Project study have been described. Many stroke participants received prophylaxis for deep-vein thrombosis, but 65 cases occurred, almost all in patients with moderate to severe stroke and many within the first day or two of admission. Thirty-three percent of participants received no antiplatelet or anticoagulant medication, suggesting possibilities for increased secondary stroke prevention. Antihypertensive medications were used in 73% of patients, and their blood pressures were on average higher than those of nonhypertensive patients during the entire rehabilitation stay, despite medication use (mean systolic at discharge 146.6 versus 131 mm/Hg). More aggressive blood pressure lowering is indicated during rehabilitation, if tolerated by patients, given the proven benefits of secondary stroke prevention. Neurostimulant medications were used in 20% of participants and were not associated with any differences in length of stay or cognitive or motor recovery. Pain medications were frequently used, and sites of pain, in order of decreasing frequency, were the head, leg, back, shoulder and hip.[147]

Other new research is studying constraint-induced movement therapy that improves motor function in specific types of patients.[148–150] One mechanism is having patients overcome learned disuse. A recent multicenter randomized study included 222 patients who had mostly ischemic strokes in the prior 3 to 9 months and noted that 106 who underwent constraint-induced motor therapy demonstrated clinically relevant improvements in arm motor function that persisted for at least 1 year.[151] Researchers are studying the potential benefits of robotics in stroke rehabilitation with promising approaches.[152,153]

The interactions of family function, caregiver health, and stroke survivor function were evaluated in a trial of 132 patients who had had strokes 3 to 9 months earlier. Thirty-two percent of the families scored positively for ineffective family functioning. Some family conflict was reported by 66% of the caregivers. Predictors of worse caregiver mental health (measured from the Medical Outcomes Study Short Form 36) included ineffective family functioning as well as poorer memory and behavior function in the stroke survivor. High family conflict was associated with poorer caregiver mental health, even if the stroke survivor had lesser memory and behavior problems.[31] In another study evaluating caregivers, a randomized controlled trial of early supported discharge to home for stroke survivors included education and support. Caregivers receiving this intervention consistently experienced a lower caregiver burden than caregivers receiving usual care.[154]

Effective stroke rehabilitation care, in the form of adherence with the stroke rehabilitation guidelines, is associated with better functional outcomes.[155] These are among the first data that validate the recommendations made by the national post-stroke rehabilitation guidelines.[156]

Stroke rehabilitation continues to need to focus on longer term outcomes. In a study that evaluated participation at 6 months after stroke onset, a significant number of people were found to have problems with travel, social activities, recreational activities, moving around the community, and having an important activity to fill the day.[157] Studies for effective interventions to help in these areas are needed.

Modification of This Question in Light of New Research: We recommend keeping this question on the research agenda without modification, as findings of such research are still needed.

***Rehab 24 (Level A)*: Randomized controlled trials of exercise-based cardiac rehabilitation, as a function of age and comorbid conditions, would be very valuable and are urgently needed.**

New Research Addressing This Question: Cardiac rehabilitation programs in older adults will need to adapt to increased activity limitations and chronic comorbidities. In evaluation of two nationally representative cross-sectional surveys (the Health and Retirement Survey and the Assets and Health Dynamics of the Oldest Old study), Oldridge and Stump identified an increased likelihood of mobility and other activity limitation among those with heart disease and especially those with multiple comorbidities.[158] Cardiac rehabilitation programs need to be aware of these issues, both to determine optimal programming and to be sure patients are not unnecessarily excluded from beneficial cardiac rehabilitation. This may be especially important, given preliminary data from a descriptive study of 6-month cardiac rehabilitation program outcomes. The patients studied had a mean age of approximately 76 and had all undergone coronary bypass surgery; they had self-selected to participate in a cardiac rehabilitation program or not. These two groups were generally comparable as a result of the use of strict exclusion criteria. Lower-extremity function and balance were clearly better at 6 months in patients who had participated in the rehabilitation program.[159]

A randomized controlled trial of cardiac rehabilitation for patients with significant cardiac disease is ongoing in Denmark. Forty-nine percent of the 770 subjects are 65 years or older. The researchers noted, however, that the percentage of eligible older patients who consent to participation drops as patients get older. For example, only 17% of eligible patients aged 85 years and older agreed to participate in the study.[160] Nonetheless, this study will contribute to understanding the value of cardiac rehabilitation in older adults.

Modification of This Question in Light of New Research: We recommend keeping this question on the research agenda without modification, as findings of such research are still needed.

Rehab 25 (Level A): **Randomized controlled trials are needed to test the efficacy and safety for elderly patients of early, high-intensity physical therapy following hip fracture surgery and of postoperative restrictions on ambulation.**

New Research Addressing This Question: Outcomes from hip fractures are highly variable—from full recovery of walking abilities and activities to survival at wheelchair level to death. If we understood patient prognoses better, it would be clearer for whom the hip fracture represented disability at the end of life where little or no recovery would be possible, for whom recovery would be total without residual problems, or for whom outcomes would fall in between. Clinically appropriate and cost-effective therapies could then be better targeted. One creative analytic approach to this issue used cluster analysis. By collecting known and suspected predictive variables, the researchers used cluster analysis to identify four typological categories, or profiles, of patients with different 1-year outcomes. For example, those patients who died during 1-year follow-up were found to have had significantly diminished prefracture leisure activities, increased disorientation, more comorbidities, greater use of drugs, and unfavorable levels of prefracture ADL scores and relative perceived health.[161] Additional work on this approach may help clinicians more explicitly target appropriate disability management strategies.

Other studies have identified risk factors for mortality and decreased walking ability after hip fracture in individual patients and in comparison with age-matched community-dwelling populations.[162,163] Active medical issues play a role.[164] Neurologic comorbidity complicates hip fracture rehabilitation and is associated with longer lengths of stay and overall lower functional scores in comparison with controls (hip fracture patients without neurologic impairment). However, no difference was found in the amount of functional gain between the two groups.[165]

Rehabilitation outcomes have been known to depend on social supports in certain situations. In hip fracture patients, a standardized rehabilitation and discharge planning protocol during acute care hospitalization was found to yield better results only in those patients with low social supports (assessed as number of contacts outside the home and the size of patients' social networks). Three-month Barthel Index scores were better, and more patients were living in the community at 6 months.[166]

Rehabilitation services have usually been provided for the few weeks or months after a fracture. However, in a randomized controlled trial, a duration of 6 months of physical therapy (three times a week) that included resistance training was found to result in improved physical function and mobility in more frail community-dwelling patients. Quality-of-life reports were better at 9 to 12 months as well.[167] This finding underscores the potential of structured strength training and exercise in recovery. The next issue is practical implementation, and payment for, such a relatively extensive intervention.

Optimal settings for hip fracture rehabilitation have been evaluated. In Finland, a randomized controlled trial (N = 243) compared outcomes for patients with dementia and hip fractures who were rehabilitated on a geriatric inpatient service with outcomes for patients who received usual local hospital care. Patients with moderate dementia, a Mini-Mental State Examination (MMSE) score of 12 to 17, had shorter inpatient rehabilitation stays (47 versus 147 days, $P = .042$), and a higher percentage were living at home at 3 months (63% versus 17%). Patients with mild dementias (MMSE scores 18 to 23) also had shorter rehabilitation inpatient stays (29 versus 46 days, $P = .002$), and more were living at home at 3 months (91% versus 67%).[168]

One summary review of best practices for older hip fracture patients concluded that evidence has identified some peri-operative practices with consistent benefits.[169] However, types of surgical management, postoperative wound drainage, and even multidisciplinary care do not have consistent evidence for improving outcomes.[170] In combination with some of the work described above, more detailed research is required to determine optimal interventions for specific subcategories of hip fracture patients.

Modification of This Question in Light of New Research: We recommend keeping this question on the research agenda without modification, as findings of such research are still needed.

***Rehab 26 (Levels B, A)*: Observational and cohort studies should be performed to compare the costs and benefits of using newer prostheses in younger and older persons; factors found to be associated with better outcomes for older persons should then be tested in controlled trials.**

New Research Addressing This Question: A detailed descriptive study of a 5% sample of Medicare patients who had index amputations in 1996 (N = 3565) documented considerable 1-year morbidity and mortality. Reamputation rates for persons with initial amputations at the toe, at the foot or ankle (or both), transtibial, transfemoral, and bilateral sites were 35%, 39%, 23%, 14%, and 29%, respectively. One-year mortality rates for these levels were, respectively, 23%, 29%, 36%, 50%, and 53%. [171] In a study using Massachusetts Hospital Case Mix and Charge Data from 1997, discharge locations after amputation were as follows: only 33% home, 32% to SNFs, 16% to inpatient rehabilitation, and 15% to other sites. [172]

Better evaluation methods for level of amputation would be very helpful. Out-of-pocket costs and health insurance benefits for care can accumulate significantly for patients and families with each amputation episode. Reasons for high mortality are likely due to diffuse vascular disease and merit further research. Rehabilitation programs, in collaboration with primary care physicians, need to consider this significant mortality in planning appropriate rehabilitation approaches. On a systems level, the rate of dysvascular amputation increased 27% between 1988 and 1996. [173] With the increasing age of the population, the number of patients experiencing amputations will likely increase and require improved systems of care. [174]

Modification of This Question in Light of New Research: We recommend keeping this question on the research agenda without modification, as findings of such research are still needed.

***Rehab 27 (Levels B, A)*: Basic laboratory research is needed to determine the factors that cause sarcopenia or that interact to cause it in older persons. Findings from this research should then be used in clinical trials of interventions to prevent or treat sarcopenia.**

New Research Addressing This Question: Our literature search found no articles on sarcopenia. However, several articles discussed aspects of bed rest, which we include under this rehabilitation question.

Bed rest, an acute form of inactivity, causes a series of physiologic changes usually referred to as *deconditioning*. In order to truly constitute deconditioning, these changes must be reversible once activity is renewed. Little study has been done measuring specifically the effects of bed rest on older healthy adults. It has been assumed, however, that physiologic decrements are likely to be similar to those experienced by younger persons. Functional decrements have long been assumed to be related to bed rest. The association of bed rest and functional decrements has been confirmed in a study of 680 nondisabled, community-living persons aged 70 years or older. Study participants were asked about "taking to bed" and were surveyed again at 18 months. The loss at 18 months from baseline in instrumental ADLs, mobility, physical activity, and social activity was found to be greater with increasing self-reported days of bed rest in nonfrail individuals than in frail ones. Of note, the nonfrail group always performed better than the frail group. [175]

Special challenges exist for keeping people active once they have lost the ability to be active on their own. One assessment of a bedfast quality indicator report found that SNF residents spend an average of 17 hours in bed, indicating significant disability. [176]

For especially frail elderly patients recovering from acute illness, a very slow inpatient rehabilitation program may be necessary to get them home. A Canadian study of 154 patients described outcomes of "slow stream rehabilitation." Eighty percent of patients came from acute care hospitals and 14% from "fast stream" rehabilitation sites. Fifty-three percent of the patients were discharged to their preferred discharge goal location (the great majority were home) with a long rehabilitation program of up to 9 months. Markers distinguishing these 53% from those who remained in a nursing home included expert clinician opinion, good vision, better ADL function, and help at home.[60]

Modification of This Question in Light of New Research: We recommend keeping this question on the research agenda, as findings of such research are still needed, but with the addition of research that focuses on deconditioning as well as on sarcopenia.

***Rehab 28 (Level A)*: Randomized trials are needed to examine the merits of specific falls-prevention interventions (eg, types or duration or frequency of exercise, mobility aids, home safety interventions) and for specific subgroups of elderly patients (eg, cognitively impaired, hospitalized) and to examine the cost-effectiveness of various falls-prevention strategies.**

New Research Addressing This Question: Fear of falling, an independent risk factor for functional decline and decrease in recreational physical activity, has been evaluated in older hospitalized patients, patient with hip fractures, patients with amputations, older adults transitioning to frailty, and community-dwelling seniors.[177] Fear of falling is associated with history of falls (but not always), a lower Falls Efficacy Scale score (feeling less confident of ability to do activities without falling), use of a walking aid, and more ADL dependency.[178] Fear of falling, even in the absence of any fall history, can be associated with a greatly increased risk of institutionalization. In one study of rehabilitation for hip fractures, Falls Efficacy Scale score was found to improve, but this did not correlate with improvements in the FIM score.[179] This suggests that falls efficacy could be targeted for treatment in more comprehensive hip fracture rehabilitation. Fear of falling is present in patients with amputation, especially if overall perceived health is fair to poor.[180] Even healthy older women without a history of falls can have a fear of falling. This fear of falling is present in active women but is greater in less active women.[177] Falls are independent predictors of the development of the fear of falling. In turn, fear of falling is a predictor of falling.[181] Interventions that help reduce the fear of falling include a physical activity or education program and Tai Chi.[182,183] For rehabilitation patients, a unidimensional fear of falling measure was developed through Rasch analysis. It includes 16 items and rates people's fear of falling on the basis of a hierarchy of activities.[184] This may provide a newer fear-of-falling instrument for research and clinical use.

Risk factors for falls have been extensively studied. Dual tasking of cognitive and physical tasks becomes harder to do in older patients. Maximal motor performance was found to decline significantly with concurrent cognitive tasks, especially in older adults with a history of injurious falls and cognitive impairment.[185] This may be the link between cognitive impairment and higher risk of falls.

A measure of gait stride length variability in ambulatory community-living adults aged 70 years and over is predictive of falls during the following year.[186] In patients admitted to home health care, risk factors include gait and balance difficulties, wandering, depression, and living in unsafe dwellings with environmental hazards.[187] The development and use of normative standards on common objective measures like the Six-Minute Walk Test, Berg Balance Scale, Timed Up and Go Test, and comfortable- and fast-speed walking may help in assessing older adults.[188]

Recurrent falls are an especially challenging rehabilitation problem. For example, one study found that of 100 hip fracture patients, 53% fell at least once in the 6 months following the initial hip fracture.[189] A cluster of risk factors for these is not surprising—lower performance on balance and mobility measures, prefracture falls history, and use of a gait device.

One small randomized trial used a bilateral separated treadmill to train frail older adults, most of whom had fallen once already. The control group received usual care. Gait parameters improved, but falls over the next 6 months were similar in the exercised and control group.[190]

In the past, multiple types of interventions—either single interventions or several concurrent interventions—have been tested for falls reduction. Some exercise programs and multidimensional interventions have most effectively prevented falls.[191] A randomized factorial trial tested three interventions (exercise, vision, home hazard management) separately and in combination in 1090 participants. The home hazard assessment was included because these are readily available at low cost in Australia. Results showed that the greatest reduction in falls occurred when all three interventions were combined. Exercise alone yielded benefit (14% estimated reduction in annual fall rate, number needed to treat of 7), but neither vision or home hazard management alone reduced falls.[192] Another study, a randomized controlled trial of clinic-based 6-week exercise program for community-dwelling older adults, demonstrated modest reductions in falls at 6 months.[193] One limitation on generalizing such an intervention is that a significant number of participants did not complete the full exercise program. Interventions to reduce falls therefore seem to be more feasible when done at home, but they require sufficient exercise to improve aspects of balance and mobility.

Risk factors for falls were successfully decreased in a study of women with thoracic kyphosis of 50 to 65 degrees (Cobb angle). These women were compared with age-matched controls and showed significantly worse balance and gait by objective measures. The women then received a 4-week spinal proprioceptive extension exercise dynamic program with the use of a spinal weighted kypho-orthosis. Significant improvements occurred in balance, muscle strength in the back, and in the falls efficacy score (from 32.4 ± 13.8 to 13.5 ± 3.5, $P < .001$ with score of 10 normal). Mean physical activity improved as well.[194]

Modification of This Question in Light of New Research: We recommend keeping this question on the research agenda without modification, as findings of such research are still needed.

> *Rehab 29 (Levels B, A)*: **Observational and cohort studies are needed to clarify the natural history of pain syndromes, identify risk factors, and describe the effects of treatment approaches. Ultimately, the most promising approaches should be identified and tested in controlled trials.**

New Research Addressing This Question: Pain always has been a huge clinical issue, especially in older patients. One community survey of older adults found that 72% had experienced as least some musculoskeletal pain in the prior 2 weeks. Severe pain was associated with disability.[195] In the rehabilitation process, pain is common, and management challenges are similar to those with pain in other areas of medicine. Pain treatment always requires a comprehensive, whole-person approach. Current recommendations point to the areas requiring research in rehabilitation in general, especially in postoperative geriatric pain management, cancer, and persistent pain.[196–199]

Modification of This Question in Light of New Research: We recommend keeping this question on the research agenda without modification, as findings of such research are still needed.

NEW HORIZONS IN GERIATRIC REHABILITATION

THEORETICAL UNDERPINNINGS FOR GERIATRIC REHABILITATION

Patient Assessments

Appropriate patient assessments to target rehabilitation therapies and management need further development. For example, on an inpatient rehabilitation unit, OTs and PTs were found to have difficulty detecting both cognitive abnormalities and symptoms of depression in older patients (mean age 73).[200] In a survey of more than 1700 rehabilitation inpatients with musculoskeletal and cardiovascular diseases, 369 patients were identified as appropriate for an in-depth psychologic interview. Chart reviews were done on the interviewed patients. Rehabilitation staff correctly detected mental disorders only 48% of the time in the orthopedic patients and only 32% of the time in cardiovascular patients.[201] The use of clock drawing and clock copying may be an easy way to screen for cognitive problems. Results correlate well with other general cognitive measures, and they do correlate with poorer functional outcomes during inpatient rehabilitation.[202]

New dimensions of assessment that are predictive of functional outcomes will potentially become important for assessment. For example, poor participation in inpatient therapies is associated with both longer lengths of inpatient rehabilitation and poorer functional outcomes.[203] Researchers have created a tool to measure geriatric rehabilitation that assesses mobility, basic ADLs, independent living, leisure, physical functioning, psychologic function, social function, and caregiver status.[204]

Comprehensiveness of assessments may be required in some clinical circumstances. One meta-analysis found that prevention of functional decline in older adults living in the community occurred only if assessments were multidimensional.[4] Where successes have occurred in inpatient and outpatient geriatric evaluation (and management), assessments have been comprehensive.[205] Continued work is needed to best identify the when, where, and how of comprehensive assessment of older adults with disabilities.

> *Rehab 30 (Levels B, A)*: **Careful observational and longitudinal studies are needed to identify the optimal timing of comprehensive assessments that lead to significant clinical benefit. Comparative studies are needed to identify the most effective and efficient types of assessments. Information from these studies can lead to interventional trials that compare different comprehensive assessment methodologies with clinical outcomes.**

Prehabilitation

The term *prehabilitation* is appearing in the literature now that clinicians and researchers are shifting emphasis toward preventing disability. It began in the sports medicine literature. Athletes prehabilitate, or condition or train, to prevent injuries. Now, in the medical literature the concept is used in several contexts beyond reference to athletes and sports medicine. Initially, in the late 1980s, the focus was on improving care for older adults.[206] Papers describing prehabilitation discuss preoperative exercise to hasten recovery and improve functional outcome, exercise prior to elective intensive rehabilitation care unit admissions to prevent the consequences of deconditioning, and in-home exercise programs for older adults living in the community.[207–209] Gill et al used a randomized controlled trial to demonstrate less decline in function at 7 and 12 months from a 6-month, home-based, PT-prescribed exercise program in moderately, but not severely, frail persons aged 75 years or older.[210] Another randomized controlled exercise study, preoperatively, of total hip replacement patients yielded less stiffness and better physical function, as well as better self-rated improvement in health in the intervention group than in the control group.[211]

> *Rehab 31 (Levels B, A)*: **Observational studies are needed to identify feasible prehabilitation activities for elective surgical patients. Observational and longitudinal studies are needed of aging adults with a range of musculoskeletal symptoms, including mild, to identify interventions that prevent worsening of symptoms and onset of disability. More interventional studies are needed to assess the effectiveness of promising prehabilitation activities.**

Spirituality

Medical articles and books increasingly address issues of spirituality, religion, and health.[212,213] Religion and spirituality are being studied with various research methods and research instruments. Religious practices are rooted in the beliefs and traditions of specific religions. Spirituality refers to a sense of connectedness with something beyond and can include a sense of power, meaning, or purpose either from within or from a transcendent source.[214]

In one study of geriatric outpatients, self-report of greater spirituality, but not greater religious activity, was found to be associated with better self-reported health status.[215] A detailed study evaluated persons with musculoskeletal disabilities and recent hospitalization (rheumatology or rehabilitation services). The mean age was 56 but included some individuals as old as 82 years. Using a qualitative study design, the researchers found self-reported health to be very dependent on spiritual awareness. A Self Attributes Model was developed to show what internal processes are required for good health.[216]

A cross-cultural study of spirituality, religion, and personal beliefs included 5087 persons who reported belonging to a variety of religions: Christianity, animism, Islam, Judaism, Buddhism, and Hinduism. Differences were found between younger (< 45 years old) and older people. Results showed a correlation between spirituality, religion, and personal beliefs and all quality-of-life domains measured (physical, psychologic, independence, social support, environment). The authors suggested that spirituality and religion could be especially important as a component of quality of life for patients reporting very poor health.[217]

This sampling of recent work suggests that future geriatric rehabilitation research will need to assess aspects of spirituality and health in individuals with mild, moderate, and severe disability, as well as those with disability at the end of life.

Rehab 32 (Levels B, A): **More observational studies on spirituality, disability, and rehabilitation are needed to augment our understanding of their relationship. Innovative intervention studies are needed to understand how to enhance healing aspects in the relationships of spirituality, disability, and rehabilitation.**

THE COMPONENTS OF REHABILITATION

Outcomes of Care

Studies of rehabilitation outcomes for older patients comparing care settings have been hampered by the lack of uniform functional measures for use in these varied settings. [218] Setting-specific measures do not have adequate breadth to assess the wide range of functional abilities of persons receiving rehabilitation across multiple health care and community settings. They lack the precision in content, and important functional tasks are excluded. Floor and ceiling effects are common. Computer adaptive testing uses item response theory or Rasch models to determine a hierarchy of items within a questionnaire along a hierarchical unidimensional scale. It uses computer interfaces allowing items to be selected on the basis of the individual ability of each patient. Research with this technology is showing that group scores on three domains—physical and movement, personal care and instrumental, and applied cognition—can be derived for older patients receiving rehabilitation in different settings. [219] This approach works also for complex medical patients who require rehabilitation for cardiac, pulmonary, medical, or surgical complications, and other conditions. [220] Ongoing research on this approach will lead to clinical applications.

There has been a need to better understand longer term functional outcomes in social and community activities in patients who have had either acute onset of disability or more chronic, slowly progressive disability. In the World Health Organization's ICF framework, participation (defined as a person's involvement in a life situation) is conceived as the result of a complex interaction among a person's disease, the person's body structure and function (anatomic parts and physiologic functions), and the person's activity performance (execution of a task or action). Participation is also influenced by personal characteristics and the environmental context, including social and physical elements. Through the use of a newly developed Participation Measure for Post-Acute Care, community participation at 1, 6, and 12 months was assessed for patients receiving rehabilitation in both inpatient and outpatient rehabilitation settings. Personal and social environmental factors were found to play a major role in predicting levels of social and home participation. At 6 months, some participation components in community function were improved. These "community participation" items reflect a person's mobility, functioning in work, and other daily activities. Activities that were being performed less well were social and home participation. These activities reflect communication, social relationships, and home management roles. [221] Ongoing work in this area, using participation measures for patients who have recently received rehabilitation services, will help answer questions in all the rehabilitation agenda items regarding components of care.

Some significant changes have occurred, however, in outcomes of medical rehabilitation programs between 1994 and 2001. Lengths of stay have decreased from 20 to 12 days. Functional status as measured by the FIM score at discharge remained somewhat similar over this 8-year period. However, increases in standard deviations and decreases in absolute values ranging from 3.1 to 6.4 FIM units in all impairment groups, except orthopedic conditions, does raise the question of poorer function at discharge on average.[222] These changes in FIM scores, while small, are likely significant given the large sample sizes (eg, 48,055 stroke survivors, 8871 patients with other neurologic conditions). Possibly, a greater range of patients—from very medically stable to less stable—is now receiving inpatient rehabilitation. The increase in mortality from less than 1% in 1994 to 4.7% in 2001 is not explained by variables in the data set but would be consistent with an increase in the number of sicker patients being admitted to inpatient rehabilitation units.

Rehab 33 (Levels B, A): **Analyses of rehabilitation outcomes in currently collected rehabilitation outcomes databases are needed to better define the relationship of medical conditions and rehabilitation outcomes. Observational studies are needed that use functional and medical outcome measures that cover a broader range of outcomes. Innovative interventional studies are needed that can test these new rehabilitation outcome measures.**

Patient Satisfaction

Patient satisfaction with health care services has now become a routine outcome measure. For people with disabilities and insured through Medicare, dissatisfaction with health care services was greater as the number of ADL limitations increased. The aspects of care most highly associated with dissatisfaction included difficulty in getting to the doctor, availability of medical services at night and on weekends, availability of care by specialists, and follow-up care received.[223] Patient satisfaction has also been shown to be greater for stroke patients in centers that have complied more completely with post-stroke rehabilitation guidelines.[224] Amount of functional recovery has been associated with satisfaction in some, but not other, studies of stroke patients.[225]

Rehab 34 (Levels B, A): **Both observational and interventional studies are required to understand components of dissatisfaction with care and cost-effective interventions that work for patients with activities of daily living limitations.**

REHABILITATION FOR SPECIFIC CONDITIONS

Traumatic Brain Injury

There is a bimodal peak in traumatic brain injury (TBI), with peaks in persons ages 15 to 24 and in those 70 years of age and older. The most frequent cause of TBI in older adults is falling. Evidence suggests that functional impairments in older patients with TBI are more severe and that an age threshold for poor outcomes exists between ages 50 to 60. In a study with an inception cohort of 195 patients with mild, moderate, and severe TBI, older patients (50 to 89 years of age) were found to be more likely than younger patients to become financially dependent and require help of others. However, many of the 49 older patients were still able to live independently and reported being independent in some kind of work (80% and 49%, respectively, compared with 93% and 61%, pre-injury).[226] A large study of 45,982 cases of ICD-9 TBI in the New York State Trauma Registry (excluding New York City) from 1994 through 1995 documented higher mortality in older patients. Higher mortality occurred in older patients at even mild Glasgow Coma Scores of 13 to 15.[227] Ongoing work will better define the cluster of prognostic factors that may help clinical decision making on both aggressiveness of acute medical care as well as optimal rehabilitation approaches given different levels of injury severity.

***Rehab 35 (Levels B, A)*: More observational studies are required to understand the range of severity of head injury in older patients who fall, as well as all of the consequences. Different interventional studies need to address the range of traumatic brain injury disability, from mild to moderate to severe and to end-stage.**

REFERENCES

1. Hoenig H, Siebens H. Geriatric rehabilitation. In Solomon DH, LoCicero J, 3rd, Rosenthal RA (eds): New Frontiers in Geriatrics Research: An Agenda for Surgical and Related Medical Specialties. New York: American Geriatrics Society, 2004, pp. 339-367 (online at http://www.frycomm.com/ags/rasp).
2. Hoenig H, Siebens H. Research agenda for geriatric rehabilitation. Am J Phys Med Rehabil 2004;83:858-866.
3. Fletcher AE, Price GM, Ng ES, et al. Population-based multidimensional assessment of older people in UK general practice: a cluster-randomised factorial trial. Lancet 2004;364:1667-1677.
4. Stuck AE, Egger M, Hammer A, et al. Home visits to prevent nursing home admission and functional decline in elderly people: systematic review and meta-regression analysis. JAMA 2002;287:1022-1028.
5. World Health Organization. International Classification of Functioning, Disability and Health (ICF). Geneva, Switzerland: 2001 (online at http://www.who.int/classifications/icf/en/).
6. Stucki G, Grimby G. Applying the ICF in medicine. J Rehabil Med 2004;44:5-6.
7. Weigl M, Cieza A, Andersen C, et al. Identification of relevant ICF categories in patients with chronic health conditions: a Delphi exercise. J Rehabil Med 2004;44:12-21.
8. Brockow T, Cieza A, Kuhlow H, et al. Identifying the concepts contained in outcome measures of clinical trials on musculoskeletal disorders and chronic widespread pain using the International Classification of Functioning, Disability and Health as a reference. J Rehabil Med 2004;44:30-36.
9. DeJong G, Horn SD, Gassaway JA, et al. Toward a taxonomy of rehabilitation interventions: using an inductive approach to examine the "black box" of rehabilitation. Arch Phys Med Rehabil 2004;85:678-686.
10. DeJong G, Horn SD, Conroy B, et al. Opening the black box of post-stroke rehabilitation: stroke rehabilitation patients, processes, and outcomes. Arch Phys Med Rehabil 2005;86:S1-S7.
11. Boyd CM, Xue QL, Guralnik JM, Fried LP. Hospitalization and development of dependence in activities of daily living in a cohort of disabled older women: the Women's Health and Aging Study I. J Gerontol A Biol Sci Med Sci 2005;60:888-893.
12. Gill TM, Allore HG, Holford TR, Guo Z. Hospitalization, restricted activity, and the development of disability among older persons. JAMA 2004;292:2115-2124.

13. McCusker J, Kakuma R, Abrahamowicz M. Predictors of functional decline in hospitalized elderly patients: a systematic review. J Gerontol A Biol Sci Med Sci 2002;57:M569-M577.
14. Bean J, Kiely DK, Leveille SG, Morris J. Associating the onset of motor impairments with disability progression in nursing home residents. Am J Phys Med Rehabil 2002;81:696-704; quiz 705-697, 720.
15. Hardy SE, Gill TM. Recovery from disability among community-dwelling older persons. JAMA 2004;291:1596-1602.
16. Onder G, Penninx BW, Ferrucci L, et al. Measures of physical performance and risk for progressive and catastrophic disability: results from the Women's Health and Aging Study. J Gerontol A Biol Sci Med Sci 2005;60:74-79.
17. Lenze EJ, Schulz R, Martire LM, et al. The course of functional decline in older people with persistently elevated depressive symptoms: longitudinal findings from the Cardiovascular Health Study. J Am Geriatr Soc 2005;53:569-575.
18. Freedman VA, Martin LG, Schoeni RF. Recent trends in disability and functioning among older adults in the United States: a systematic review. JAMA 2002;288:3137-3146.
19. Fries JF. Reducing disability in older age. JAMA 2002;288:3164-3166.
20. Wan H, Sengupta M, Velkoff VA, DeBarros KA. 65+ in the United States. Washington, D.C.: U.S. Census Bureau, Current Population Reports. U.S. Government Printing Office, 2005, pp. 23-209 (available online: http://www.census.gov/prod/2006pubs/p23-209.pdf).
21. Chan L, Houck P, Prela CM, MacLehose RF. Using medicare databases for outcomes research in rehabilitation medicine. Am J Phys Med Rehabil 2001;80:474-480.
22. Chan L, Beaver S, Maclehose RF, et al. Disability and health care costs in the Medicare population. Arch Phys Med Rehabil 2002;83:1196-1201.
23. Chan L, Shumway-Cook A, Yorkston KM, et al. Design and validation of a methodology using the International Classification of Diseases, 9th Revision, to identify secondary conditions in people with disabilities. Arch Phys Med Rehabil 2005;86:1065-1069.
24. Bronfenbrenner U. Toward an experimental ecology of human development. Am Psychologist 1977;32:513-530.
25. Whiteneck GG, Harrison-Felix CL, Mellick DC, et al. Quantifying environmental factors: a measure of physical, attitudinal, service, productivity, and policy barriers. Arch Phys Med Rehabil 2004;85:1324-1335.
26. Keysor J, Jette A, Haley S. Development of the home and community environment (HACE) instrument. J Rehabil Med 2005;37:37-44.
27. Shumway-Cook A, Patla A, Stewart A, et al. Environmental components of mobility disability in community-living older persons. J Am Geriatr Soc 2003;51:393-398.
28. Lansley P, McCreadie C, Tinker A. Can adapting the homes of older people and providing assistive technology pay its way? Age Ageing 2004;33:571-576.
29. Bogardus ST, Bradley EH, Williams CS, et al. Goals for the care of frail older adults: do caregivers and clinicians agree? Am J Med 2001;110:97-102.
30. Clark PC, King KB. Comparison of family caregivers: stroke survivors vs. person with Alzheimer's disease. J Gerontol Nurs 2003;29:45-53.
31. Clark PC, Dunbar SB, Shields CG, et al. Influence of stroke survivor characteristics and family conflict surrounding recovery on caregivers' mental and physical health. Nurs Res 2004;53:406-413.
32. Levine C. Family Caregivers on the Job: Moving beyond ADLs and IADLs. New York, NY: United Hospital Fund of New York, 2004, pp. 1-166.
33. Caregiving in the U.S. Bethesda, MD: National Alliance for Caregiving and AARP, 2004, pp. 1-85.
34. Iezzoni LI. When Walking Fails: Mobility Problems of Adults with Chronic Conditions. Berkeley, CA: University of California Press, 2003, pp. 1-355.

35. Levy BR, Slade MD, Kasl SV. Longitudinal benefit of positive self-perceptions of aging on functional health. J Gerontol B Psychol Sci Soc Sci 2002;57:P409-P417.
36. Phillips EM, Schneider JC, Mercer GR. Motivating elders to initiate and maintain exercise. Arch Phys Med Rehabil 2004;85:S52-S57; quiz S58-S59.
37. Harter M, Reuter K, Weisser B, et al. A descriptive study of psychiatric disorders and psychosocial burden in rehabilitation patients with musculoskeletal diseases. Arch Phys Med Rehabil 2002;83:461-468.
38. Stineman MG. A model of health environmental integration. Top Stroke Rehabil 2001;8:34-45.
39. Siebens H. Applying the domain management model in treating patients with chronic diseases. Jt Comm J Qual Improv 2001;27:302-314.
40. Siebens H. The domain management model: organizing care for stroke survivors and other persons with chronic diseases. Top Stroke Rehabil 2002;9:1-25.
41. Siebens H. The domain management model—a tool for teaching and management of older adults in emergency departments. Acad Emerg Med 2005;12:162-168.
42. Bode RK, Heinemann AW, Semik P, Mallinson T. Patterns of therapy activities across length of stay and impairment levels: peering inside the "black box" of inpatient stroke rehabilitation. Arch Phys Med Rehabil 2004;85:1901-1908.
43. Horn SD, DeJong G, Ryser DK, et al. Another look at observational studies in rehabilitation research: going beyond the holy grail of the randomized controlled trial. Arch Phys Med Rehabil 2005;86:S8-S15.
44. Maulden SA, Gassaway J, Horn SD, et al. Timing of initiation of rehabilitation after stroke. Arch Phys Med Rehabil 2005;86:S34-S40.
45. Latham NK, Jette DU, Slavin M, et al. Physical therapy during stroke rehabilitation for people with different walking abilities. Arch Phys Med Rehabil 2005;86:S41-S50.
46. Richards LG, Latham NK, Jette DU, et al. Characterizing occupational therapy practice in stroke rehabilitation. Arch Phys Med Rehabil 2005;86:S51-S60.
47. Hatfield B, Millet D, Coles J, et al. Characterizing speech and language pathology outcomes in stroke rehabilitation. Arch Phys Med Rehabil 2005;86:S61-S72.
48. James R, Gines D, Menlove A, et al. Nutrition support (tube feeding) as a rehabilitation intervention. Arch Phys Med Rehabil 2005;86:S82-S92.
49. Conroy B, Zorowitz R, Horn SD, et al. An exploration of central nervous system medication use and outcomes in stroke rehabilitation. Arch Phys Med Rehabil 2005;86:S73-S81.
50. Horn SD, DeJong G, Smout RJ, et al. Stroke rehabilitation patients, practice, and outcomes: is earlier and more aggressive therapy better? Arch Phys Med Rehabil 2005;86:S101-S114.
51. Donabedian A. The quality of care: how can it be assessed? JAMA 1988;260:1743-1748.
52. Horn SD, Hopkins DSP. Clinical Practice Improvement: A New Technology for Developing Cost-Effective Quality Health Care. New York: Faulkner & Gray, Inc., 1994, pp. 1-271.
53. Ward D, Severs M, Dean T, Brooks N. Care home versus hospital and own home environments for rehabilitation of older people. Cochrane Database Syst Rev 2003:CD003164.
54. Chen CC, Heinemann AW, Granger CV, Linn RT. Functional gains and therapy intensity during subacute rehabilitation: a study of 20 facilities. Arch Phys Med Rehabil 2002;83:1514-1523.
55. Jette DU, Warren RL, Wirtalla C. The relation between therapy intensity and outcomes of rehabilitation in skilled nursing facilities. Arch Phys Med Rehabil 2005;86:373-379.
56. Munin MC, Seligman K, Dew MA, et al. Effect of rehabilitation site on functional recovery after hip fracture. Arch Phys Med Rehabil 2005;86:367-372.
57. Leach LS, Yip JY, Myrtle RC, Wilber KH. Outcomes among orthopedic patients in skilled nursing facilities: does managed care make a difference? J Nurs Adm 2001;31:527-533.
58. Walsh MB, Herbold J. Outcome after rehabilitation for total joint replacement at IRF and SNF: a case-controlled comparison. Am J Phys Med Rehabil 2006;85:1-5.

59. Horn S, Dejong G. Joint replacement outcomes in inpatient rehabilitation facilities and nursing treatment sites (JOINTS). Institute for Clinical Outcomes Research, ISIS Inc. (Salt Lake City, UT) and National Rehabilitation Hospital (Washington, D.C.), 2007: Study in progress. Information available online: http://jointsstudy.net.
60. Blackman-Weinberg C, Crook J, Roberts J, Weir R. Longitudinal study of inpatients admitted to a general activation service: variables that predict discharge to a patient's discharge goal location. Arch Phys Med Rehabil 2005;86:1782-1787.
61. Murray PK, Love TE, Dawson NV, et al. Rehabilitation services after the implementation of the nursing home prospective payment system: differences related to patient and nursing home characteristics. Med Care 2005;43:1109-1115.
62. Strasser DC, Falconer JA, Herrin JS, et al. Team functioning and patient outcomes in stroke rehabilitation. Arch Phys Med Rehabil 2005;86:403-409.
63. Bean JF, Vora A, Frontera WR. Benefits of exercise for community-dwelling older adults. Arch Phys Med Rehabil 2004;85:S31-S42; quiz S43-S44.
64. Hunter GR, McCarthy JP, Bamman MM. Effects of resistance training on older adults. Sports Med 2004;34:329-348.
65. Meuleman JR, Brechue WF, Kubilis PS, Lowenthal DT. Exercise training in the debilitated aged: strength and functional outcomes. Arch Phys Med Rehabil 2000;81:312-318.
66. Sousa N, Sampaio J. Effects of progressive strength training on the performance of the Functional Reach Test and the Timed Get-Up-and-Go Test in an elderly population from the rural north of Portugal. Am J Hum Biol 2005;17:746-751.
67. Brandon LJ, Gaasch DA, Boyette LW, Lloyd AM. Effects of long-term resistive training on mobility and strength in older adults with diabetes. J Gerontol A Biol Sci Med Sci 2003;58:740-745.
68. Capodaglio P, Ferri A, Scaglloni G. Effects of a partially supervised training program in subjects over 75 years of age. Aging Clin Exp Res 2005;17:174-180.
69. Latham NK, Bennett DA, Stretton CM, Anderson CS. Systematic review of progressive resistance strength training in older adults. J Gerontol A Biol Sci Med Sci 2004;59:48-61.
70. Seynnes O, Fiatarone Singh MA, Hue O, et al. Physiological and functional responses to low-moderate versus high-intensity progressive resistance training in frail elders. J Gerontol A Biol Sci Med Sci 2004;59:503-509.
71. Symons TB, Vandervoort AA, Rice CL, et al. Effects of maximal isometric and isokinetic resistance training on strength and functional mobility in older adults. J Gerontol A Biol Sci Med Sci 2005;60:777-781.
72. Galvao DA, Taaffe DR. Resistance exercise dosage in older adults: single- versus multiset effects on physical performance and body composition. J Am Geriatr Soc 2005;53:2090-2097.
73. Barrett CJ, Smerdely P. A comparison of community-based resistance exercise and flexibility exercise for seniors. Aust J Physiother 2002;48:215-219.
74. Newton RU, Hakkinen K, Hakkinen A, et al. Mixed-methods resistance training increases power and strength of young and older men. Med Sci Sports Exerc 2002;34:1367-1375.
75. Hagerman FC, Walsh SJ, Staron RS, et al. Effects of high-intensity resistance training on untrained older men. I. Strength, cardiovascular, and metabolic responses. J Gerontol A Biol Sci Med Sci 2000;55:B336-B346.
76. Humphries B, Newton RU, Bronks R, et al. Effect of exercise intensity on bone density, strength, and calcium turnover in older women. Med Sci Sports Exerc 2000;32:1043-1050.
77. Vincent KR, Braith RW. Resistance exercise and bone turnover in elderly men and women. Med Sci Sports Exerc 2002;34:17-23.
78. Vincent KR, Braith RW, Feldman RA, et al. Improved cardiorespiratory endurance following 6 months of resistance exercise in elderly men and women. Arch Intern Med 2002;162:673-678.

79. Latham NK, Anderson CS, Lee A, et al. A randomized, controlled trial of quadriceps resistance exercise and vitamin D in frail older people: the Frailty Interventions Trial in Elderly Subjects (FITNESS). J Am Geriatr Soc 2003;51:291-299.
80. Bean JF, Leveille SG, Kiely DK, et al. A comparison of leg power and leg strength within the InCHIANTI study: which influences mobility more? J Gerontol A Biol Sci Med Sci 2003;58:728-733.
81. Bean JF, Herman S, Kiely DK, et al. Increased Velocity Exercise Specific to Task (InVEST) training: a pilot study exploring effects on leg power, balance, and mobility in community-dwelling older women. J Am Geriatr Soc 2004;52:799-804.
82. Fielding RA, LeBrasseur NK, Cuoco A, et al. High-velocity resistance training increases skeletal muscle peak power in older women. J Am Geriatr Soc 2002;50:655-662.
83. Miszko TA, Cress ME, Slade JM, et al. Effect of strength and power training on physical function in community-dwelling older adults. J Gerontol A Biol Sci Med Sci 2003;58:171-175.
84. Keysor JJ, Jette AM. Have we oversold the benefit of late-life exercise? J Gerontol A Biol Sci Med Sci 2001;56:M412-M423.
85. Whelton SP, Chin A, Xin X, He J. Effect of aerobic exercise on blood pressure: a meta-analysis of randomized, controlled trials. Ann Intern Med 2002;136:493-503.
86. Lee IM, Sesso HD, Oguma Y, Paffenbarger RS, Jr. Relative intensity of physical activity and risk of coronary heart disease. Circulation 2003;107:1110-1116.
87. Duncan GE, Anton SD, Sydeman SJ, et al. Prescribing exercise at varied levels of intensity and frequency: a randomized trial. Arch Intern Med 2005;165:2362-2369.
88. Short KR, Vittone JL, Bigelow ML, et al. Impact of aerobic exercise training on age-related changes in insulin sensitivity and muscle oxidative capacity. Diabetes 2003;52:1888-1896.
89. Haykowsky M, McGavock J, Vonder Muhll I, et al. Effect of exercise training on peak aerobic power, left ventricular morphology, and muscle strength in healthy older women. J Gerontol A Biol Sci Med Sci 2005;60:307-311.
90. Morio B, Barra V, Ritz P, et al. Benefit of endurance training in elderly people over a short period is reversible. Eur J Appl Physiol 2000;81:329-336.
91. King MB, Whipple RH, Gruman CA, et al. The Performance Enhancement Project: improving physical performance in older persons. Arch Phys Med Rehabil 2002;83:1060-1069.
92. Hatch J, Gill-Body KM, Portney LG. Determinants of balance confidence in community-dwelling elderly people. Phys Ther 2003;83:1072-1079.
93. Hirsch MA, Toole T, Maitland CG, Rider RA. The effects of balance training and high-intensity resistance training on persons with idiopathic Parkinson's disease. Arch Phys Med Rehabil 2003;84:1109-1117.
94. Nelson ME, Layne JE, Bernstein MJ, et al. The effects of multidimensional home-based exercise on functional performance in elderly people. J Gerontol A Biol Sci Med Sci 2004;59:154-160.
95. Kerrigan DC, Xenopoulos-Oddsson A, Sullivan MJ, et al. Effect of a hip flexor-stretching program on gait in the elderly. Arch Phys Med Rehabil 2003;84:1-6.
96. Lee LW, Zavarei K, Evans J, et al. Reduced hip extension in the elderly: dynamic or postural? Arch Phys Med Rehabil 2005;86:1851-1854.
97. Brown M, Sinacore DR, Ehsani AA, et al. Low-intensity exercise as a modifier of physical frailty in older adults. Arch Phys Med Rehabil 2000;81:960-965.
98. de Vreede PL, Samson MM, van Meeteren NL, et al. Functional-task exercise versus resistance strength exercise to improve daily function in older women: a randomized, controlled trial. J Am Geriatr Soc 2005;53:2-10.
99. Thielman GT, Dean CM, Gentile AM. Rehabilitation of reaching after stroke: task-related training versus progressive resistive exercise. Arch Phys Med Rehabil 2004;85:1613-1618.

100. Salbach NM, Mayo NE, Robichaud-Ekstrand S, et al. The effect of a task-oriented walking intervention on improving balance self-efficacy poststroke: a randomized, controlled trial. J Am Geriatr Soc 2005;53:576-582.
101. Dunn AL, Marcus BH, Kampert JB, et al. Comparison of lifestyle and structured interventions to increase physical activity and cardiorespiratory fitness: a randomized trial. JAMA 1999;281:327-334.
102. Andersen RE, Wadden TA, Bartlett SJ, et al. Effects of lifestyle activity vs structured aerobic exercise in obese women: a randomized trial. JAMA 1999;281:335-340.
103. Heyn P, Abreu BC, Ottenbacher KJ. The effects of exercise training on elderly persons with cognitive impairment and dementia: a meta-analysis. Arch Phys Med Rehabil 2004;85:1694-1704.
104. Hoeksma HL, Dekker J, Ronday HK, et al. Comparison of manual therapy and exercise therapy in osteoarthritis of the hip: a randomized clinical trial. Arthritis Rheum 2004;51:722-729.
105. Gur H, Cakin N, Akova B, et al. Concentric versus combined concentric-eccentric isokinetic training: effects on functional capacity and symptoms in patients with osteoarthrosis of the knee. Arch Phys Med Rehabil 2002;83:308-316.
106. Scandalis TA, Bosak A, Berliner JC, et al. Resistance training and gait function in patients with Parkinson's disease. Am J Phys Med Rehabil 2001;80:38-43; quiz 44-36.
107. Ouellette MM, LeBrasseur NK, Bean JF, et al. High-intensity resistance training improves muscle strength, self-reported function, and disability in long-term stroke survivors. Stroke 2004;35:1404-1409.
108. Cornman JC, Freedman VA, Agree EM. Measurement of assistive device use: implications for estimates of device use and disability in late life. Gerontologist 2005;45:347-358.
109. Ivanoff SD, Sonn U. Changes in the use of assistive devices among 90-year-old persons. Aging Clin Exp Res 2005;17:246-251.
110. Wolff JL, Agree EM, Kasper JD. Wheelchairs, walkers, and canes: what does Medicare pay for, and who benefits? Health Aff (Millwood) 2005;24:1140-1149.
111. Fuchs RH, Gromak PA. Wheelchair use by residents of nursing homes: effectiveness in meeting positioning and mobility needs. Assist Technol 2003;15:151-163.
112. Hoenig H, Landerman LR, Shipp KM, et al. A clinical trial of a rehabilitation expert clinician versus usual care for providing manual wheelchairs. J Am Geriatr Soc 2005;53:1712-1720.
113. Best KL, Kirby RL, Smith C, MacLeod DA. Wheelchair skills training for community-based manual wheelchair users: a randomized controlled trial. Arch Phys Med Rehabil 2005;86:2316-2323.
114. Levy CE, Chow JW, Tillman MD, et al. Variable-ratio pushrim-activated power-assist wheelchair eases wheeling over a variety of terrains for elders. Arch Phys Med Rehabil 2004;85:104-112.
115. Rogers JC, Holm MB, Perkins L. Trajectory of assistive device usage and user and non-user characteristics: long-handled bath sponge. Arthritis Rheum 2002;47:645-650.
116. Jannink MJ, Ijzerman MJ, Groothuis-Oudshoorn K, et al. Use of orthopedic shoes in patients with degenerative disorders of the foot. Arch Phys Med Rehabil 2005;86:687-692.
117. Bohannon RW. Gait performance with wheeled and standard walkers. Percept Mot Skills 1997;85:1185-1186.
118. Brandt A, Iwarsson S, Stahl A. Satisfaction with rollators among community-living users: a follow-up study. Disabil Rehabil 2003;25:343-353.
119. Mann WC, Ottenbacher KJ, Fraas L, et al. Effectiveness of assistive technology and environmental interventions in maintaining independence and reducing home care costs for the frail elderly: a randomized controlled trial. Arch Fam Med 1999;8:210-217.

120. Hoenig H, Taylor DH, Jr., Sloan FA. Does assistive technology substitute for personal assistance among the disabled elderly? Am J Public Health 2003;93:330-337.
121. Agree EM, Freedman VA, Cornman JC, et al. Reconsidering substitution in long-term care: when does assistive technology take the place of personal care? J Gerontol B Psychol Sci Soc Sci 2005;60:S272-S280.
122. Steultjens EM, Dekker J, Bouter LM, et al. Occupational therapy for community dwelling elderly people: a systematic review. Age Ageing 2004;33:453-460.
123. Lenker JA, Scherer MJ, Fuhrer MJ, et al. Psychometric and administrative properties of measures used in assistive technology device outcomes research. Assist Technol 2005;17:7-22.
124. Jutai JW, Fuhrer MJ, Demers L, et al. Toward a taxonomy of assistive technology device outcomes. Am J Phys Med Rehabil 2005;84:294-302.
125. Nagi SZ. A study in the evaluation of disability and rehabilitation potential: concepts, methods and procedures. In Pope AM, Tarlov AR (eds): Disability in America—Toward a National Agenda for Prevention. Washington, D.C.: National Academy Press, 1991, pp. 309-327.
126. Stanhope S. Scientific areas and emerging technologies. Bethesda MD: Musculoskeletal Research Conference, 2006.
127. Mazza C, Benvenuti F, Bimbi C, Stanhope SJ. Association between subject functional status, seat height, and movement strategy in sit-to-stand performance. J Am Geriatr Soc 2004;52:1750-1754.
128. Verbrugge LM, Jette AM. The disablement process. Soc Sci Med 1994;38:1-14.
129. Magaziner J. Epidemiology of musculoskeletal conditions. Bethesda, MD: Interagency Committee on Disability Research, 2006.
130. Pope AM, Tarlov AR. A model for disability and disability prevention. In Pope AM, Tarlov AR (eds): Disability in America: Toward a National Agenda for Prevention. Washington, D.C.: Institute of Medicine. National Academy Press, 1991, pp. 76-108.
131. Golant SM. Do impaired older persons with health care needs occupy U.S. assisted living facilities? An analysis of six national studies. J Gerontol B Psychol Sci Soc Sci 2004;59:S68-S79.
132. Fried LP, Ferrucci L, Darer J, et al. Untangling the concepts of disability, frailty, and comorbidity: implications for improved targeting and care. J Gerontol A Biol Sci Med Sci 2004;59:255-263.
133. Rozzini R, Frisoni GB, Ferrucci L, et al. Geriatric Index of Comorbidity: validation and comparison with other measures of comorbidity. Age Ageing 2002;31:277-285.
134. Lawrence RC, Helmick CG, Arnett FC, et al. Estimates of the prevalence of arthritis and selected musculoskeletal disorders in the United States. Arthritis Rheum 1998;41:778-799.
135. Penninx BW, Messier SP, Rejeski WJ, et al. Physical exercise and the prevention of disability in activities of daily living in older persons with osteoarthritis. Arch Intern Med 2001;161:2309-2316.
136. AGS Panel on Osteoarthritis and Exercise. Exercise prescription for older adults with osteoarthritis pain: consensus practice recommendations. A supplement to the AGS Clinical Practice Guidelines on the management of chronic pain in older adults. J Am Geriatr Soc 2001;49:808-823.
137. Berger RA, Jacobs JJ, Meneghini RM, et al. Rapid rehabilitation and recovery with minimally invasive total hip arthroplasty. Clin Orthop Relat Res 2004:239-247.
138. Fortin PR, Clarke AE, Joseph L, et al. Outcomes of total hip and knee replacement: preoperative functional status predicts outcomes at six months after surgery. Arthritis Rheum 1999;42:1722-1728.
139. Fitzgerald JD, Orav EJ, Lee TH, et al. Patient quality of life during the 12 months following joint replacement surgery. Arthritis Rheum 2004;51:100-109.

140. Bischoff-Ferrari HA, Lingard EA, Losina E, et al. Psychosocial and geriatric correlates of functional status after total hip replacement. Arthritis Rheum 2004;51:829-835.
141. Wang AW, Gilbey HJ, Ackland TR. Perioperative exercise programs improve early return of ambulatory function after total hip arthroplasty: a randomized, controlled trial. Am J Phys Med Rehabil 2002;81:801-806.
142. Kramer JF, Speechley M, Bourne R, et al. Comparison of clinic- and home-based rehabilitation programs after total knee arthroplasty. Clin Orthop Relat Res 2003;410:225-234.
143. Cheville A, Chen A, Oster G, et al. A randomized trial of controlled-release oxycodone during inpatient rehabilitation following unilateral total knee arthroplasty. J Bone Joint Surg Am 2001;83-A:572-576.
144. Beaupre LA, Davies DM, Jones CA, Cinats JG. Exercise combined with continuous passive motion or slider board therapy compared with exercise only: a randomized controlled trial of patients following total knee arthroplasty. Phys Ther 2001;81:1029-1037.
145. Mukand JA, Cai C, Zielinski A, et al. The effects of dehydration on rehabilitation outcomes of elderly orthopedic patients. Arch Phys Med Rehabil 2003;84:58-61.
146. Marcinkowski K, Wong VG, Dignam D. Getting back to the future: a grounded theory study of the patient perspective of total knee joint arthroplasty. Orthop Nurs 2005;24:202-209.
147. Zorowitz RD, Smout RJ, Gassaway JA, Horn SD. Outcomes in stroke rehabilitation. Top Stroke Rehabil 2005;12:1-49.
148. Alberts JL, Butler AJ, Wolf SL. The effects of constraint-induced therapy on precision grip: a preliminary study. Neurorehabil Neural Repair 2004;18:250-258.
149. Bonifer NM, Anderson KM, Arciniegas DB. Constraint-induced movement therapy after stroke: efficacy for patients with minimal upper-extremity motor ability. Arch Phys Med Rehabil 2005;86:1867-1873.
150. Dettmers C, Teske U, Hamzei F, et al. Distributed form of constraint-induced movement therapy improves functional outcome and quality of life after stroke. Arch Phys Med Rehabil 2005;86:204-209.
151. Wolf SL, Winstein CJ, Miller JP, et al. Effect of constraint-induced movement therapy on upper extremity function 3 to 9 months after stroke: the EXCITE randomized clinical trial. JAMA 2006;296:2095-2104.
152. Fasoli SE, Krebs HI, Stein J, et al. Robotic therapy for chronic motor impairments after stroke: follow-up results. Arch Phys Med Rehabil 2004;85:1106-1111.
153. Volpe BT, Krebs HI, Hogan N, et al. A novel approach to stroke rehabilitation: robot-aided sensorimotor stimulation. Neurology 2000;54:1938-1944.
154. Teng J, Mayo NE, Latimer E, et al. Costs and caregiver consequences of early supported discharge for stroke patients. Stroke 2003;34:528-536.
155. Duncan PW, Horner RD, Reker DM, et al. Adherence to postacute rehabilitation guidelines is associated with functional recovery in stroke. Stroke 2002;33:167-177.
156. Post-stroke rehabilitation. Rockville, MD: Agency for Health Care Policy and Research, 1995: AHCPR Publication No. 95-0062.
157. Mayo NE, Wood-Dauphinee S, Cote R, et al. Activity, participation, and quality of life 6 months poststroke. Arch Phys Med Rehabil 2002;83:1035-1042.
158. Oldridge NB, Stump TE. Heart disease, comorbidity, and activity limitation in community-dwelling elderly. Eur J Cardiovasc Prev Rehabil 2004;11:427-434.
159. Dolansky MA, Moore SM. Effects of cardiac rehabilitation on the recovery outcomes of older adults after coronary artery bypass surgery. J Cardiopulm Rehabil 2004;24:236-244.
160. Zwisler AD, Schou L, Soja AM, et al. A randomized clinical trial of hospital-based, comprehensive cardiac rehabilitation versus usual care for patients with congestive heart failure, ischemic heart disease, or high risk of ischemic heart disease (the DANREHAB trial)—design, intervention, and population. Am Heart J 2005;150:899.

161. Michel JP, Hoffmeyer P, Klopfenstein C, et al. Prognosis of functional recovery 1 year after hip fracture: typical patient profiles through cluster analysis. J Gerontol A Biol Sci Med Sci 2000;55:M508-M515.
162. Hannan EL, Magaziner J, Wang JJ, et al. Mortality and locomotion 6 months after hospitalization for hip fracture: risk factors and risk-adjusted hospital outcomes. JAMA 2001;285:2736-2742.
163. Magaziner J, Fredman L, Hawkes W, et al. Changes in functional status attributable to hip fracture: a comparison of hip fracture patients to community-dwelling aged. Am J Epidemiol 2003;157:1023-1031.
164. Halm EA, Magaziner J, Hannan EL, et al. Frequency and impact of active clinical issues and new impairments on hospital discharge in patients with hip fracture. Arch Intern Med 2003;163:108-113.
165. Di Monaco M, Vallero F, Di Monaco R, et al. Functional recovery and length of stay after hip fracture in patients with neurologic impairment. Am J Phys Med Rehabil 2003;82:143-148; quiz 149-151, 157.
166. Beaupre LA, Cinats JG, Senthilselvan A, et al. Does standardized rehabilitation and discharge planning improve functional recovery in elderly patients with hip fracture? Arch Phys Med Rehabil 2005;86:2231-2239.
167. Binder EF, Brown M, Sinacore DR, et al. Effects of extended outpatient rehabilitation after hip fracture: a randomized controlled trial. JAMA 2004;292:837-846.
168. Huusko TM, Karppi P, Avikainen V, et al. Randomised, clinically controlled trial of intensive geriatric rehabilitation in patients with hip fracture: subgroup analysis of patients with dementia. BMJ 2000;321:1107-1111.
169. Beaupre LA, Jones CA, Saunders LD, et al. Best practices for elderly hip fracture patients: a systematic overview of the evidence. J Gen Intern Med 2005;20:1019-1025.
170. Cameron ID, Handoll HH, Finnegan TP, et al. Co-ordinated multidisciplinary approaches for inpatient rehabilitation of older patients with proximal femoral fractures. Cochrane Database Syst Rev 2001:CD000106.
171. Dillingham TR, Pezzin LE, Shore AD. Reamputation, mortality, and health care costs among persons with dysvascular lower-limb amputations. Arch Phys Med Rehabil 2005;86:480-486.
172. Dillingham TR, Pezzin LE. Postacute care services use for dysvascular amputees: a population-based study of Massachusetts. Am J Phys Med Rehabil 2005;84:147-152.
173. Dillingham TR, Pezzin LE, MacKenzie EJ. Limb amputation and limb deficiency: epidemiology and recent trends in the United States. South Med J 2002;95:875-883.
174. Fletcher DD, Andrews KL, Hallett JW, Jr., et al. Trends in rehabilitation after amputation for geriatric patients with vascular disease: implications for future health resource allocation. Arch Phys Med Rehabil 2002;83:1389-1393.
175. Gill TM, Allore H, Guo Z. The deleterious effects of bed rest among community-living older persons. J Gerontol A Biol Sci Med Sci 2004;59:755-761.
176. Bates-Jensen BM, Alessi CA, Cadogan M, et al. The Minimum Data Set bedfast quality indicator: differences among nursing homes. Nurs Res 2004;53:260-272.
177. Bruce DG, Devine A, Prince RL. Recreational physical activity levels in healthy older women: the importance of fear of falling. J Am Geriatr Soc 2002;50:84-89.
178. Cumming RG, Salkeld G, Thomas M, Szonyi G. Prospective study of the impact of fear of falling on activities of daily living, SF-36 scores, and nursing home admission. J Gerontol A Biol Sci Med Sci 2000;55:M299-M305.
179. Petrella RJ, Payne M, Myers A, et al. Physical function and fear of falling after hip fracture rehabilitation in the elderly. Am J Phys Med Rehabil 2000;79:154-160.
180. Miller WC, Speechley M, Deathe B. The prevalence and risk factors of falling and fear of falling among lower extremity amputees. Arch Phys Med Rehabil 2001;82:1031-1037.

181. Friedman SM, Munoz B, West SK, et al. Falls and fear of falling: which comes first? A longitudinal prediction model suggests strategies for primary and secondary prevention. J Am Geriatr Soc 2002;50:1329-1335.
182. Brouwer BJ, Walker C, Rydahl SJ, Culham EG. Reducing fear of falling in seniors through education and activity programs: a randomized trial. J Am Geriatr Soc 2003;51:829-834.
183. Sattin RW, Easley KA, Wolf SL, et al. Reduction in fear of falling through intense Tai Chi exercise training in older, transitionally frail adults. J Am Geriatr Soc 2005;53:1168-1178.
184. Velozo CA, Peterson EW. Developing meaningful fear of falling measures for community dwelling elderly. Am J Phys Med Rehabil 2001;80:662-673.
185. Hauer K, Marburger C, Oster P. Motor performance deteriorates with simultaneously performed cognitive tasks in geriatric patients. Arch Phys Med Rehabil 2002;83:217-223.
186. Hausdorff JM, Rios DA, Edelberg HK. Gait variability and fall risk in community-living older adults: a 1-year prospective study. Arch Phys Med Rehabil 2001;82:1050-1056.
187. Cesari M, Landi F, Torre S, et al. Prevalence and risk factors for falls in an older community-dwelling population. J Gerontol A Biol Sci Med Sci 2002;57:M722-M726.
188. Steffen TM, Hacker TA, Mollinger L. Age- and gender-related test performance in community-dwelling elderly people: Six-Minute Walk Test, Berg Balance Scale, Timed Up & Go Test, and gait speeds. Phys Ther 2002;82:128-137.
189. Shumway-Cook A, Ciol MA, Gruber W, Robinson C. Incidence of and risk factors for falls following hip fracture in community-dwelling older adults. Phys Ther 2005;85:648-655.
190. Shimada H, Obuchi S, Furuna T, Suzuki T. New intervention program for preventing falls among frail elderly people: the effects of perturbed walking exercise using a bilateral separated treadmill. Am J Phys Med Rehabil 2004;83:493-499.
191. Tinetti ME. Clinical practice: preventing falls in elderly persons. N Engl J Med 2003;348:42-49.
192. Day L, Fildes B, Gordon I, et al. Randomised factorial trial of falls prevention among older people living in their own homes. BMJ 2002;325:128.
193. Means KM, Rodell DE, O'Sullivan PS. Balance, mobility, and falls among community-dwelling elderly persons: effects of a rehabilitation exercise program. Am J Phys Med Rehabil 2005;84:238-250.
194. Sinaki M, Brey RH, Hughes CA, et al. Significant reduction in risk of falls and back pain in osteoporotic-kyphotic women through a Spinal Proprioceptive Extension Exercise Dynamic (SPEED) program. Mayo Clin Proc 2005;80:849-855.
195. Scudds RJ, Robertson JM. Pain factors associated with physical disability in a sample of community-dwelling senior citizens. J Gerontol A Biol Sci Med Sci 2000;55:M393-M399.
196. Burris JE. Pharmacologic approaches to geriatric pain management. Arch Phys Med Rehabil 2004;85:S45-S49; quiz S50-S51.
197. Karani R, Meier DE. Systemic pharmacologic postoperative pain management in the geriatric orthopaedic patient. Clin Orthop Relat Res 2004;425:26-34.
198. Rao A, Cohen HJ. Symptom management in the elderly cancer patient: fatigue, pain, and depression. J Natl Cancer Inst Monogr 2004;32:150-157.
199. Fine PG. Pharmacological management of persistent pain in older patients. Clin J Pain 2004;20:220-226.
200. Ruchinskas R. Rehabilitation therapists' recognition of cognitive and mood disorders in geriatric patients. Arch Phys Med Rehabil 2002;83:609-612.
201. Harter M, Woll S, Reuter K, et al. Recognition of psychiatric disorders in musculoskeletal and cardiovascular rehabilitation patients. Arch Phys Med Rehabil 2004;85:1192-1197.
202. Ruchinskas RA, Singer HK, Repetz NK. Clock drawing, clock copying, and physical abilities in geriatric rehabilitation. Arch Phys Med Rehabil 2001;82:920-924.

203. Lenze EJ, Munin MC, Quear T, et al. Significance of poor patient participation in physical and occupational therapy for functional outcome and length of stay. Arch Phys Med Rehabil 2004;85:1599-1601.
204. Demers L, Desrosiers J, Ska B, et al. Assembling a toolkit to measure geriatric rehabilitation outcomes. Am J Phys Med Rehabil 2005;84:460-472.
205. Cohen HJ, Feussner JR, Weinberger M, et al. A controlled trial of inpatient and outpatient geriatric evaluation and management. N Engl J Med 2002;346:905-912.
206. Regenstrief DI. As the senior program project officer in 1988, Dr. Regenstrief used the term as part of the John A. Hartford Foundation research initiative on Hospital Outcomes Project for the Elderly (HOPE).
207. Carli F, Zavorsky GS. Optimizing functional exercise capacity in the elderly surgical population. Curr Opin Clin Nutr Metab Care 2005;8:23-32.
208. Topp R, Ditmyer M, King K, et al. The effect of bed rest and potential of prehabilitation on patients in the intensive care unit. AACN Clin Issues 2002;13:263-276.
209. Gill TM, Baker DI, Gottschalk M, et al. A prehabilitation program for the prevention of functional decline: effect on higher-level physical function. Arch Phys Med Rehabil 2004;85:1043-1049.
210. Gill TM, Baker DI, Gottschalk M, et al. A program to prevent functional decline in physically frail, elderly persons who live at home. N Engl J Med 2002;347:1068-1074.
211. Gilbey HJ, Ackland TR, Wang AW, et al. Exercise improves early functional recovery after total hip arthroplasty. Clin Orthop Relat Res 2003;408:193-200.
212. Puchalski CM. Walking together—physicians, chaplains and clergy caring for the sick. Washington, D.C.: George Washington Institute for Spirituality and Health, 2003.
213. Schlitz M, Amorok T, Micozzi M. Consciousness and Healing. Philadelphia, PA: Elsevier Churchill Livingstone, 2005, pp. 1-583.
214. Wulff DH. Psychology of Religion: Classic and Contemporary. New York: John Wiley & Sons, 1997.
215. Daaleman TP, Perera S, Studenski SA. Religion, spirituality, and health status in geriatric outpatients. Ann Fam Med 2004;2:49-53.
216. Faull K, Hills MD, Cochrane G, et al. Investigation of health perspectives of those with physical disabilities: the role of spirituality as a determinant of health. Disabil Rehabil 2004;26:129-144.
217. WHOQOL SRPB Group. A cross-cultural study of spirituality, religion, and personal beliefs (SRPB) as components of quality of life (QOL). Soc Sci Med 2006;62:1486-1497.
218. Haley SM, Coster WJ, Andres PL, et al. Activity outcome measurement for postacute care. Med Care 2004;42:I49-I61.
219. Haley SM, Coster WJ, Andres PL, et al. Score comparability of short forms and computerized adaptive testing: simulation study with the activity measure for post-acute care. Arch Phys Med Rehabil 2004;85:661-666.
220. Siebens H, Andres PL, Pengsheng N, et al. Measuring physical function in patients with complex medical and postsurgical conditions: a computer adaptive approach. Am J Phys Med Rehabil 2005;84:741-748.
221. Jette AM, Keysor J, Coster W, et al. Beyond function: predicting participation in a rehabilitation cohort. Arch Phys Med Rehabil 2005;86:2087-2094.
222. Ottenbacher KJ, Smith PM, Illig SB, et al. Trends in length of stay, living setting, functional outcome, and mortality following medical rehabilitation. JAMA 2004;292:1687-1695.
223. Jha A, Patrick DL, MacLehose RF, et al. Dissatisfaction with medical services among Medicare beneficiaries with disabilities. Arch Phys Med Rehabil 2002;83:1335-1341.
224. Reker DM, Duncan PW, Horner RD, et al. Postacute stroke guideline compliance is associated with greater patient satisfaction. Arch Phys Med Rehabil 2002;83:750-756.

225. Tooth LR, Ottenbacher KJ, Smith PM, et al. Effect of functional gain on satisfaction with medical rehabilitation after stroke. Am J Phys Med Rehabil 2003;82:692-699; quiz 700-691, 715.
226. Testa JA, Malec JF, Moessner AM, Brown AW. Outcome after traumatic brain injury: effects of aging on recovery. Arch Phys Med Rehabil 2005;86:1815-1823.
227. Susman M, DiRusso SM, Sullivan T, et al. Traumatic brain injury in the elderly: increased mortality and worse functional outcome at discharge despite lower injury severity. J Trauma 2002;53:219-223; discussion 223-214.

INDEX

Page references followed by *t* and *f* indicate tables and figures, respectively. Page references in **bold** indicate agenda items and key research questions. References followed by (S1) indicate pages in this first supplement.

E

G

H

U

V

W

X

Z